MW00677851

Scaling Up
Treatment for the
Global AIDS Pandemic
CHALLENGES AND OPPORTUNITIES

Committee on Examining the Probable Consequences of
Alternative Patterns of Widespread Antiretroviral Drug Use
in Resource-Constrained Settings

Board on Global Health

James Curran, Haile Debas, Monisha Arya,
Patrick Kelley, Stacey Knobler, and Leslie Pray, *Editors*

INSTITUTE OF MEDICINE
OF THE NATIONAL ACADEMIES

THE NATIONAL ACADEMIES PRESS
Washington, D.C.
www.nap.edu

THE NATIONAL ACADEMIES PRESS 500 Fifth Street, N.W. Washington, DC 20001

NOTICE: The project that is the subject of this report was approved by the Governing Board of the National Research Council, whose members are drawn from the councils of the National Academy of Sciences, the National Academy of Engineering, and the Institute of Medicine. The members of the committee responsible for the report were chosen for their special competences and with regard for appropriate balance.

This study was supported by Contract No. N01-OD-4-2319 between the National Academy of Sciences and the U.S. Department of Health and Human Services, and contract 32467 between the National Academy of Sciences and the Bill and Melinda Gates Foundation. Any opinions, findings, conclusions, or recommendations expressed in this publication are those of the author(s) and do not necessarily reflect the view of the organizations or agencies that provided support for this project.

Library of Congress Cataloging-in-Publication Data

Institute of Medicine (U.S.). Committee on Examining the Probable Consequences of Alternative Patterns of Widespread Antiretroviral Drug Use in Resource-Constrained Settings.
  Scaling up treatment for the global AIDS pandemic : challenges and opportunities / Committee on Examining the Probable Consequences of Alternative Patterns of Widespread Antiretroviral Drug Use in Resource-Constrained Settings, Board on Global Health ; James Curran . . . [et al.], editors.
     p. ; cm.
  Includes bibliographical references.
  ISBN 0-309-09264-7 (pbk.)
  1. AIDS (Disease) 2. AIDS (Disease)—Developing countries. 3. Antiretroviral agents—Developing countries.
  [DNLM: 1. HIV Infections—drug therapy. 2. Antiretroviral Therapy, Highly Active. 3. Disease Outbreaks—prevention & control. 4. Health Planning—organization & administration. WC 503.2 I59s 2004] I. Curran, James W. II. Title.
  RA643.8.I57 2004
  362.196'9792'0091724—dc22
                                        2004023710

Additional copies of this report are available from the National Academies Press, 500 Fifth Street, N.W., Lockbox 285, Washington, DC 20055; (800) 624-6242 or (202) 334-3313 (in the Washington metropolitan area); Internet, http://www. nap.edu.

For more information about the Institute of Medicine, visit the IOM home page at: **www.iom.edu.**

Cover: Detail of "Women's Faces" by Lilian Nabulime, wood and metal, 2002. Lilian Nabulime is a respected Ugandan artist whose works focus on HIV and AIDS awareness and African women. Photograph by Alexander Calder, Curator, The Art Room, San Francisco, CA.

Printed in the United States of America.

The serpent has been a symbol of long life, healing, and knowledge among almost all cultures and religions since the beginning of recorded history. The serpent adopted as a logotype by the Institute of Medicine is a relief carving from ancient Greece, now held by the Staatliche Museen in Berlin.

"Knowing is not enough; we must apply.
Willing is not enough; we must do."
—Goethe

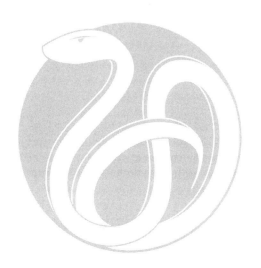

INSTITUTE OF MEDICINE
OF THE NATIONAL ACADEMIES

Adviser to the Nation to Improve Health

THE NATIONAL ACADEMIES
Advisers to the Nation on Science, Engineering, and Medicine

The **National Academy of Sciences** is a private, nonprofit, self-perpetuating society of distinguished scholars engaged in scientific and engineering research, dedicated to the furtherance of science and technology and to their use for the general welfare. Upon the authority of the charter granted to it by the Congress in 1863, the Academy has a mandate that requires it to advise the federal government on scientific and technical matters. Dr. Bruce M. Alberts is president of the National Academy of Sciences.

The **National Academy of Engineering** was established in 1964, under the charter of the National Academy of Sciences, as a parallel organization of outstanding engineers. It is autonomous in its administration and in the selection of its members, sharing with the National Academy of Sciences the responsibility for advising the federal government. The National Academy of Engineering also sponsors engineering programs aimed at meeting national needs, encourages education and research, and recognizes the superior achievements of engineers. Dr. Wm. A. Wulf is president of the National Academy of Engineering.

The **Institute of Medicine** was established in 1970 by the National Academy of Sciences to secure the services of eminent members of appropriate professions in the examination of policy matters pertaining to the health of the public. The Institute acts under the responsibility given to the National Academy of Sciences by its congressional charter to be an adviser to the federal government and, upon its own initiative, to identify issues of medical care, research, and education. Dr. Harvey V. Fineberg is president of the Institute of Medicine.

The **National Research Council** was organized by the National Academy of Sciences in 1916 to associate the broad community of science and technology with the Academy's purposes of furthering knowledge and advising the federal government. Functioning in accordance with general policies determined by the Academy, the Council has become the principal operating agency of both the National Academy of Sciences and the National Academy of Engineering in providing services to the government, the public, and the scientific and engineering communities. The Council is administered jointly by both Academies and the Institute of Medicine. Dr. Bruce M. Alberts and Dr. Wm. A. Wulf are chair and vice chair, respectively, of the National Research Council.

www.national-academies.org

Reviewers

This report has been reviewed in draft form by individuals chosen for their diverse perspectives and technical expertise, in accordance with procedures approved by the National Research Council's Report Review Committee. The purpose of this independent review is to provide candid and critical comments that will assist the institution in making its published report as sound as possible and to ensure that the report meets institutional standards for objectivity, evidence, and responsiveness to the study charge. The review comments and draft manuscript remain confidential to protect the integrity of the deliberative process. We wish to thank the following individuals for their review of this report:

Roy M. Anderson, Imperial College, London
Stefano Bertozzi, National Institute of Public Health, Cuernavaca, México
Charles C. J. Carpenter, The Miriam Hospital, Brown University, Providence, Rhode Island
James Hakim, University of Zimbabwe, Harare, Zimbabwe
King K. Holmes, University of Washington, Seattle, Washington
Joseph-Matthew Mfutso-Bengo, University of Malawi, Chichin, Malawi
Philip C. Onyebujoh, World Health Organization, Geneva, Switzerland
George Rutherford, University of California, San Francisco
Catherine M. Wilfert, Elizabeth Glaser Pediatric AIDS Foundation, Duke University, Professor Emeritus, Durham, North Carolina
Gina Wingood, Emory University, Atlanta, Georgia

Although the reviewers listed above have provided many constructive comments and suggestions, they were not asked to endorse the report's conclusions or recommendations nor did they see the final draft of the report before its release. The review of this report was overseen by **Helen Smits**, Fulbright Lecturer, Eduardo Mondlane University, Maputo, Mozambique; and **Bernard Lo**, University of California, San Francisco. Appointed by the National Research Council and Institute of Medicine, they were responsible for making certain that an independent examination of this report was carried out in accordance with institutional procedures and that all review comments were carefully considered. Responsibility for the final content of this report rests entirely with the authoring committee and the institution.

Preface

Today humanity is faced with monumental decisions on how best to apply wealth and scientific know-how to fight the global AIDS crisis, a crisis that each day kills more than 5,000 people in the developing world.

The pandemic of HIV infection that has emerged over the last 25 years has progressed to the point where more than 40 million people are infected with a virus that is universally fatal without treatment. The vast majority of these infected individuals live in some of the poorest countries of the world. About 6 million of them are now in need of antiretroviral therapy, and over the next decade, most of the remaining persons currently infected will progress to that point as well. Perhaps most sobering is that, beyond the current burden, the incidence of HIV infection continues to surge, with about 5 million new cases per year.

Clearly, resources now being mobilized to address this crisis will have to increase steadily and be sustained for decades to come. Attention to both HIV prevention and care is urgently needed. In our rush to be humane, however, we run the risk of sowing the seeds of failure if we do not base programs on solid, evidence-based principles of medical science and public health practice. Such failures would be devastating to all those in need of treatment now and into the future. In addition, by challenging the scientific credibility and feasibility of the whole enterprise, program failure would pose a threat to the willingness of donors to sustain the heroic global response upon which they have embarked. We must, therefore, proceed with caution, while at the same time tolerating no unnecessary delay in heeding the clear moral imperative to halt the devastation caused by this terrible disease.

Typically, individuals infected with HIV are in the prime of their lives, shouldering significant responsibilities for their families and their societies. In addition, thousands of infants are born each year to infected mothers and are at risk to develop HIV infection or to become orphans as their parents die, or both. The high incidence of AIDS in some countries, moreover, is threatening their social, political, economic, and military institutions, thus posing a threat to regional and global security. In African countries with the highest HIV prevalence rates in excess of 20 percent, key societal institutions are at widespread risk of collapse. The potential consequences of this disintegration for local and international peace, prosperity, and freedom are great. Although the world community today has the resources and much of the scientific know-how to begin to stem this devastation, the earliest global responses have been slow in coming and not always well informed by current science and lessons learned from earlier efforts. Furthermore, members of the international community who are leaders in the fight against AIDS in the developing world need to coordinate and harmonize their efforts.

The most-developed countries in the world have benefited from life-extending highly active antiretroviral treatment regimens for about 8 years. Tens of thousands of afflicted persons have seen their fatal infections converted into chronic conditions such that with high-quality care, they may enjoy many more years of healthy and productive life. Costly lessons have been learned in providing this care, however, lessons that must inform newly established treatment programs in resource-constrained countries so as to ensure that they operate with maximal effectiveness and efficiency.

Antiretroviral therapy is a highly demanding form of treatment even in sophisticated medical environments with the best of resources. Complex multidrug regimens must be followed with scrupulous attention to adherence to prevent treatment failure and slow the emergence of drug resistance. Fixed-dose combinations offer significant promise for improving adherence by simplifying these regimens; at the same time, however, this form of compounding presents clinical and pharmacologic quality assurance issues that should not be underappreciated. The specter of drug resistance and treatment failure, a common consequence of imperfect adherence, looms particularly large in resource-poor settings, where the considerably greater expense of second-line regimens may limit their availability. Monitoring for the emergence of resistance and toxicity is also hampered in resource-constrained countries by limited access to laboratories with the relevant capacity. To meet these challenges, well-designed logistic, clinical, and patient support systems are critical.

With the mobilization of billions of dollars to initiate antiretroviral therapy in resource-constrained settings through such mechanisms as the Global Fund to Fight AIDS, Tuberculosis, and Malaria and the U.S. Emergency Plan, the greatest obstacle to significantly prolonging millions of lives may be less lack of access to potent antiretroviral drugs than a looming shortage of qualified persons to deliver and monitor care in a manner that will produce the long-term outcomes sought. Many of the health care systems charged with caring for those infected are seriously understaffed to do so, and the talent required to meet the projected need is just not present locally in adequate amounts. A range of mechanisms, both traditional and innovative, will have to be employed to insert the many types of needed expertise.

While we must move ahead boldly, making use of the best current knowledge, there is much to be learned in the process. Systematic learning while doing will be critical to the ultimate success of these historic initiatives to scale up antiretroviral therapy. Such learning must be accomplished through rigorous monitoring and evaluation of the diversity of programs employed from country to country and in countless villages, towns, and cities. Targeted evaluations and a rigorous program of operational and applied clinical and behavioral research to answer specific questions must be thoughtfully designed, well coordinated, and funded from the beginning with ample dedicated resources.

The legacy of the United States and its international partners, and indeed of the entire global community, in the early 21st century will depend on how we respond to the challenges of the day with the resources at our disposal. While the terrorist threat may appear to dominate, the extent of our capacity to act with a humanitarian regard for those societies being devastated by AIDS may ultimately define the history of our time. We have recognized the inexorable march of HIV for over 20 years and have until recently placed relatively little emphasis on our capacity to deal with its worst manifestations—the decimation being experienced by some the poorest nations of the world. Today, at last, the international medical community has at its disposal the political backing, the know-how, and the resources to begin to meet the challenge of HIV prevention and care in the developing world. We must not abandon those we start on therapy, nor can we ignore the pleas of the millions more who will subsequently make a claim on our humanity. We must act now, and we must act well.

James Curran, M.D., M.P.H.
Haile Debas, M.D.
Cochairs

Acknowledgments

The committee was aided in its deliberations by the testimony and advice of many knowledgeable and experienced individuals, and the efforts of dedicated committee members and staff. Consultants to the committee contributed ideas and report materials. The committee thanks consultants Owen Smith, Abt Associates, Inc.; and Angela Wasunna, The Hastings Center, for their submission of commissioned papers that appear in the appendixes of this report.

The committee acknowledges with appreciation the testimony of many individuals committed to addressing the needs of individuals and communities affected by HIV/AIDS around the world. These individuals are: Diane Bennett, World Health Organization; Stefano Bertozzi, National Institute of Public Health, Cuernavaca, Mexico; Yasmin Chandani, John Snow, Inc.; Rachel Cohen, Campaign for Access to Essential Medicines, Médecins sans Frontières; Steven Deeks, University of California, San Francisco; Victor DeGruttola, Harvard School of Public Health; Paul DeLay, UNAIDS; Sam Dooley, Centers for Disease Control and Prevention; Wafaa El-Sadr, Columbia University and Harlem Hospital; Daniel Fitzgerald, Cornell University Medical College; Eric Goosby, Pangea Global AIDS Foundation; John Idoko, Jos University Teaching Hospital, Jos Nigeria; Brooks Jackson, Johns Hopkins University School of Medicine; Jim Kim, World Health Organization; Mark Kline, Baylor College of Medicine/Texas Children's Hospital; Ronaldo Lima, International AIDS Vaccine Initiative; Emi MacLean, Médecins sans Frontières; Lynn Margherio, The Clinton Foundation HIV/AIDS Initiative; Rashad Massoud, Quality and Performance Institute, University Research Co., LLC; Anthony Mbewu, Medical Research Council of South Africa; John McNeil, National Minority AIDS Education and Training Center, Howard University; Lynne Mofenson, National Institute of Child Health and Human Development, National Institutes of Health; Carla Makhlouf Obermeyer, World Health Organization; Joseph O'Neil, Office of Global AIDS, U.S. Department of State; Mead Over, The World Bank;

Thomas Quinn, Johns Hopkins University School of Medicine; Robert Redfield, University of Maryland, Baltimore; Mauro Schechter, Universidade Federal do Rio de Janeiro, Brazil; Bernhard Schwartlander, The Global Fund to Fight AIDS, Tuberculosis, and Malaria; and Angela Wasunna, The Hastings Center. The agenda for the information-gathering workshop in which these individuals participated appears in Appendix A of the report.

Finally, and in particular, the committee would like to express its deep appreciation of the Institute of Medicine (IOM) staff who facilitated its work. We especially thank Monisha Arya, Patrick Kelley, Stacey Knobler, and Leslie Pray for translating and transforming the discussions and deliberations of the committee into final prose. The committee is grateful to Karl Galle, Katherine Oberholtzer, and Dianne Stare, for their efforts in addressing the information and research verification needs of the study and preparing the final manuscript for publication. Special thanks to Allison Berger and Amy Giamis for their extra efforts and repeated attention to the logistical support of the study. Others within the IOM and the National Academies who were instrumental in seeing the project to completion were Harriet Banda, Jennifer Bitticks, Tim Brennan, Rachel Cohen, Janice Mehler, Jennifer Otten, Bronwyn Schrecker, Laura Sivitz, and Sally Stanfield. Thanks are also expressed to editorial consultants Rona Briere and Alisa Decatur.

This report was made possible by the generous support of the Fogarty International Center (FIC), the Office of AIDS Research at the National Institutes of Health (OAR), and the Bill and Melinda Gates Foundation (GF). Additional support for funding international travel of workshop speakers was provided by the Global Fund to Fight AIDS, Tuberculosis, and Malaria; UNAIDS; and the Centers for Disease Control and Prevention Global AIDS Program. The committee is appreciative of their support and of the commitment and productive efforts of Jerry Keusch and Sharon Hrynkow (FIC); Jack Whitescarver (OAR); and Helene Gayle (GF).

Synopsis

Approximately 40 million people worldwide are infected with HIV, and 6 million suffering from AIDS need antiretroviral therapy (ART) now. Yet only about 400,000 people in resource-poor nations have access to treatment, despite the fact that these countries often have the highest infection rates of HIV. The largely unchecked pace of the infection and its impact on the social, political, and economic dimensions of individuals and communities continue to undermine the development of entire countries and regions of the world.

Therefore, what must be emphasized is the need for the global community to act now. Growing recognition of this human and societal catastrophe, combined with the increased understanding and availability of technical tools necessary to halt its devastating progress, have mobilized political will and financial resources worldwide to bring treatment options within the reach of those most in need.

Equally important to scaling-up the global response to HIV/AIDS will be the need to act well. The availability of inexpensive drugs alone will not ensure the successful prolongation of millions of lives. Experience with ART in wealthy nations has led many experts to heed concerns over the suboptimal introduction of these drugs. Considerable attention to strategies that promote the highest levels of patient adherence to drug regimens will be needed to avoid treatment failure and the more rapid development of drug-resistant strains of the virus.

Key to implementing these adherence strategies, as well as to delivering effective ART, will be tens of thousands of health care and management personnel with the experience and training to treat millions of people with a disease that requires a complicated and long-term regimen. A workforce of this magnitude does not currently exist in most resource-poor nations, and its mobilization could have negative collateral effects on existing health programs through diversion of scarce resources. Significant shortages in trained personnel must be addressed immediately and energetically through innovative governmental and private-sector programs. Such efforts to address carefully defined weaknesses should seek to bring health care and other professionals from resource-rich nations into developing countries, while supporting robust efforts to train and educate a national workforce that will continue to expand sustainable HIV/AIDS treatment and prevention initiatives well into the future.

Promoting a culture of learning by doing will be an essential component of the success of ART scale-up. As a first priority, ongoing monitoring and evaluation of the many aspects of ART programs should be viewed as being as fundamental to scale-up as the antiretroviral drugs themselves.

In moving forward rapidly to stem the tragic progress of HIV/AIDS, it must be recognized that there is still much to be revealed about the most effective ways to operate large-scale ART. Existing guidelines and treatment regimens will need to be improved and adapted to meet the highly variable needs of populations with significantly different cultural, economic, epidemiological, and technical profiles.

It bears emphasizing that the global problem of HIV/AIDS will be present for decades despite prevention and treatment interventions. With a projected 5 million additional people infected by HIV each year, the numbers needing treatment will continue to increase. Once ART has been initiated, we must not abandon the millions started on therapy or ignore the pleas of the tens of millions more who will soon need these medicines. Even short-term interruptions in support could be clinically disastrous and ethically unconscionable by allowing successfully suppressed HIV infections to emerge in drug-resistant forms against which no affordable interventions would be successful. Thus, ART must not be seen simply as a short-term goal or the end point of a 5-year plan. Scale-up of HIV/AIDS treatment and prevention is an urgently needed public health endeavor of unprecedented scale. Its noble intentions must be matched by an equally unprecedented commitment to sustained action against one of the worst plagues in human history.

Contents

xvii

Executive Summary

The HIV/AIDS[1] pandemic has evolved into the greatest global public health crisis, one that has progressed virtually unchecked in many of the poorest regions of the world for over two decades. Of the 40 million people worldwide infected with HIV, an estimated 6 million are in need of immediate, life-sustaining antiretroviral (ARV) therapy (ART). Yet fewer than 400,000 people in low- and middle-income countries have access to such treatment (WHO, 2003b). Most HIV-infected individuals live in severely resource-constrained settings, where the HIV epidemic continues to grow at a rate of 5 million infections per year, compounding the already enormous treatment challenge. The high AIDS mortality rate in sub-Saharan Africa, which remains the worst-affected region of the world, contrasts sharply with the decreasing HIV-related death rate in high-income countries where ARVs are widely available and affordable. Those acutely affected by a pervasive lack of treatment in resource-constrained environments include not only the millions of infected individuals, but also the millions of children orphaned when their parents die from HIV-related illness for want of these drugs. Moreover, because HIV-related deaths occur disproportionately among young, economically productive adults, the epidemic is undermining the economic development and social fabric of entire countries.

---

[1]Human immunodeficiency virus/acquired immunodeficiency syndrome.

1

Growing recognition of the unprecedented nature and momentum of this human catastrophe, coupled with the increased understanding and growing availability of technical tools needed to halt its devastating progress, has mobilized political will and financial resources worldwide to bring treatment options to those most in need. Three initiatives highlight recent financial and operational steps being taken to accelerate access to ART and other HIV/AIDS care and prevention programs in resource-constrained settings. On December 1, 2003, also World AIDS Day, the World Health Organization (WHO) and Joint United Nations Programme on HIV/AIDS (UNAIDS) launched the "3-by-5" campaign, with a global target of providing ART to 3 million people with HIV/AIDS in developing countries by the end of 2005 (WHO, 2003b). In November 2003, the government of South Africa approved its landmark Operational Plan for Comprehensive HIV and AIDS Care, Management and Treatment for South Africa (South Africa Department of Health, 2003). One of the goals of the plan is to administer ARVs to more than 1 million people with HIV infection by 2008–2009; this goal is to be accomplished by negotiating with multiple competing drug suppliers and eventually producing the drugs locally. Finally, in January 2003, during his State of the Union address, U.S. President George W. Bush promised $15 billion to international AIDS activities over the course of the next 5 years as part of the President's Emergency Plan for AIDS Relief (U.S. Department of State, 2003). One of the goals of the plan is to provide ART to 2 million HIV-infected people in the poorest, most afflicted countries in Africa, the Caribbean, and Vietnam.

The clinical, financial, and epidemiological effects of implementing such widespread treatment and prevention programs must be considered, and rational methods for informing such efforts developed. One major concern is that of fostering the premature emergence of widespread resistance to ARVs, thereby reducing the long-term viability of ART regimens in developing countries.

In this context, the Institute of Medicine was asked to provide an independent review and assessment of ART scale-up programs currently under way and in development. The Committee on Examining the Probable Consequences of Alternative Patterns of Widespread Antiretroviral Drug Use in Resource-Constrained Settings was formed to conduct this study. The committee was charged to provide (1) an examination and evaluation of current ART implementation programs, efficacy studies, infrastructure costing models, existing guidelines for program implementation, and models that demonstrate successful scale-up of ART programs; (2) a study of the role of ongoing well-developed operations research in the field and in parallel with treatment implementation to establish sustainability outcome measures; (3) a determination of the components necessary for a systematic, structured framework to achieve a balance between resistance development and transmission and the need to provide treatment in resource-constrained settings; and (4) an assessment of current research on ARV resistance and toxicity, and the likely effects on the malnourished individuals with high disease burden found in resource-poor settings.

In response to this charge, the committee developed its findings, conclusions, and recommendations using evidence derived from the scientific literature, commissioned papers, and unpublished data drawn from workshop presentations made by individuals currently researching and implementing ART programs in resource-constrained environments. The combined weight of this evidence contributed to the committee's formulation of strategies that require immediate attention and action, as well as recommendations regarding programs, policies, and research that must continue to evolve if efforts aimed at treating millions of individuals in need are to be improved and sustained.

MOVING FORWARD NOW:
FINDINGS AND RECOMMENDATIONS

ART scale-up in resource-constrained settings worldwide must proceed immediately. Although there may be no definitive single solution regarding how best to introduce ART into such settings, the committee identified a rational framework and key principles to guide the people and institutions that are providing resources for and leading ART scale-up programs worldwide. The committee undertook this effort with a keen awareness of the potential dangers of the suboptimal introduction of ARVs on a large scale, as well as the complex ethical challenges stemming from the reality that there will not be enough treatment for everyone who needs it. Recognizing these challenges, there remains an urgency to provide ART as rapidly as is feasible in order to extend the duration of as many lives as possible and reverse the course of social collapse in many countries heavily afflicted by HIV/AIDS.

Coordinating and Sustaining the Global Response

The widespread introduction of ARVs into resource-constrained settings worldwide is expected to result in exciting and life-extending successes. The much-anticipated influx of funds and resources to be made available by initiatives such as those noted earlier—including the U.S. President's Emergency Plan for AIDS Relief; WHO's 3-by-5 campaign; and continued efforts of the Global Fund to Fight AIDS, Tuberculosis, and Malaria—as well as the World Bank's Multi-Country HIV/AIDS Program

for the Africa Region and a growing number of national HIV/AIDS programs worldwide, are generating great enthusiasm and hope that this human tragedy can be abated. The reach of these investments will continue to
be enhanced by the efforts of global health and political leaders to achieve
maximal efficiencies through innovative price reduction mechanisms, such
as the procurement strategies for drugs and equipment developed by the
William J. Clinton Foundation and Médicins sans Frontières (MSF). As
these programs develop and expand, it will be essential for all people involved, including international and national leaders and those living with
HIV/AIDS, to remain aware of the medical, social, and ethical challenges,
complexities, and risks associated with taking on a global problem of such
enormous proportions.

A considerable challenge for ART scale-up is that unreliable or interrupted drug supplies, combined with poor treatment procedures and program management, could promote treatment failure as well as the emergence of ARV-resistant virus, thereby reducing the long-term durability of
more-affordable first-line drug regimens. Therefore, paramount to the long-
term success of these programs will be recognition on the part of international and national leaders of the lifelong nature of ART and the need to
sustain a constant supply of quality drugs and services in the context of
quality supportive care. Both clinical success and ethical imperatives will
demand lifelong therapy. Unlike most interventions deployed for infectious
diseases (e.g., vaccines and short-course drug therapy), then, ART is a
lifelong treatment that will require resources, clinical management, and
patient adherence consistent with chronic disease management strategies
not often appreciated in developing countries. Therefore, new attitudes,
training, and programmatic approaches will be needed (WHO, 2002).

In addition, the natural progression of untreated HIV infections will
result in a growing call to place millions of new patients on treatment
within the next few years. These growing needs will demand long-term
commitments from the international donor community and countries bur-
dened with a high HIV prevalence. To ensure the sustainability of ART
scale-up for the next generation, these commitments must be accompanied
by new strategies for promoting self-sufficiency in countries with a high
HIV/AIDS disease burden.

> **Antiretroviral therapy scale-up in resource-constrained settings should
> proceed immediately through coordinated, aggressive action by na-
> tional governments, donors, international agencies, and nongovern-
> mental organizations.** *Donors must attempt to maximize the distribu-
> tion of scarce resources—human, financial, and technical—for people
> in need within and among all resource-constrained countries and areas.
> To this end, multiple HIV/AIDS prevention and treatment initiatives
> need to be coordinated and integrated through national leadership and*

entitities that best meet the needs of their populations and of all individuals. (Recommendation 2-1)[2]

Donors should commit to continuous funding of antiretroviral therapy scale-up for decades to ensure the sustainability necessary to avert the medical hazard of interruptions in the continuity of treatment. *Delays in donor funding after treatment programs are initiated will jeopardize the long-term durability of treatment regimens. Because it is estimated that 40 million people are currently infected with HIV, and 5 million new infections occur each year, donors should plan now for increasing support in the future. To this end, innovative mechanisms should continue to be pursued by national governments and donors in partnership with industry to ensure the continuous procurement of quality drugs, diagnostics, and other commodities at the lowest possible cost. At the same time, national governments in countries severely affected by HIV/ AIDS must begin to invest in and develop priorities for prevention and treatment programs to ensure those programs' long-term sustainability and effectiveness.* (Recommendation 2-2)

Developing and Managing Treatment Strategies

The lack of robust data and evidence-based evaluation makes it difficult to use best practices to guide initial program design within these countries. ART programs in middle- and low-income countries provide some important lessons (Galvao, 2002; Weidle et al., 2002), but population- and resource-specific guidelines tailored to individual country needs will ultimately prove most effective.

Program Design

WHO's 2003 guidelines (WHO, 2003a, presented in Appendix C) may simplify and make feasible an otherwise prohibitively complex therapy, but there are still many unanswered clinical questions regarding the most effective, safe use of ARVs in resource-constrained settings. In particular, although the guidelines include recommendations for pregnant women, patients coinfected with tuberculosis,[3] and infants and children, WHO acknowledges the guidelines' limitations given the critical lack of knowl-

---

[2]The numbers in parentheses after each recommendation correspond to the numbering scheme used in the main text. Thus, for example, Recommendation 2-1 is the first recommendation in Chapter 2.

[3]In 2002, 42 million people were living with HIV/AIDS, and 11 million adults living with HIV/AIDS were estimated to be coinfected with *Mycobacterium* tuberculosis.

edge and urgent need for research in these areas. Nonetheless, the WHO guidelines are endorsed in this report for use as a working template that should be modified according to specific country needs and the findings of ongoing operational research.

Before countries develop their own directives, the World Health Organization's 2003 guidelines for the treatment of adults, children, and pregnant women should serve as an initial template for the design of antiretroviral therapy programs with respect to when to start therapy, which regimens to use, how to monitor the progress of therapy, and when to switch drugs or terminate therapy. *As new evidence becomes available through the efforts of international, national, and local research, the WHO guidelines, particularly with regard to pregnant women and those coinfected with tuberculosis, may require refinement or modification.* (Recommendation 4-2)

Program managers, international donors, and national policy makers should ensure that strong tuberculosis control programs continue in parallel with antiretroviral treatment scale-up programs, given that nearly one-third of HIV-infected persons in the world are coinfected with tuberculosis. *Because dual infection with HIV and tuberculosis poses a life-threatening diagnostic and therapeutic dilemma, strong HIV care programs must include capabilities for diagnosis, treatment, and prophylaxis of tuberculosis. Tuberculosis treatment programs should be supported as an important point of entry for HIV testing and consideration for ART. It is critical to overall treatment success that these coexisting epidemics be addressed in parallel.* (Recommendation 4-6)

Integration of Prevention and Treatment Strategies

ART can and should serve a critical secondary role in the prevention of HIV/AIDS, both clinically and behaviorally. It may be hoped that, beyond reducing both sexual and maternal-to-infant transmission of infection by decreasing patient viral load (Quinn et al., 2000; Gray et al., 2001; Ometto et al., 2000; John et al., 2001) in those being treated, the availability of ART will motivate many millions more people to seek voluntary counseling and testing—a critical component of any prevention or care intervention—and help diminish the stigma associated with HIV/AIDS (Nierengarten, 2003).

National and international program planners should coordinate and integrate stronger and more effective HIV/AIDS prevention initiatives concurrently with the scale-up of antiretroviral therapy programs. *Pre-*

*vention initiatives should focus on those at risk for acquiring or trans-
mitting HIV infection, in addition to those receiving treatment. To be
optimally successful, voluntary counseling and testing programs and
programs to prevent mother-to-child transmission should encompass
both preventive and therapeutic dimensions. National and community
leaders should be strong advocates for effective HIV prevention efforts
and engage government agencies and community groups in sectors
beyond health, including education and public relations, as well as
legislative leaders (to prevent discrimination).* (Recommendation 4-8)

**Governmental and community leaders at all levels of civic life should
spearhead an effort to create a culture of openness and support in
order to eliminate stigma and ensure the successful continuance of
antiretroviral treatment and HIV prevention programs.** (Recommendation 4-1)

Adherence and Drug Quality

Adherence to drug regimens will be a critical factor in determining the
success of ART programs, but it is also expected to be one of the greatest
clinical challenges of ART scale-up. Although studies have shown that good
adherence is quite feasible in resource-constrained settings under certain
circumstances (e.g., in clinical settings where the studies are conducted)
(Laniece et al., 2003; Orrell et al., 2003), the reproducibility of these results
in other settings involving widespread scale-up cannot be assured. The
challenge is made more difficult by the lack of conclusive evidence on what
factors contribute to poor adherence and what interventions would likely
be most effective at maximizing adherence in resource-constrained settings.
It has been suggested that ease of administration, timing and dosing requirements, drug efficacy, improved well-being, and patient education are
all important elements contributing to adherence.

**Antiretroviral therapy program managers, international donors, and
national planners should take the necessary measures and provide
resources to ensure the strict adherence to therapy that is fundamental
to program success. Such measures should include timely and adequate
provision of drugs and health care, knowledgeable and available providers, and appropriate patient education.** *ART programs should encourage community involvement in the development of adherence interventions. This involvement should include people living with HIV/
AIDS, family members, and community and religious leaders. Additionally, in special populations—such as migrant workers, trucking
and transportation workers, and the military—special multisite and*

transnational program links may need to be established. (Recommendation 4-7)

Some experts have called for the use of fixed-dose combinations (FDCs) to improve adherence. There is controversy, however, regarding how to best measure the quality and effectiveness of FDCs. It is not well understood whether adequate procedures are in place to ensure ongoing drug quality after initial qualification (surveillance and specimen inspection) or to identify the emergence of drug-related adverse events (postmarket). The benefits of high levels of adherence to ARV regimens would not be realized if those drugs were not themselves efficacious, safe, and of consistent quality. Therefore, ongoing, rigorous quality assurance throughout the manufacturing and distribution chain will be essential to ensure that cost savings are not routinely or intermittently sought at the expense of quality.

> **The committee endorses as critical the use of the cheapest, safest, most effective high-quality antiretroviral drugs that can be procured. Fixed-dose combinations are recommended as most desirable if they are also of high quality, safe, effective, and inexpensive. The committee also strongly endorses a rigorous, standardized international mechanism to support national quality assurance programs for antiretroviral drugs. This mechanism should be timely, transparent, and independent of conflicts of interest; employ evidence-based standards; and provide ongoing assurance of consistent high-quality manufacture and handling. In particular, the pharmacological issues associated with fixed-dose combinations must be rigorously and rapidly addressed.** (Recommendation 5-6)

Initiation and Monitoring of Treatment

As medically, fiscally, and logistically challenging as the consequences of treatment failure due to toxicity or drug resistance may be, they should not be construed as a reason to discourage or unnecessarily delay the introduction of responsibly designed ART scale-up programs in resource-limited settings. On the other hand, the risk of widespread treatment failure due to resistance and other factors demands a careful, rational, evidence-based public health approach to ART scale-up and the capacity to know when therapeutic and programmatic changes are needed. To this end, the immediate application of basic longitudinal clinical care, surveillance, and laboratory tools will be necessary. Although many patients in resource-rich countries have continued to derive immunological and clinical benefit from ART even after the emergence of highly resistant viral strains (Deeks et al., 2000), the more-expensive drug options, monitoring tools, sequential therapeutic schemes, and provider expertise that allow for this continuing benefit are lacking in most resource-constrained settings.

Antiretroviral therapy programs should be designed to optimize the balance between individual efficacy and population effectiveness while minimizing toxicity and resistance. *ART regimens or programs shown to be significantly less effective or ineffective—such as mono- or dual-therapy and nucleoside-only regimens—must be avoided. Because resources and population and patient needs will vary considerably among different countries and regions, countries should develop population-specific guidelines.* (Recommendation 4-5)

For individual patients about to embark on therapy, general clinical screening for resistance to antiretroviral drugs is not recommended at this time for two reasons: because the prevalence of resistance in HIV-infected individuals not previously exposed to antiretroviral therapy is expected to be undetectable or low, and because the proportion of total persons with HIV who are receiving therapy in a given country will also be relatively small in the short term. Coordinated, systematic testing for resistance to antiretroviral drugs should, however, be conducted among a subset of patients failing treatment. *These latter results will be critical in evaluating ART programs and in determining whether and when routine population-based resistance testing might eventually prove effective. Sentinel surveillance of treatment-naïve HIV-positive persons may also be indicated in the future.* (Recommendation 3-1)

Donors and program managers should plan and budget for laboratory activities that will foster more accurate and effective HIV diagnosis and management, using the World Health Organization's 2003 guidelines as the initial template. *Incorporating emerging evidence and resources into their decision-making process, countries should consider developing population-specific guidelines reflective of the best possible practices in their particular circumstances. In those localities where it is possible to go beyond the WHO guidelines, treatment failure should be defined through viral RNA determination; otherwise, it should be defined by means of clinical or other laboratory markers consistent with the guidelines.* (Recommendation 4-3)

Under the leadership of their ministries of health and national reference laboratory experts, all countries should develop hierarchical laboratory networks that integrate the local, district, and referral hospital levels through tiered quality assurance programs and provide referral support for increasingly complex laboratory assays. Full development of these networks is not required before the initiation of scaled-up antiretroviral therapy programs, however. *National reference laboratories should promulgate tier-specific quality assurance protocols, and donors supporting ART programs should provide the means to properly ensure acceptable technical performance by these laboratory networks. Dedi-*

cated funds, training, and other resources to ensure the maintenance of the laboratory equipment employed in these networks should be provided. To better facilitate the diagnosis and treatment of HIV infection in infants less than 18 months of age, the laboratory networks should put in place a capacity for the direct detection of HIV, such as HIV DNA, HIV RNA, or HIV p24 antigen. (Recommendation 4-4)

Building a Comprehensive Infrastructure for Scaling Up

While the declining costs of ARVs have removed a significant impediment to ART scale-up, successful efforts will depend on much more than inexpensive drugs. The drugs must be delivered into an infrastructure with the capacity to distribute them and other commodities rapidly and securely while also ensuring the readiness of facilities and personnel to provide complex lifelong medical treatment and associated monitoring to millions of people. Success will require serious attention to address critical shortcomings in infrastructure, particularly with regard to human resource capacity.

Ensuring Equitable Care

Even in countries such as South Africa, which is not as severely resource-constrained as most of its sub-Saharan neighbors, the vast health and wealth disparities that exist between the "urban poor" and the "rural poorer" create extraordinary logistical and ethical challenges to delivering equitable ART. Resolving such disparities will require immediate investments in rural areas in the basic infrastructure needed for ART programs. By ensuring that contributions can be used for infrastructure and workforce development, international and national decision makers will enhance the equitable delivery of ART.

Mobilizing a Workforce

The shortage of workers in *all* areas of the health care sector has been identified as a rate-limiting constraint to rolling out large, countrywide ART programs. The progress of scale-up in many, if not most, areas will require signficantly greater workforce capacity; without this increased capacity, scale-up could potentially fail on these grounds alone. WHO has estimated that its 3-by-5 campaign will require an additional 100,000 health providers and community treatment supporters trained to deliver ARVs in accordance with national standards (WHO, 2003b). Care must be taken to maintain existing health care services and not to weaken current infrastructures. Of concern is that as health care systems receive an infusion of fiscal resources for new HIV prevention and treatment programs, there could be a migration of already scarce workers to these new programs and away from other critical public health endeavors, such as maternal and child health and malaria control.

Efforts should be made to augment mechanisms that can be used to mobilize larger numbers of trained professionals from resource-rich countries with extensive and relevant expertise to provide technical assistance and training to countries in need. *Such an HIV/AIDS corps would serve to strengthen long-term ties among health professionals working to fight HIV/AIDS in all countries. A variety of innovative governmental and private-sector mechanisms should be designed and expanded to bring qualified volunteer medical professionals into both urban and rural areas to support prevention, care, and training programs relevant to ART scale-up. The required expertise and skills and the areas for placement in country should be determined by local programs.* (Recommendation 5-1)

In addition to the immediate human resource needs that must be addressed to initiate ART, a well-trained and sufficiently populated workforce will be needed to provide care through the next several decades. Improved educational opportunities and training programs will be necessary to build a critical mass of health care professionals, program managers, and technology professionals to meet the continuing needs of programs for HIV/AIDS prevention, treatment, and care. Methods and tools for assessing and monitoring human resource needs will improve and inform decision making in the areas of both investment and training.

Donors and organizations with relevant expertise (e.g., academia, industry, public health agencies, nongovernmental organizations) should support active partnerships among all institutions possessing such expertise and those seeking to acquire the benefits of training; mentoring; and the transfer of antiretroviral therapy–related medical, technical, and managerial knowledge and skills. Partnerships among medical institutions within and across national borders should be encouraged by donors and governmental authorities. *These twinning relationships should support the transfer of appropriate technology; expertise in medicine, monitoring and evaluation, and applied and operations research; and lessons learned. Physical and electronic means should be used to provide ongoing support for these partnerships.* (Recommendation 5-2)

Expertise within the AIDS Education and Training Center networks sponsored by the U.S. government and similar initiatives by other countries should be utilized to support the development of effective training programs in HIV care in order to prepare local physicians, nurses, community health workers, laboratory professionals, pharmacists, and logisticians in heavily HIV-afflicted countries facing severe human resource shortages. (Recommendation 5-3)

Countries should establish information systems at the regional and national levels so they can regularly assess and coordinate their evolving human resource needs. *Both countries with relatively adequate human resources and those that are more resource-constrained should pursue appropriate policies and programs to stem the "brain drain" of local expertise that is critically needed for the scale-up of ART programs. The current shortage of trained, dedicated personnel for monitoring and evaluation programs should be rectified in conjunction with meeting other training and personnel needs.* (Recommendation 5-4)

Securing the Delivery of Effective Drugs

In addition to clinical and human resource issues surrounding ART scale-up, the logistics of drug delivery pose a complex challenge. An interruption in the drug supply line—whether caused by transportation, financial, corruption, or other problems—will increase the risk of treatment failure regardless of how adherent a patient is or how knowledgeable providers are about HIV/AIDS treatment and care.

To provide continuous, secure delivery of quality drugs, diagnostics, and other products, national and international program managers of antiretroviral scale-up efforts should ensure that well-coordinated commodity and logistics systems are in place from the outset of program initiation. *Technical leadership, governmental commitment, and institutional support are needed to ensure the secure delivery of quality drugs and supplies. Methods to avert the interruption of drug supplies include information systems to facilitate the projection of needs and track the distribution of available stocks. Such planning and investment should also account for the consequences of civil disruption or natural disasters, which would require adequate contingencies to avoid disruption to the supply and treatment systems.* (Recommendation 5-5)

Learning by Doing:
The Essential Role of Monitoring and Evaluation

As much as ART scale-up can and should be founded in evidence-based public health knowledge, it will also depend largely on a learn-by-doing approach. Global efforts to control the pandemic in severely resource-constrained environments are still too new to have yielded extensive evidence-based best practices. Much of the medical and public health knowledge garnered to date is based on research conducted in the context of the United States and other resource-rich countries. Although some of this knowledge is transferable to a multitude of settings, much will need to be reassessed. In this process, mistakes and setbacks should be construed as learning experiences, not excuses to withhold treatment from those in need. In fact, formal methods for recognizing program success and failure and then effecting change as a result of what is observed should be incorporated into all clinical care and management strategies.

Improving Effectiveness and Sustainability Through Monitoring and Evaluation

There are concerns about whether and how dedicated ART scale-up funds will be allocated to the often-overlooked but vitally important monitoring and evaluation components of program design. Monitoring and evaluation are based on intensive data collection and analysis and assessment of programmatic outcomes, not simply process indicators; both are vital to the long-term sustainability of ART scale-up.

Monitoring and evaluation involves the routine assessment of ongoing activities and progress and the episodic assessment of overall achievements. Given that there are serious short- and long-term risks associated with widespread treatment failure and resistance, it is critical that the future direction of national ART programs be continuously informed by a robust monitoring and evaluation system. National program leaders must know when their treatment guidelines are failing and when changes need to be made.

Monitoring and evaluation can be used to assure the global community, including funders and decision makers, that ART scale-up is achieving its intended goals. Such assurance will be vital to the long-term fiscal sustainability of ART programs.

Monitoring and evaluation processes should be put in place by program managers at all levels at the start of scale-up initiatives. *A fixed percentage (approximately 5–10 percent) of ART program funding should be budgeted strictly for monitoring and evaluation (exclusive of support for hypothesis-driven operations research).* (Recommendation 5-7)

Program managers should measure the effectiveness of HIV prevention and treatment efforts by means of scientifically valid and systematically conducted surveys of HIV prevalence and incidence, HIV morbidity and mortality, and risk behaviors. *ART programs should be designed* *to improve the quality of life and add many years of productivity for as many people as possible. The success of ART scale-up should be evaluated on the basis of the extent to which these specific goals are achieved.* (Recommendation 5-8)

Monitoring and evaluation measures and requirements, as directed by various donors and other stakeholders, should be harmonized across programs to minimize time-consuming inefficiencies in data collection and program management. *Additional efficiencies would be achieved if these efforts were coordinated by a single national ministry or agency. Donors should avoid attempting to ascribe results solely to individual funding sources in order to minimize the in-country confusion and inefficiency created by mandates to conduct multiple, uncoordinated monitoring and evaluation efforts in the midst of rapid scale-up.* (Recommendation 5-9)

IMPROVING FUTURE OUTCOMES

Recognizing the limited infrastructure, tools, knowledge, and personnel currently available in resource-constrained settings, it is clear that future efforts in the provision of ART will benefit from expanded investments and research. Given the limited experience with large-scale ART programs in resource-constrained countries, the capturing of lessons learned from newly implemented programs will be essential to informing the direction and priorities that will ensure long-term sustainability, quality, and success. Gaps in knowledge still inhibit our efforts to prevent, diagnose, and treat HIV/AIDS more effectively. Such discoveries will ultimately facilitate not only more cost-effective care, but also the saving of millions of lives.

Formulating a Research Agenda

Operations Research

Operations research involves the planned, systematic experimental design, testing, and analysis of different processes or practices. A well-designed operations research program will be critical to gathering as much information as possible during what will of necessity be learning by doing. Lessons learned can be used to establish national guidelines specific to a country's needs, to correct mistakes, and to inform changes and new initiatives. Well-designed programs based on the best available objective evidence stand a better chance of success—not only because of the direct benefit to those patients receiving treatment, but also because of the greater number of people that can be treated as a result of the cost savings realized by such programs. At the same time, it is essential not to become paralyzed by the desire to have all of the details in place before beginning. The HIV/AIDS tragedy demands urgent action.

Operations research should begin at the initiation of scale-up and continue to inform the future direction and sustainable success of antiretroviral treatment and HIV prevention programs in resource-constrained settings. *Priorities for operations research should be identified by national programs and funded by donors through an explicit allocation that will address the need for rapid development of evidence for policy. Input from national authorities working with donors should be supplemented by consultation with WHO and other multilateral agencies to obtain technical advice and to help maximize regional synergies, share information, and avoid unnecessarily duplicative studies within a given region.* (Recommendation 6-1)

Research priorities should be informed by the perspectives of local researchers, health workers, and community representatives and reflect respect for the cultures of affected communities. *Just as every pilot initiative functions uniquely, every scale-up initiative and national program will have its own way of functioning and should be shaped by the perspectives of those with a stake in its success. Ideally, if a well-developed operations research agenda is established early on, these different ways of functioning can be objectively evaluated in a timely fashion and the results used to inform managers of other scale-up programs about newly identified best practices. Collaborative partnerships and endeavors between the research and health care communities should be encouraged.* (Recommendation 6-2)

Applied Clinical and Behavioral Research

In addition to operations research that will identify and optimize clinical and management processes, it will be important to address the numerous gaps in knowledge and tools that still limit our ability to respond effectively to the global HIV/AIDS pandemic. Support for applied clinical and behavioral research is of fundamental importance. Rapid and inexpensive diagnostic tools and laboratory tests would greatly improve the clinician's ability to determine when to initiate and how to monitor therapy, including making important decisions about the selection of and changes in drug regimens to avoid treatment failure. A better understanding of the impact of the nutritional status of patients on drug effectiveness and toxicity will be critical in populations plagued by chronic malnutrition and often by the lack of adequate quantities of food. The social and behavioral dimensions of ART scale-up are complex. Responding to these challenges will be greatly facilitated by a better understanding of the factors that improve adherence to drug therapy, the most effective methods for reducing risk behaviors that contribute to HIV transmission, and effective measures for reducing stigma related to HIV/AIDS.

> **Development and field evaluation of simple, rapid, inexpensive laboratory tests for diagnosing HIV infection and for monitoring therapeutic responses should be a high priority.** *The shortage of laboratories and laboratory technicians in resource-poor countries, together with the millions in need of HIV testing and treatment monitoring, underlies the priority of developing tests with these characteristics. In relatively well-resourced countries, critical monitoring for toxicity and viral response utilizes generally expensive assays, whose annual costs could themselves be comparable to those of the antiretroviral drugs to be used. For resource-constrained countries, less-costly measurement tools, such as viral load and CD4 counts, are needed to stretch limited budgets and enable technicians trained at a more basic level to perform the tests.* (Recommendation 6-3)

Box ES-1 lists some priority topics for applied research to support ART scale-up initiatives.

BOX ES-1
Some Applied Research Priorities for ART Scale-up Initiatives

- Simple, rapid, inexpensive laboratory tests for diagnosing and monitoring HIV/AIDS, to include the particular case of infants under 18 months of age.
- Culturally appropriate adherence interventions for both adult and pediatric populations.
- Randomized trials quantifying the effects of FDCs on health outcomes and adherence, along with relative benefits compared with blister packages and loose drugs, to better inform decisions about drug selection and delivery.
- The pharmacokinetics of ARVs in chronically malnourished populations and effects related to drug toxicity.
- The evidence-based development of pediatric ARV formulations.
- The optimal means of integrating ARV initiatives with other health services so as to minimize the negative collateral effects of these new large-scale programs.

CONCLUSION

Sustained action for scaling up treatment for the HIV epidemic presumes solutions to numerous scientific and management challenges. At the same time, as wealthy, middle-income, and poor nations join together to tackle the overarching challenge of bringing the pandemic under control, it bears emphasizing that the global problem of HIV/AIDS will likely be present for decades despite research findings and optimized interventions. In a few years, when it may be hoped that the initial objectives of WHO's 3-by-5 campaign and the U.S. Emergency Plan will have been met, we must not abandon the millions started on therapy or ignore the pleas of the tens of millions more who will soon need these medicines. Even short-term interruptions in support could be clinically disastrous and ethically unconscionable by allowing successfully suppressed HIV infections to emerge in drug-resistant forms. Thus, ART must not be seen simply as a short-term goal or the end point of a 5-year plan. The world is indeed at the beginning of a very long path forward that will require vigilant and sustained support.

REFERENCES

Deeks SG, Barbour JD, Martin JN, Swanson MS, Grant RM. 2000. Sustained CD4+ T cell response after virologic failure of protease inhibitor-based regimens in patients with human immunodeficiency virus infection. *Journal of Infectious Diseases* 181:946–953.

Galvao J. 2002. Access to antiretroviral drugs in Brazil. *Lancet* 360(9348):1862–1865.

Gray R, Wawer MJ, Brookmeyer R, Sewan Kambo NK, Serwadda D, Wabwire-Mangen F, Lutalo T, Li X, VanCott T, Quinn TC, Rakai Project Team. 2001. Probability of HIV-1 transmission per coital act in monogamous, heterosexual, HIV-1 discordant couples in Rakai, Uganda. *Lancet* 357:1149–1153.

John GC, Nduati RW, Mbori-Ngacha DA, Richardson BA, Panteleeff D, Mwatha A, Overbaugh J, Bwayo J, Ndinya-Achola JO, Kreiss JK. 2001. Correlates of mother-to-child human immunodeficiency virus type 1 (HIV-1) transmission: Association with maternal plasma HIV-1 RNA load, genital HIV-1 DNA shedding, and breast infections. *Journal of Infectious Diseases* 183:206–212.

Laniece I, Ciss M, Desclaux A, Diop K, Mbodj F, Ndiaye B, Sylla O, Delaporte E, Ndoye I. 2003. Adherence to HAART and its principle determinants in a cohort of Senegalese adults. *AIDS* 17:S103–S108.

Nierengarten MB. 2003. Haiti's HIV equity initiative, *Lancet* 3:266.

Ometto L, Zanchetta M, Mainardi M, DeSalvo GL, Garcia-Rodriguez MC, Chieco-Bianchi L, Gray L, Newell ML, DeRossi A. 2000. Co-receptor usage of HIV-1 primary isolates, viral burden, and CCR5 genotype in mother-to-child HIV-1 transmission. *AIDS* 14: 1721–1729.

Orrell C, Bangsberg DR, Badri M, Wood R. 2003. Adherence is not a barrier to successful antiretroviral therapy in South Africa. *AIDS* 17:1369–1375.

Quinn TC, Wawer MJ, Sewankambo N, Serwadda D, Li C, Wabwire-Mangen F, Meehan MO, Lutalo T, Gray RH. 2000. Viral load and heterosexual transmission of human immunodeficiency virus type 1. Rakai Project Study Group. *New England Journal of Medicine* 342:921–929.

South Africa Department of Health. 2003. Operational Plan for Comprehensive HIV and AIDS care, management, and Treatment for South Africa. [Online]. Available: http://www.gov.za/issues/hiv/careplan19nov03.htm [accessed July 26, 2004].

U.S. Department of State. 2003. The President's Emergency Plan for AIDS Relief. [Online]. Available: http://www.state.gov/documents/organization/29831.pdf [accessed July 26, 2004].

Weidle PJ, Malamba S, Mwebaze R, Sozi C, Rukundo G, Downing R, Hanson D, Ochola D, Mugyenyi P, Mermin J, Samb B, Lackritz E. 2002. Assessment of a pilot antiretroviral drug therapy programme in Uganda: patients' response, survival, and drug resistance. *Lancet* 360(9326):4–40.

WHO. 2002. Innovative Care for Chronic Conditions: Building Blocks for Action. [Online]. Available: http://www.who.int/chronic_conditions/icccreport/en/ [accessed July 26, 2004].

WHO. 2003a. Scaling Up Antiretroviral Therapy in Resource-Limited Settings: Treatment Guidelines for a Public Health Approach. [Online]. Available: http://www.who.int/3by5/publications/documents/arv_guidelines/en/ [accessed July 26, 2004].

WHO. 2003b. Treating 3 Million by 2005. Making it Happen. The WHO Strategy. Geneva: WHO. [Online]. Available: http://www.who.int/3by5/en/ [accessed July 26, 2004].

1

Introduction

There is no question that the pandemic can be defeated. No matter how terrible the scourge of AIDS, no matter how limited the capacity to respond, no matter how devastating the human toll, it is absolutely certain that the pandemic can be turned around with a joint and Herculean effort between the African countries themselves and the international community.

—Stephen Lewis

The discovery of highly active antiretroviral (ARV) therapy (ART) and its introduction in developed countries is considered by many to be one of the greatest success stories of modern medicine—this despite still-critical concerns regarding toxicity, adherence, and the widespread development of viral resistance. These concerns cannot negate the dramatic reductions in HIV-associated morbidity and mortality that have resulted from the widespread introduction of triple-combination ART in the mid-1990s. Two decades ago, it was common for HIV-infected patients to present in U.S. clinics and hospitals with only a 10-month survival as their prognosis. Today, ARV-treated patients can generally anticipate leading a good-quality life for many years.

The provision of safe, effective ART to the millions of individuals in need in resource-constrained settings is likewise expected to dramatically reduce HIV/AIDS-related morbidity and mortality, improve quality of life, and increase social and political stability. The challenge is great, however, as HIV/AIDS has progressed largely unchecked in many parts of the world where the epidemic has been underestimated and shrouded in denial and stigma (see Figure 1-1).

Of the 40 million people worldwide infected with HIV, an estimated 6 million are in need of immediate, life-sustaining ART. Yet only around 400,000 people in low- and middle-income countries have access to such treatment (WHO, 2003) (see Table 1-1). Most HIV-infected individuals live in severely resource-constrained settings, where the HIV epidemic continues to grow at a rate of 5 million infections per year, compounding the

20

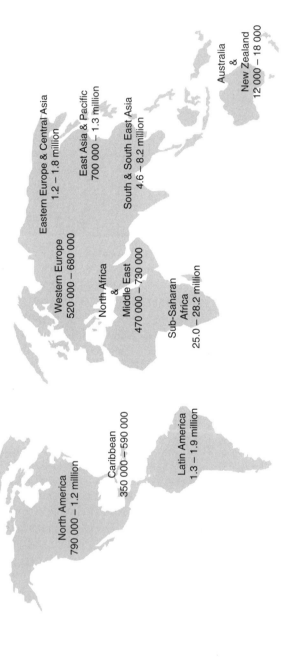

FIGURE 1-1 Adults and children estimated to be living with HIV/AIDS at the end of 2003.
SOURCE: UNAIDS, 2003.

TABLE 1-1 Coverage of ART in Developing Countries, 2003 (adults by WHO region)

Region	Number of People on ART	Estimated Need	Coverage
Africa	100,000	4,400,000	2%
Americas	210,000	250,000	84%
Europe (Eastern Europe, Central Asia)	15,000	80,000	19%
Eastern Mediterranean	5,000	100,000	5%
Southeast Asia	60,000	900,000	7%
Western Pacific	10,000	170,000	6%
All WHO Regions	400,000	5,900,000	7%

SOURCE: WHO, 2003.

already enormous treatment challenge. The high AIDS mortality rate in sub-Saharan Africa, which remains the worst-affected region in the world, contrasts sharply with the decreasing HIV-related death rate in high-income countries where ARVs are widely available and affordable. Those acutely affected by the widespread lack of treatment include not only the millions of infected individuals, but also the millions of children orphaned when their parents die from HIV-related illness. Because HIV-related deaths occur disproportionately among young, economically productive adults, moreover, the epidemic is undermining the economic development and social fabric of entire countries (Bell et al., 2003; Dixon et al., 2001).

CHALLENGES AND OPPORTUNITIES: ANTIRETROVIRAL THERAPY IN RESOURCE-CONSTRAINED SETTINGS

Most of the clinical, epidemiological, behavioral, and other aspects of the HIV/AIDS pandemic have been addressed predominantly within the United States and other resource-rich settings. As a result, there are a multitude of unanswered questions regarding how best to introduce ARVs on a broad scale in resource-constrained settings, where the public health and drug delivery infrastructures are often weak or nonexistent and operational capacity is largely lacking. Although several pilot initiatives worldwide have garnered early success and proven the feasibility of implementing ART programs in resource-poor settings, we have yet to determine how these pilot initiatives can be scaled up to meet larger needs. No one program or country can provide all the answers.

The urgent demand to provide free or affordable ARVs to the millions of people in need must be tempered by awareness of the crucial importance of acting rationally and making decisions based on the best scientific evidence so that the long-term durability of individual patient regimens and the sustainability of ART programs will not be jeopardized. A lack of careful planning could create conditions conducive to treatment failure and the development of drug-resistant virus, leading ultimately to disillusionment and demoralization. While avoiding delays in delivering treatment, the international and national communities of donors, planners, and providers must remain vigilant in seeking continued improvements and necessary course corrections to maximize treatment benefits and extend as many lives as possible. Failed programs using first-line regimens, regardless of the reasons for failure, necessitate much more costly and less-sustainable second-line regimens or result in the termination of ART for affected patients; they also limit treatment opportunities for others afflicted today and for the tens of millions of additional HIV-infected persons anticipated over the next decade or so.

Ultimately, the best lessons may be learned from ART scale-up itself. Critical to the long-term success of these programs will be their ability to recognize where both desired outcomes and failures are encountered. These programs, their leaders, and their funders will require sufficient flexibility and commitment to quality to ensure that changes, when necessary, are made.

For now, ART programs already in various stages of implementation throughout the developing world provide advice worth heeding (see Figure 1-2). Some of these programs have met with success, others with high rates

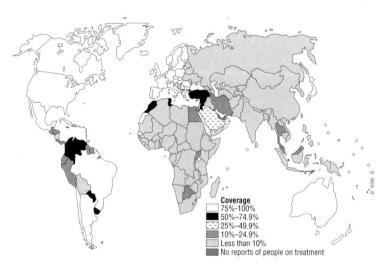

Coverage
- 75%–100%
- 50%–74.9%
- 25%–49.9%
- 10%–24.9%
- Less than 10%
- No reports of people on treatment

FIGURE 1-2 Estimated worldwide coverage with antiretroviral treatment at the end of 2003.
SOURCE: WHO, 2004.

of drug resistance. Suboptimal introduction of ART in both Cote d'Ivoire (Adje et al., 2001) and Gabon (Vergne et al., 2002), for example, has led to high levels of drug resistance in treated patients, as well as treatment failure due to unsustainable drug supplies (and consequent inadequate dosing) and health care infrastructures without the capacity to detect resistance. ART programs in Uganda (Weidle et al., 2002), Senegal (Laurent et al., 2002), and Haiti (Mukherjee et al., 2003; Farmer et al., 2001), on the other hand, have shown preliminary success, with clinical, biological, and therapeutic results similar to those seen in developed-country cohorts—this despite variable HIV-1 subtypes and advanced stages of disease at treatment outset.

Questions remain about the impact—positive or negative—that major investments in ART will have overall on health care systems in developing countries (Benatar, 2004; Walton et al., 2004). Evidence-based assessments are still needed to determine the effects of large-scale ART programs on HIV/AIDS prevention efforts and other health care initiatives. It will be important to determine in different settings the extent to which integration of ART programs into the general health care system will be most appropriately balanced with other needs. This is of particular concern because of the already strained and often inadequate overall health care infrastructure and workforce in many developing countries for the delivery of effective medical care and treatment (Narasimhan et al., 2004; USAID, 2003).

Despite these challenges and unresolved issues, recent ARV price cuts due to international competition among generic and proprietary drug manufacturers have led to a conviction that it is possible to provide universal, comprehensive HIV/AIDS treatment and care. In fact, general consensus exists today that minimization of resistance can be achieved by accelerating the introduction of ARVs worldwide *in a rational manner.*

This conviction, coupled with growing political, ethical, and humanitarian concerns, has elevated HIV/AIDS to the top of the political and financial agendas of many national governments and international organizations. Increased domestic and external funding for HIV/AIDS programs and continuing drug price negotiations are enabling a growing number of low- and middle-income countries to provide or promise affordable ARVs and other HIV-related medications to at least some of their citizens (Pogge, 2002).

BEYOND THE BIOMEDICAL MODEL

HIV/AIDS, like many other emerging infectious diseases, is symptomatic of major changes in the ways people live in today's world. The pandemic has arisen in the wake of complex social and economic forces that have widened disparities in health and wealth, disrupted living conditions, and created new ecological niches for the emergence or reemergence of disease (Garrett, 1995). While the biomedical approach to responding to the global HIV/AIDS crisis is a necessary first step and has already demonstrated its strength by prolonging the lives of tens of thousands of people, a sustainable response will require addressing the upstream social, economic, and environmental events and factors that have led to the emergence of this pandemic and will likely influence the emergence of future pandemics as well (Benatar, 2002). As with tuberculosis, for example, HIV/AIDS has largely become a disease of the poor, so understanding and addressing threats that perpetuate and aggravate poverty and marginalize the millions of HIV-infected people worldwide is especially important (Houweling et al., 2001; Katz, 2002; Murray and Lopez, 1999; *The Return of the White Plague*, 2003; Wood et al., 2002).

ART scale-up in resource-constrained settings will depend on the generous support of wealthy nations, at least in the near future (see Table 1-2). Yet sustaining improved health care and population health in the distant future will ultimately require new, ambitious ways of thinking about how to enhance the capabilities of people and nations so they can become self-sufficient and independent of philanthropy. For example, debt roll-back or a shift toward fairer trade rules could be implemented concurrently with the introduction of ART to boost the capacity of local governments in poor countries to provide the education and health care needed to promote greater self-sufficiency (Benatar, 2003). The importance of sustainability and the need to address upstream economic, social, and ecological factors that to date have received inadequate consideration are now beginning to receive the scholarly attention they deserve (Ferraro and Rosser, 1994; Pettifor, 2003a,b; Labonte et al., 2004; Sreenivasan, 2002).

Long-term sustainability aside, even a successful short-term response requires addressing social and behavioral aspects of HIV/AIDS that lie outside the traditional realm of epidemiological and biomedical modeling of infectious disease transmission. Improving patient adherence to therapy, for example, involves more than patient education. It also requires addressing social problems that contribute to program dropout, such as AIDS-related stigma and familial dysfunction (e.g., the disruption that ensues when more than one family member is infected with HIV). Likewise, minimizing increased risky behavior once ARVs become widely available will involve more than patient or public education: it will require addressing the underlying, pervasive social conditions that generate such behavior.

Global disparities in health, disease, and behavior and, most particularly, the forces that generate these disparities pose great threats to the implementation of medical interventions that offer hope for the future. Understanding and acknowledging these forces that imperil global health and having the will to address them are essential complements to the introduction of modern treatments.

TABLE 1-2 Income and Health Resources of Selected Countries

Country	Gross National Income per Capita ($) 2002[a]	Health Expenditures per Capita ($) 1997–2000	Physicians per 1,000 People 1995–2000
United States	35,060	4,499	2.8
Brazil	2,850	267	1.3
PEPFAR Countries[b]			
Botswana	2,980	191	NA[c]
Cote d'Ivoire	610	16	0.1
Ethiopia	100	5	NA[c]
Guyana	NA[c]	NA[c]	NA[c]
Haiti	440	21	0.2
Kenya	360	28	0.1
Mozambique	210	9	NA[c]
Namibia	1,780	136	0.3
Nigeria	290	8	NA[c]
Rwanda	230	12	NA[c]
South Africa	2,600	255	0.6
Tanzania	280	12	0.0
Uganda	250	10	NA[c]
Vietnam	430	21	0.5
Zambia	330	18	0.1

[a]Following current statistical practice, the World Bank recently adopted new terminology in line with the 1993 System of National Accounts (SNA). Therefore, gross national product per capita is now called gross national income per capita. (See http://www.worldbank.org/data/changinterm.html for more information.)

[b]PEPFAR = The President's Emergency Plan for AIDS Relief.

[c]NA = not available.

SOURCE: World Bank, 2004.

GOALS OF THE STUDY

In consideration of the issues outlined above, the Institute of Medicine was asked to provide a rapid, independent review and assessment of ART scale-up programs under way and in development. This fast-track study was initiated in late November 2003 to provide guidance and establish a framework of principles for decision making in anticipation of the growing number of investments in ART scale-up programs. The Committee on Examining the Probable Consequences of Alternative Patterns of Widespread Antiretroviral Drug Use in Resource-Constrained Settings was charged to provide (1) an examination and evaluation of current ART implementation programs, efficacy studies, infrastructure costing models, existing guidelines for program implementation, and models that demonstrate successful scale-up of ART programs; (2) a study of the role of ongoing well-developed operations research in the field and in parallel with treatment implementation to establish sustainability outcome measures; (3) a determination of the components necessary for a systematic, structured framework to achieve a balance between resistance development and transmission and the need to provide treatment in resource-constrained settings; and (4) an assessment of current research on ARV resistance and toxicity, including the likely effects on the malnourished individuals with high disease burden found in resource-poor settings.

STUDY APPROACH

The committee formed to conduct this study encompassed broad international expertise in the clinical and basic research aspects of HIV/AIDS, epidemiology, virology, pathology, ethics, behavioral science, community medicine, health care financing and policy, and public health. The members of the committee were also chosen for their first-hand experience with HIV/AIDS in a wide range of middle- and low-income countries. The committee members are listed at the beginning of the report and are briefly profiled in Appendix G.

The data needed for this study were identified by the committee members and other experts representing disciplines relevant to the committee's charge. Although a large proportion of the findings on HIV/AIDS in developing countries has been published in international and national journals and reports, many important findings have appeared in local journals, the proceedings of meetings, and unpublished reports prepared for the World Health Organization (WHO) and other international organizations. To tap this knowledge base, the committee enlisted a broad range of experts with recent research or service experience in developing countries. Data and supportive evidence were provided by these experts through workshop presentations, commissioned papers, and technical consultation on chapters of this report (for additional information, see Appendix A). The framework for the committee's deliberations included an overview of the available epidemiological parameters; a review of the existing knowledge base on interventions; and projections of the feasibility, cost, and impact of proposed interventions.

The combined weight of such evidence, the committee believes, has produced an accurate account of the state of knowledge concerning the introduction of ARVs in resource-constrained settings and the capacity of local health care systems to provide such treatment. Evaluation of the available evidence enabled the committee to identify gaps in knowledge and to propose strategies for a research agenda that would fill these gaps. The findings, strategies, and recommendations presented in this report were developed from this broad base of evidence.

ORGANIZATION OF THE REPORT

This report reviews the issues surrounding the large-scale introduction of ART into resource-constrained settings; conditions necessary for the long-term sustainability of quality ART programs; and steps that must be taken to achieve an appropriate and adequate balance among the priorities, benefits, and risks of introducing ART into these settings. The report is organized into six chapters.

Following this introduction, Chapter 2 describes some of the most recent initiatives and investments by international donors and national governments that will provide the foundational elements of large-scale ART programs in the developing world. In highlighting these efforts, the committee describes issues that will require further resolution as ART programs evolve, such as the need for global and national coordination of financial, technical, and human resource investments; ethical considerations at the international, national, and local levels; and, the importance of ensuring the long-term fiscal sustainability of these programs to avert the dire medical consequences of treatment interruption or termination. (Additional ethical issues for consideration are presented in Appendix D.)

Chapter 3 responds to the committee's charge to examine and evaluate current ART programs and to assess what these programs and additional research reveal about the potential implications of the emergence of drug-resistant strains of HIV. To this end, it describes the phenomenon of the evolution of drug-resistant viruses, tools for anticipating the magnitude of drug resistance among populations, and the current and potential implications of such developments for ART scale-up in resource-constrained settings. The chapter also includes a collection of lessons learned from ART programs in developing countries with varying degrees of resource constraints, disease burden, and overall health care infrastructure. (Additional background information on ARV-resistant viruses is contained in Appendix B.)

In setting forth the principles to be applied in scaling up ART programs, Chapter 4 outlines a set of framework components that the committee believes to be essential for establishing effective, quality care that can respond to the overwhelming burden of HIV/AIDS in many resource-constrained environments. In responding to its charge in this area, the committee built its findings and recommendations upon extant knowledge from the field and the outcomes of operations research related to ART programs in developed and developing countries. Informed by these lessons learned, Chapter 4 identifies the obstacles and opportunities involved in developing

ART programs that encompass the reduction of stigma and discrimination, as well as the identification of points of entry for treatment, such as programs for voluntary counseling and testing and tuberculosis treatment and control. A guiding set of clinical principles is described that is grounded in an assessment of existing program implementation guidelines. Strategies are included for selecting treatment regimens; for using laboratories to diagnose, initiate, and monitor therapies; and for meeting the treatment needs of special populations, such as pregnant women, children, and those suffering also from opportunistic infections, especially tuberculosis. Emphasis is placed on the benefits of treatment programs that are synergized with prevention efforts, and on the critical importance of adherence to treatment to ensure the life-sustaining effects of the therapy and prevent the emergence of drug-resistant virus that not only would result in individual treatment failure, but also might jeopardize the long-term durability of select drug regimens at the population level.

Additional essential components of ART scale-up are described in Chapter 5. Inextricably linked to the success of drug interventions will be logistics systems that ensure the safe and timely procurement and delivery of the drugs and include effective information and data collection systems. This chapter emphasizes the paramount importance of a properly trained workforce that comprises not only those who will administer ART, but also those who will effectively manage, monitor, and continuously optimize the scale-up of ART programs and ensure the adequate training and allocation of human and technical resources. (Further analysis of these issues is presented in Appendix E.) Barriers to be overcome in developing these multidimensional resources include the lack of adequate training programs and access to education in most resource-constrained countries, the effects of "brain drain" that usurps talented yet limited in-country resources, and the inability to sustain and secure a robust supply chain of drugs because of unreliable funding sources.

In all of its findings and recommendations throughout Chapters 2 through 5 regarding the components of a system for scaling up ART, the committee emphasizes the critical need for a learn-by-doing approach and the current paucity of data to support such efforts. The unprecedented nature of the scale-up of ART programs to treat many millions of people in resource-constrained settings leaves decision makers and practitioners without a well-evaluated, evidence-based strategy at the outset of program implementation. Thus, Chapter 5 concludes by detailing how discretely and adequately funded monitoring and evaluation of new and expanding ART programs can provide multiple benefits, including the ongoing realignment and optimization of ART programs and systems with regard to their effectiveness, quality, and allocation of human, technical, and financial resources; the development of an evidence base and scientific knowledge that can inform the design and implementation of new programs in the future (identifying earlier programs or elements that worked and should be expanded and those that should be abandoned); and the provision of data and evaluation results that establish accountability and allow for the measurement of intended outcomes essential to securing continued funding by international donors and national and local governments.

In the report's final chapter, the committee continues to highlight the need to know more and to develop better strategies and more effective tools so as to improve the effectiveness of treatment programs for HIV/AIDS. The chapter sets forth priorities for an operations, clinical, and behavioral research agenda that will enable both iterative and breakthrough improvements for ART. The report concludes with a sobering call to the many decision makers, researchers, and practitioners who will take up arms against this deadly plague to heed the crucial lesson learned from ongoing investigations: that within the imperative to act now, it will also be important to act well.

Defining a Country's Wealth

Low income = a country having an annual gross national income (GNI) per capita equivalent to $735 or less in 2002.

Middle income = a country having an annual GNI per capita between $736 and $9,075 in 2002.

High income = a country having an annual GNI per capita equivalent to $9,076 or greater in 2002.

Note: Gross national income is equivalent to gross national product according to the new World Bank terminology.

SOURCE: World Bank, 2004.

REFERENCES

Adje C, Cheingsong R, Roels TH, Maurice C, Djomand G, Verbiest W, Hertogs K, Larder B, Monga B, Peeters M, Eholie S, Bissagene E, Coulibaly M. 2001. High prevalence of genotypic and phenotypic HIV-1 drug-resistant strains among patients receiving antiretroviral therapy in Abidjan, Cote d'Ivoire. *Journal of Acquired Immune Deficiency Syndromes* 26:501–506.
Bell C, Devarajan S, Gersbach H. 2003. *The Long-Run Economic Costs of AIDS: Theory and an Application to South Africa.* Washington, DC: World Bank.
Benatar SR. 2002. The HIV/AIDS pandemic: A sign of instability in a complex global system. *Journal of Medicine and Philosophy* 27:163–177.
Benatar SR. 2003. Ethics and tropical disease: Some global considerations. In: Manson P, ed. *Tropical Diseases.* 21st Edition. London, UK: Saunders. Pp. 85–93.
Benatar SR. 2004. Health care reform and the crisis of HIV and AIDS in South Africa. *New England Journal of Medicine* 351(1):81–92.
Dixon S, McDonald S, Roberts J. 2001. The impact of HIV and AIDS on Africa's economic development. *British Medical Journal* 324(7331):232–234.
Farmer P, Leandre F, Mukherjee JS, Claude M, Nevil P, Smith-Fawzi MC, Koenig SP, Castro A, Becerra MC, Attaran A, Kim JY. 2001. Community based approaches to HIV treatment in resource-poor settings. *Lancet* 358:404–409.
Ferraro V, Rosser M. 1994. Global debt and third world development. In: *World Security: Challenges for a New Century.* Klare M, Thomas D, eds. New York: St. Martin's Press. Pp. 332–355.
Garrett L. 1995. *The Coming Plague: Newly Emerging Diseases in a World Out of Balance.* New York: Penguin Books.
Houweling TA, Kunst AE, Malkenbach JP. 2001. World Health Report 2000: Inequality index and socioeconomic inequalities in mortality. *Lancet* 357:1671–1672.
Katz A. 2002. AIDS, individual behavior and unexplained remaining variation. *African Journal of AIDS Research* 1:125–142.
Labonte R, Schrecker T, Sanders D, Mecus W. 2004. *Fatal Indifference: The G8, Africa, and Global Health.* Ottawa, Canada: University of Cape Town Press.
Laurent C, Diakhate N, Gueye NF, Toure MA, Sow PS, Faye MA, Gueye M, Laniece I, Toure Kane C, Liegeois F, Vergne L, Mboup S, Badiane S, Ndoye I, Delaporte E. 2002. The Senegalese government's highly active antiretroviral therapy initiative: An 18-month follow-up study. *AIDS* 16:1363–1370.
Mukherjee J, Colas M, Farmer P, Leandre F, Lambert W, Raymonville M, Koenig S, Walton D, Nevil P, Louissant N, Orelus S. 2003. *Access to Antiretroviral Treatment and Care: The Experience of the HIV Equity Initiative.* Cange, Haiti: WHO.
Murray CJ, Lopez AD. 1999. Mortality by cause for eight regions of the world: Global burden of disease study. *Lancet* 349:1269–1276.
Narasimhan V, Brown H, Pablos-Mendez A, Adams O, Dussault G, Elzinga G, Nordstrom A, Habte D, Jacobs M, Solimano G, Sewankambo N, Wilbulpolprasert S, Evans T, Chen L. 2004. Responding to the global human resources crisis. *Lancet* 363(9419):1469–1472.
Pettifor A. 2003a. *The Legacy of Globalization: Debt and Deflation.* Pettifor A, ed. New York: Palgrave Press.
Pettifor A. 2003b. Resolving international debt crises fairly. *Ethics and International Affairs* 17(2)2–9.
Pogge T. 2002. *World Poverty and Human Rights: Cosmopolitan Responsibilities and Reforms.* Cambridge, UK: Polity Press.
Sreenivasan G. 2002. International justice and health. *Ethics and International Affairs* 16(2)81–90.

The Return of the White Plague. 2003. Gandy M, Zumla Z, eds. New York: Oxford University Press.

UNAIDS. 2003. *AIDS Epidemic Update.* Geneva: UNAIDS.

USAID (U.S. Agency for International Development). 2003. *The Health Sector Human Resource Crisis in Africa: An Issues Paper.* [Online]. Available: http://www.aed.org/ToolsandPublications/upload/healthsector.pdf [accessed August 23, 2004].

Vergne L, Malonga-Mouellet G, Mistoul I, Mavoungou R, Peeters M, Monsaray H, Delaporte E. 2002. Resistance to antiretroviral treatment in Gabon: Need for implementation of guidelines on antiretroviral therapy use and HIV-1 drug resistance monitoring in developing countries. *Journal of Acquired Immune Deficiency Syndromes* 29:154–158.

Walton DA, Farmer PE, Lambert W, Leandre F, Koenig SP, Mukherjee JS. 2004. Integrated HIV prevention and care strengthens primary health care: Lessons from rural Haiti. *Journal of Public Health Policy* 25(2):137–158.

Weidle P, Malamba S, Mwebaze R, Sozi C, Rukundo G, Downing R, Hanson D, Ochola D, Mugyenyi P, Mermin J, Samb B, Lackritz E. 2002. Assessment of a pilot antiretroviral drug therapy programme in Uganda: Patients' response, survival, and drug resistance. *Lancet* 360:34–40.

WHO (World Health Organization). 2003. *Treating 3 Million by 2005. Making it Happen. The WHO Strategy.* Geneva: WHO. [Online]. Available: http://www.who.int/3by5/en/ [accessed July 26, 2004].

WHO. 2004. *The World Health Report 2004: Changing History.* Geneva: WHO.

Wood E, Montaner JS, Chan K, Tyndall MW, Schechter MT, Bangsberg D, O'Shaughnessy MV, Hogg RS. 2002. Socioeconomic status, access to triple therapy, and survival from HIV-disease since 1996. *AIDS* 16:2065–2072.

World Bank. 2004. *World Development Report 2004: Making Services Work for Poor People.* Washington, DC: World Bank.

2

Opportunities and Challenges

The remarkable focus and unprecedented funding currently being directed toward providing affordable antiretrovirals (ARVs) to resource-poor countries and accelerating HIV/AIDS treatment and prevention programs worldwide reflect an admirable and ambitious shift in humanitarian, political, and economic perspectives on what is arguably the worst pandemic ever to hit humankind (see Box 2-1).

Many initiatives, organizations, and governments—including the Global Fund to Fight AIDS, Tuberculosis and Malaria (The Global Fund); U.S. funding for global HIV/AIDS efforts, in particular the President's Emer-

---

BOX 2-1
The Global AIDS Pandemic at a Glance

- Leading infectious cause of adult death in the world
- Leading cause of death in adults aged 15–59
- First case of AIDS recognized in 1981
- 40 million persons now living with HIV/AIDS, 50% of them women
- More than 70% of HIV-infected persons living in Africa
- 14,000 new infections daily
- Sexual transmission responsible for more than 85% of infections
- 6 million in need of immediate treatment and fewer than 8% receiving it

SOURCES: Quinn and Chaisson, 2004; WHO, 2003a,b.

---

gency Plan for AIDS Relief (PEPFAR); the World Health Organization's (WHO) 3-by-5 campaign; the William J. Clinton Presidential Foundation; the World Bank's Multi-Country HIV/AIDS Program for the Africa Region (MAP); and the courageous efforts of the afflicted countries themselves, such as ART scale-up in South Africa—have contributed to this historic opportunity to develop and implement the global scale-up of ARV therapy (ART). Each of these efforts is briefly reviewed in turn below. Issues related to coordinating these and other elements of the global response to the HIV/ AIDS pandemic are then examined. Next, the crucial issue of fiscal sustainability is addressed. The final section examines the ethical issues and challenges at both the local and international levels.

CURRENT EFFORTS

The Global Fund: Scale-Up of Antiretroviral Therapy in Action

The Global Fund to Fight AIDS, Tuberculosis, and Malaria, sponsored by the United Nations (UN), is a performance-based financing mechanism and network whose purpose is to provide countries with substantial resources that can be used at the national level and in a way that promotes country ownership. The goal is to help launch programs designed to combat these three devastating diseases. Although the Global Fund has been operating legally for nearly 2 $^1/_2$ years, it has been functional for only about 2 years. Thus far the program has pledged $4.8 billion to fund 214 proposals among 121 countries through 2008; however, only $2.1 billion of these funds had been received from donors as of November 2003 (see Figure 2-1) (The Global Fund, 2003a). The proposals include specific plans for HIV/ AIDS, tuberculosis (TB), and malaria, as well as joint efforts (e.g., HIV/ AIDS–TB), and both country-specific and cross-border initiatives. Of these 214 proposals, 135 have moved forward in terms of having a specific work plan in place, and about $250 million had been dispersed as of January 2004 (Schwartlander et al., 2004) (see Box 2-2).

Global Fund monies are expected to provide enough ARVs to treat approximately 700,000 people over the course of the next several years. About 60 percent of Global Fund resources have gone or will go to sub-Saharan Africa, and about 60 percent toward HIV/AIDS (The Global Fund, 2003b). Of the amount dedicated to HIV/AIDS, a little less than half is dedicated to commodities, and about half of that amount to ARVs. The majority of project plans that have HIV/AIDS components include prevention elements, although the primary focus of most is treatment (i.e., ART).

After technical review and negotiations, the majority of funded HIV/ AIDS projects in African countries spend, on average, about US$400 per patient per year for ART (Schwartlander et al., 2004). Global Fund–sup-

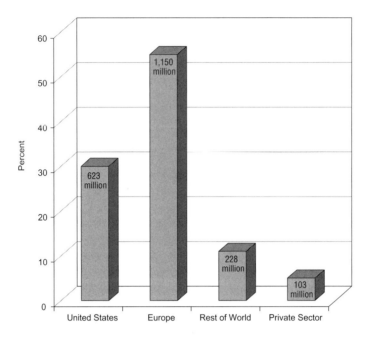

FIGURE 2-1 Contributions to the global fund to date.
SOURCE: The Global Fund, 2004c.

ported ARVs are a bit more expensive in Latin America, where income
levels are slightly higher and resource constraints somewhat less pronounced, although negotiations are in progress to lower drug prices there as
well. The drug prices are higher in Eastern Europe as well, where the annual
cost of ART per patient can run as high as US$1,000. These figures include
only commodities (e.g., drugs, very simple diagnostics) and not costs for
health care workers and other basic infrastructure.

    Many are concerned that the Global Fund monies have been slow to
roll out and that, despite agreements being in place, some countries do not
yet have the promised funds or ARVs. Total global funding budgeted for
the fund in 2003 for HIV/AIDS was an estimated US$4.2 billion (including
funding from all donor governments and UN agencies and disbursements
from The World Bank, foundations, and major nongovernmental organizations [NGOs]). However, estimates from the Joint United Nations Program
on HIV/AIDS (UNAIDS) indicate that actual spending in 2003 totaled only
about US$3.6 billion (UNAIDS, 2003). It is believed that much of the
discrepancy is due to the lag time between the receipt and disbursement of
contributions to the Global Fund, as well as to differences between bud-

BOX 2-2
The Global Fund to Fight AIDS, Tuberculosis, and Malaria

Created in 2002 by Kofi Annan, Secretary General of the United Nations, the Global Fund to Fight AIDS, Tuberculosis, and Malaria is an independent, nonprofit foundation. It is governed by an international board that is currently chaired by the U.S. Secretary of Health and Human Services. The foundation's goal is to act quickly and effectively to mobilize resources for combating HIV/AIDS, tuberculosis, and malaria. The foundation is governed by an international board that consists of representatives of donor and recipient governments, nongovernmental organizations, the private sector (including businesses and philanthropic organizations), and affected communities.

In mobilizing resources, the Global Fund operates as a financial instrument to attract, manage, and disburse funding to fight HIV/AIDS, tuberculosis, and malaria worldwide through a competitive grant support mechanism. It seeks to fund projects that will form new or innovative alliances with governments, civil society, the private sector, and affected communities, which in turn will create local ownership of programs. The fund's existence is based on strong public–private partnerships, results-based management, and a focus on local capacity building.

Grant applications are evaluated by an independent technical review panel of disease-specific and cross-cutting health and development experts. In the evaluation process, funding priority is given to countries with the highest incidence of disease and the fewest financial resources and to programs that can coordinate and strengthen existing health systems. Additional weight is given to applications built on proven best practices that incorporate the principles of results-based management and strong mechanisms of accountability for both in-country and fund project managers. Funded projects cannot replace or reduce existing sources of funding.

Since its inception, the Global Fund has attracted over US$5 billion in pledges from donor nations, foundations, corporations, and individuals; the total paid to the fund to date is just over US$2 billion. Since the review of three proposal rounds in April 2002 and January and October 2003, project grants total US$2 billion over 2 years to support 224 programs in 121 countries and 3 territories worldwide.

With Global Fund resources, approved local programs will support an unprecedented scale-up of ART. Over 5 years, an estimated 700,000 people will receive ART, more than tripling current coverage in poor countries (including a 10-fold increase in Africa). The Global Fund will also reach 1 million children orphaned by AIDS; provide treatment for nearly 3 million people with infectious tuberculosis, tripling the coverage of treatment of multidrug-resistant tuberculosis; and finance 22 million combination drug treatments for resistant malaria. The Global Fund proves that with cooperation, goals can be achieved.

SOURCES: The Global Fund, 2003a,b; 2004a,b; U.S. Department of State, 2004.

geted amounts and actual spending by donor governments (Henry J. Kaiser Family Foundation, 2004a). This lag time points to the need to include funding mechanisms in all ART scale-up monitoring and evaluation programs so that any such problems can be identified and addressed. (See Chapter 5 for further discussion of monitoring and evaluation.)

If broad-based financing mechanisms for the procurement of ARVs are not in place (directly linked to some of the major donor sources), monies can often be slow to trickle in. Such financial uncertainty does not allow for the development or implementation of effective ART programming and places those who are relying on promised drugs and other essentials at risk for treatment failure. (See the discussion of fiscal sustainability later in this chapter.) Erratic provision of treatment caused by interruptions in the drug supply can lead to treatment failure regardless of how adherent patients may be or how experienced their health care providers are. Thus it is crucial that organizations providing global funding for HIV/AIDS act more expeditiously in getting the funds to countries so their programs can meet the needs of people on ART, as well as programmatic expectations and global expectations for scale-up.

The World Bank's Multi-Country HIV/AIDS Program

In 2000, the World Bank began the US$500 million MAP to bolster existing national-level HIV/AIDS programs in sub-Saharan Africa. The MAP seeks to enhance prevention, care, and treatment programs, with particular emphasis on at-risk groups, including youth and women of childbearing age. Each aid package is multisectorial, providing money to both national and community-level programs and NGOs. In 2002, the Bank approved an additional US$500 million for MAPII. As of September 2003, US$848 million had been committed to African countries (see Table 2-1).

The following criteria must be met for MAP participation (The World Bank Group, 2001):

• Satisfactory evidence of a strategic approach to HIV/AIDS, developed in a participatory manner
• Existence of a high-level HIV/AIDS coordinating body, with broad representation of key stakeholders from all sectors, including people living with HIV/AIDS
• Government commitment to quick implementation arrangements, including channeling grant funds for HIV/AIDS activities directly to communities, civil society, and the private sector
• Agreement by the government to use multiple implementation agencies, especially NGOs/community based organizations

TABLE 2-1 World Bank HIV/AIDS
Projects by Country

Country	Commitment (US$millions)
Benin	23.0
Burkina Faso	22.0
Burundi	36.0
Cameroon	50.0
Cape Verde	9.0
Central Africa Republic	17.0
Eritrea	40.0
Ethiopia	59.7
Gambia	15.0
Ghana	25.0
Guinea	20.3
Kenya	50.0
Madagascar	20.0
Malawi	35.0
Mauritania	21.0
Mozambique	55.0
Niger	25.0
Nigeria	90.3

U.S. Funding for Global HIV/AIDS Efforts

History of U.S. Funding

The United States has been funding international HIV/AIDS activities since 1986, when it made its first commitment of US$1.1 million. Funding levels increased slowly and steadily until 1999 ($219 million), at which point they increased substantially. The 1999 Leadership and Investment in Fighting an Epidemic (LIFE) Initiative under President Clinton and the 2001 creation of the Global Fund both significantly contributed to the increase in funding. By 2001, U.S. funding had more than tripled to $756 million, (a figure that included the first U.S. contribution to the Global Fund), and then rose again to $1.03 billion in 2002, $1.463 billion in 2003, and $2.3 billion in 2004 (Henry J. Kaiser Family Foundation, 2004b).

The money is channeled through both bilateral assistance and multilateral efforts. In 2003, for example, about 58 percent of the funding was allocated to bilateral programs, 24 percent to the Global Fund, and 18 percent to international HIV/AIDS research efforts at the National Institutes of Health (NIH) and the Centers for Disease Control and Prevention (CDC). Most of the bilateral assistance is administered by the U.S. Agency for International Development (USAID). In 2004, USAID handled $550 million (i.e., 25 percent) of the total U.S. global HIV/AIDS funding. Other bilateral administrators have included CDC's Global AIDS Program and the Departments of Commerce, Agriculture, Defense, and Labor. In 2005, the latter three departments will not be administering any U.S. funding for global HIV/AIDS; instead, the State Department will become the second-largest recipient and administrator of U.S. global HIV/AIDS funding (i.e., second to USAID).

Most of the U.S. multilateral assistance goes to the Global Fund (see above). UNAIDS, WHO, and The World Bank also receive U.S. multilateral support.

The President's Emergency Plan for AIDS Relief

On May 27, 2003, President Bush signed Public Law 108-25, the United States Leadership against HIV/AIDS, Tuberculosis, and Malaria Act of 2003. Among other provisions, the act requires that the President establish a comprehensive, integrated 5-year strategy to combat global HIV/AIDS (Office of Legislative Policy and Analysis, 2004). Although the focus of past programs has been largely on prevention, the United States has begun broadening its response to provide care and treatment as well (Henry J. Kaiser Family Foundation, 2004b). Among other goals, the new funding is intended to provide ARVs to 2 million people (see Box 2-3).

In January 2004, Congress appropriated $2.4 billion to PEPFAR for fiscal year 2004, $488 million of which was new funding for the plan. On February 23, 2004, details of the $15 billion PEPFAR were released, along with the first $350 million (Office of the United States Global AIDS Coordinator, 2003), including $189 million in funding awards. The plan targets 15 countries: Botswana, Cote d'Ivoire, Ethiopia, Guyana, Haiti, Kenya, Mozambique, Namibia, Nigeria, Rwanda, South Africa, Tanzania, Uganda, Vietnam, and Zambia. The first round of funds is expected to provide treatment for 50,000 people.

The World Health Organization's 3-by-5 Campaign: The Vision

The WHO 3-by-5 campaign, with the aim of providing ART to 3 million people by 2005, is a target, not a program. Established in 2002, 3-by-5 was based on an assessment of existing entry points in public health infrastructure (e.g., an estimated 500,000 persons needing therapy will be reached through already-functioning TB programs); an unprecedented global commitment to finally dealing with the growing enormity of a problem that had been, until then, underestimated; and accumulating evidence that the implementation of ART programs is feasible in resource-constrained settings. As part of the campaign, WHO has established a set of simplified, standardized treatment guidelines (which are discussed in more detail in Chapter 4 and presented as Appendix C). As discussed in Chapter 4, several of the recommendations are understandably nonspecific, given the critical lack of knowledge and urgent need for research in some areas. It is important to note that the limitations of the guidelines do not reflect shortcomings in WHO's 3-by-5 campaign, but rather the general state of knowledge about HIV/AIDS and the global inexperience with caring and treating for infected patients in resource-constrained settings. Box 2-4 provides more detail on the campaign.

The WHO campaign recognizes that almost all of the more than 40 million people now infected with HIV worldwide will eventually require access to therapy. Looking beyond 2005, WHO and its partners will be developing a new strategic approach to maintain the gains of 3-by-5 and to extend them, using sustainable financing and delivery mechanisms, so that ART becomes part of the primary health care package provided at every health center and clinic.

The William J. Clinton Presidential Foundation

The Clinton Foundation's HIV/AIDS initiative has established effective strategies for the procurement of affordable, high-quality ARVs and diagnostics for several African and Caribbean countries (Mozambique, Rwanda, South Africa, Tanzania, the Bahamas, the Dominican Republic, and Haiti). In October 2003, the foundation announced an agreement with several generic suppliers, including suppliers of some of the most common first-line regimens, for a fixed-dose AZT, 3TC, and nevirapine combination at $239 per person per year and a fixed-dose D4T, 3TC, and nevirapine combination at $132 per person per year. Continued negotiations are also being directed toward a number of other drugs, including pediatric formulations. The procurement strategy of the foundation's HIV/AIDS initiative is discussed in greater detail below in the section on fiscal sustainability.

Operational Plan for Comprehensive HIV and AIDS Care, Management, and Treatment for South Africa

Of the more than 5 million HIV-infected South Africans, 400,000 to 500,000 are eligible for ART based on the WHO guidelines, indicating one of the largest AIDS burdens in the world. Fully 12 percent of the general population is infected with HIV. Moreover, 21 percent of the population between the ages of 15 and 49 is infected. Although the introduction of nevirapine has decreased mother-to-child transmission over the past few years, 90,000 HIV-positive babies were at one point being born each year.

BOX 2-3
The President's Emergency Plan for AIDS Relief

Overview of Goals
- Prevent 7 million new HIV infections
- Treat 2 million HIV-infected people
- Care for 10 million HIV-infected individuals and AIDS orphans

Focus
- Focus is on 15 countries: Botswana, Cote d'Ivoire, Ethiopia, Guyana, Haiti, Kenya, Mozambique, Namibia, Nigeria, Rwanda, South Africa, Tanzania, Uganda, Vietnam, and Zambia
- These 15 countries represent 50% of all HIV-infected people in the world, including 70% of all HIV-infected individuals in sub-Saharan Africa and the Caribbean

Target Areas
- HIV/AIDS prevention initiatives focused on abstinence, behavior change and remaining faithful, and consistent use of condoms*
- ART programs for HIV-infected persons
- Safe national blood transfusion programs
- Programs for orphans and vulnerable children
- Programs to reduce transmission by unsafe medical practices, including in particular the promotion of safe medical injection practices

Management
- Coordinator for International HIV/AIDS Assistance at the U.S. Department of State

---

Life expectancy in South Africa declined over the past decade to 50.7 years in 2002, largely because of HIV/AIDS.

Although South Africa is classified as a middle-income country, with a 2002 annual per capita gross domestic product (GDP) of approximately $2,408, huge disparities exist between the rich and poor, predicated mainly on race and stemming from a 46-year system of apartheid and a 300-year legacy of colonialism. About 10 percent of the population lives in abject poverty, and another 20 percent lives in poverty with incomes of less than US$2 a day. Most of the poverty exists in rural areas.

Since the country's first democratic government came to power in 1994, national efforts have made remarkable headway through many socioeconomic, educational, and development interventions. Examples include providing clean water to 8.4 million new South Africans, providing access to electricity for 3.8 million households, building 1.46 million formal houses, increasing literacy, increasing the number of children in school, and increasing the number of people involved in an integrated nutrition program.

Resources
- $15 billion to be used over 5 years
- $10 billion in new funds and $5 billion in existing funds
- $10 billion to be used for 15 countries in Africa plus Haiti, Guyana, and Vietnam
- $5 billion to be used to support HIV/AIDS, tuberculosis, and malaria programs currently active in more than 50 countries
- $1 billion (of the $15 billion) for the Global Fund to Fight HIV/AIDS, Tuberculosis, and Malaria
- Largest commitment ever by a single nation for an international health initiative

Implementation
- Plan will integrate prevention, treatment, and care through a layered network of central medical centers that support satellite centers and mobile units
- Plan to include improving health care infrastructure, training workers, providing voluntary counseling and testing, encouraging awareness and behavior change, fighting stigma, and administering medicines
- Partners with PEPFAR may include willing host governments; NGOs (e.g., faith-based and community organizations); private corporations; donor and developing nations; and international organizations such as UNAIDS, UNICEF, and WHO

---

* The prevention initiatives will be modeled after the "ABC" model used in Uganda (U.S. Department of State, 2004).

SOURCES: American Enterprise Institute, 2004; The Foreign Press Center, 2003; The White House, 2003.

Also in the early 1990s, the South African government developed its first strategic plan for HIV/AIDS.

In terms of expenditures, the national response to the HIV epidemic was initially quite inadequate, with only US$4.4 million (2004 exchange rate) being spent in 1994. The budget gradually increased to reach some $50.7 million in 2002. Since then, expenditures have increased dramatically to approximately $444.6 million a year, and they are expected to reach $1.2 billion by 2008. This increase has been achieved during a period of modest economic growth (GDP growth was 0 percent from 1985 to 1994 and 2.8 percent from 1995 to 2002) and at a time when the government has been faced with a multitude of other health, educational, development, and socioeconomic challenges.

After acknowledging the need for an ART program in the public sector in 2002, the government established a joint health and treasury task team to investigate and determine the cost of such a program. The team delivered

---

BOX 2-4
The WHO 3-by-5 Campaign

On World AIDS Day 2003, WHO and UNAIDS released a detailed and concrete plan to reach the "3-by-5" target of providing ART to 3 million people living with AIDS in developing countries and those in transition by the end of 2005.

The 3-by-5 campaign complements the groundbreaking commitment to addressing the global AIDS pandemic made by the U.S. PEPFAR initiative (see Box 2-3), the pathfinding work of NGOs, the efforts of pharmaceutical companies to reduce the prices of ARVs, the contributions of international foundations, the initiatives and hard work of many national and international agencies, and, critically, the courageous contributions of nations increasing access to AIDS treatment for their citizens.

After 20 years of fighting the epidemic, it is now clear that a comprehensive approach to HIV/AIDS must include prevention, treatment, and care. WHO's 3-by-5 campaign supports this comprehensive goal by using best-practice theories and technical reports to guide those involved in combating the HIV/AIDS pandemic. The technical briefs and reports provided focus on general HIV/AIDS management issues such as ART, patient follow-up, resistance surveillance, emergency scale-up of support personnel and community involvement, public health approaches to prevention, and guidelines for surveillance and monitoring and evaluation. NGOs, local communities, and governmental organizations are encouraged to use WHO's comprehensive strategy and what is referred to as "the five pillars" to develop and promote programs linking treatment, prevention, care, and full social support for those affected by HIV/AIDS. The five pillars are as follows:

1. Global leadership, strong partnership, and advocacy
2. Urgent, sustained country support
3. Simplified, standardized tools to deliver ARVs
4. Effective, reliable supply of medicines and diagnostics
5. Rapid identification and reapplication of new knowledge and success

Ultimately, WHO's success will rest on the ability of NGOs, affected communities, and public health officials to implement best practices and combat the disease effectively, economically, and in a timely fashion. With focused strategies and guiding principles; however, WHO has already taken a vital step toward the ultimate goal of providing universal access to AIDS treatment.

SOURCES: Kim, 2004; WHO, 2003a.

---

its report in August 2003, after which the Ministry of Health was requested to develop a plan for ART roll-out by September 2003. A task team was convened and, with the assistance of up to 40 technical consultants from the Clinton Foundation, an operational plan was written; this plan was endorsed by the Cabinet on November 19, 2003, without reservation. On January 23, 2004, the first patient received treatment.

The overarching goals of the plan are to provide comprehensive care and treatment for people living with HIV/AIDS and to facilitate the strengthening of the national health system in South Africa. It is important to note that, while the provision and effective management of ARVs will be an integral part of this effort, so, too, will preventative (particularly with regard to sexual behavior), nutritional, opportunistic infection, and non–health sector interventions.

More specifically, the goal is to provide ART to all South Africans in need of such treatment within 5 years. The care and treatment protocols for ARVs are rigorous and standardized, and the drugs will be delivered through provincial AIDS teams working in 53 different service points (one in each of South Africa's 53 health districts) so as to maximize the equitable distribution of comprehensive care and treatment. The first-line ARV regimen is d4T/3TC/nevirapine (pregnant women) or efavirenz (all others); the second-line regimen is AZT/ddI/Kaletra (lopinavir and ritonavir).

As noted, ARVs are not the only component of the treatment plan. Ensuring access to prophylactic care and treatment for opportunistic infections is integral, as is providing nutrition-related interventions to those in need. The latter interventions are believed to be vital to slowing the progression of disease in HIV-infected persons. In recognition that some 80 percent of South Africans have recourse to traditional healers and take traditional medicines, the plan includes efforts to destigmatize traditional medicine and ensure that health professionals are aware of possible interactions and other issues surrounding the use of such medicines.

During the development of the plan, as with ART scale-up in general, human resource deficiencies were identified as the principal constraint (see Chapter 5 for further discussion), as there is approximately only one doctor for every 2,000 South Africans overall, with a remarkably skewed distribution between urban and rural areas. Thus the current plan includes forecasts of the growing numbers of trained health personnel that will be needed to implement ART effectively (see Table 2-2).

Furthermore, in February 2003, South Africa registered only one public-sector general physician per 4,829, one public-sector specialist physician per 10,403, and one public-sector professional nurse per 910 South Africans. Of most critical concern is the lack of a sufficient number of pharmacists, as there is only one public-sector pharmacist per 29,579 persons (South African National Treasury, 2003). Detailed and rigorous training manuals and processes for health professionals who will deliver HIV/AIDS interventions are being developed to extend the available expertise as much as possible. It is expected that the initiation of therapy will be by medical doctors, with nurses delivering much of the follow-up care.

A total estimated $696.5 million will be spent annually by 2007–2008, broken down as follows:

TABLE 2-2 Anticipated Personnel Needs for HIV/AIDS Care, Management, and Treatment in South Africa, by Category

Category	Phase I	Phase II	Phase III
Medical Officers	110	271	628
Professional Nurses	330	813	1,883
Enrolled Nurses	220	542	1,255
Assistant Nurses	220	542	1,255
Pharmacists	110	271	314
Pharmacist Assistants	110	271	314
Dieticians	110	136	314
Counsellors/Community Health Workers	1,100	2,710	6,275
Administrative Clerks	220	542	1,255

SOURCE: Paper presented by Dr. Anthony Mbewu on South Africa plan.

- $244.5 million to be spent on ARVs, if the prices negotiated by the Clinton Foundation can be implemented
- $148 million for recruiting of new health professionals
- $118.5 million for laboratory tests
- $96.3 million for additional nutritional supplements and support

Based on this budget and according to the plan, 1.1 million individuals will be on ART by 2008 (i.e., all individuals in need of therapy at that time), at a cost of about R600 per year per patient. An important element of the plan is about R50 million per year for research. These funds will be channeled through the Medical Research Council and overseen by a research subcommittee convened by the Department of Health.

COORDINATING THE GLOBAL RESPONSE

The ambitious ART roll-out goals of the PEPFAR initiative, the South African government, WHO, and a considerable number of countries and organizations worldwide represent a desperately needed global response to a devastating human tragedy (see Table 2-3). No single group or nation has all the fiscal, human, or intellectual resources to address these challenges, nor will a single approach or regimen be suitable for all settings. An organized culture of learning by doing will be central to identifying and refining best practices for particular settings, and the sharing of knowledge, resources, and efforts will be critical to the rapid, effective, safe delivery of ARVs to the millions of people in immediate need of life-sustaining treatment.

Coordinating global HIV/AIDS efforts in a way that maximally ben-

TABLE 2-3 Bilateral HIV/AIDS Support from Selected Countries, 2002 (in US$ millions)

Country	Projected 2002 Disbursements	% of GDP[a]
G8 Members		
United States	$413	0.00410
United Kingdom	300	0.02106
Japan	85	0.00205
Germany	55	0.00297
Canada	39	0.00561
France	25	0.00190
Italy (included in "other" below)		
Subtotal G8 Members	$917	
Other Countries		
Netherlands	$55	0.01447
Norway	35	0.02108
European Commission (EC)	25	
Other (including Italy[b])	190	
Subtotal Other Countries	$305	
Total	$1,222	

[a]GDP percentages calculated from 2004 World in Figures, The Economist.

[b]Exact figures for Italy are not available. According to UNAIDS, estimated bilateral spending by Italy is <$25 million.

NOTE: Amounts shown do not include funding for international HIV/AIDS research, and represent fiscal year (FY) 2002 budgeted/appropriated dollar amounts. Some countries are still finalizing FY 2002 figures.

SOURCE: Henry J. Kaiser Family Foundation, 2004a,b.

efits the affected countries and minimizes the diversion of resources from other critically important national health and social programs presents a great challenge. While recognizing the political complexities of a globally coordinated response of this magnitude, externally funded programs should make every effort to contribute to overall success rather than claiming organizational credit. It is imperative to maximize synergy and minimize competition among different initiatives and to ensure that the long-term potential to achieve sustainable results is not compromised by short-sighted ambitions and quick fixes. Equally imperative is the need to have a clear understanding of the local needs of affected communities and how they may differ from well-intentioned but sometimes misguided foreign perceptions.

A lack of coordination among donors and partners who enter countries with their various objectives and intentions can create confusion at the country level and make it difficult to monitor and assess the progress and impact of the respective efforts. Monitoring and evaluation (discussed in more detail in Chapter 5) is vital to knowing whether programs are succeeding and if not, to identifying problems and areas in need of improvement. At a recent WHO/UNAIDS workshop on generating strategic information for use in ART scale-up, the need to standardize monitoring and evaluation processes was identified as an urgent priority (WHO, 2004a). Yet monitoring and evaluation can become highly complicated very quickly. Although defining and monitoring input variables (i.e., what goes into a program) may be relatively easy, objectively monitoring and evaluating what becomes of those input variables (i.e., how the program proceeds and what the outcomes are) can be much more difficult. Without internationally harmonized monitoring and evaluation procedures, countries may be at a loss as to how to proceed. Duplication of effort and generation of redundant data may create unnecessary additional work for those responsible for collecting and managing monitoring and evaluation data.

Role of National Governments

The role of the governments of affected countries will be crucial to a coordinated response, since NGOs and universities, which serve as valuable sources and concentrations of expertise, do not have the mandate to scale up. The sooner the national government assumes leadership and engages in a specific scale-up effort, the more likely it is that scale-up will proceed rapidly and efficiently. Moreover, as the national government defines the standard of care for its country, so, too, does it define the continuum of medical care and support services that its HIV/AIDS population should have. Thus it is important that country plans be in place to inform allocation decisions and that procurement processes be integrally linked to country plans. Accordingly, one of the explicit policies of the Global Fund is that recipient countries must develop their own plans, which means they must have the necessary systems in place for doing so, including monitoring systems to gather information demonstrating that the funds provided are being used appropriately (Schwartlander et al., 2004).

The need to respect country processes raises important questions about the readiness of countries to implement large-scale ART programs and effectively absorb the great influx of resources being made available. There must be visible and meaningful commitment at the national level, and there should be established country mechanisms for coordinating multiple donor efforts, particularly with regard to ARV procurement (to ensure a continuous, reliable drug supply). Budgets must be designed appropriately; priorities should be realistic, based on actual resource allocations, reflective of cost-effectiveness and other value-driven considerations, and set by the countries rather than the donors; and the balance among various interventions should be founded in evidence-based knowledge, not arbitrary decisions. As important as these factors are to the short-term success and long-term sustainability of national HIV/AIDS strategic plans and global ART scale-up in general, all too often they do not receive sufficient consideration (Alban, 2002).

Assessment Tools

Quantitative assessment tools and costing analyses can be used to identify where the most absorptive capacity exists, where (e.g., in which regions, facilities) and how (e.g., which regimens) scale-up is likely to be most successful and cost-effective, and what steps need to be taken to scale up capacity in particular situations. A recent report on the cost and resource requirements associated with public-sector ART scale-up in Zambia illustrates the utility of such analyses for identifying key issues and exploring different approaches (e.g., alternative monitoring protocols and drug regimens) (Kombe and Smith, 2003).

Assessment tools may work best when the focus is on a specific geographic area. Otherwise, as the Clinton Foundation has learned from its experience conducting assessments of program readiness in several countries, the country's needs overwhelm the ability to define the standard or continuum of care and services that are impacting or available to a specific population (Goosby, 2004). Focusing on a specific population in a particular geographic area allows for a more quantitative assessment of service points (e.g., clinics, drug storage facilities, and transportation to such facilities) that intersect with a given population, as well as the steps necessary to create such links where they do not exist. It is important to emphasize that the assessment is aimed not at creating a parallel system with new clinics, laboratories, and the like, but on evaluating the current system, identifying gaps in service, and determining steps that can be taken to fill those gaps. Box 2-5 describes one example of an assessment tool.

Of note, based on its experience assessing program readiness, the Clinton Foundation has repeatedly identified human resource capacity as the major limiting factor. Not only are most sites experiencing a serious shortage of trained, qualified health care workers, but the amount of time it takes to train such workers makes it impossible to solve the problem quickly by adding new workers to a system that already exists (as can be done with other, quickly available resources, such as the ARVs themselves). Human resource capacity is discussed in detail in Chapter 5.

BOX 2-5
DELIVER: An Example of an Assessment Tool

In May 2003, DELIVER, a USAID-funded worldwide technical support contract implemented by John Snow, Inc., produced a 20-page guide for evaluating site capacity and readiness to initiate ART according to six domains: leadership and program model, services and clinical care, management and evaluation, staffing and experience, laboratory capacity, and drug management and procurement. An overall score determines which of five readiness stages characterizes a program and what steps can be taken to advance a program to a higher stage. The goal of the tool is to assess readiness based not on site type, size, or location, but rather on capacity, vision, and activities and services needed for the rational introduction and expansion of ART. The tool can also be used for site self-assessment and for the identification of areas in need of technical assistance and ways in which site programs can serve as resources for other programs.

SOURCE: Hirschhorn et al., 2002.

Importance of Engaging the Private Sector and Nongovernmental Organizations

Although the tendency when discussing and planning ART scale-up is to focus on the public sector, nongovernmental and private-sector programs may provide innovative, creative mechanisms for getting programs—including ART programs—off the ground more rapidly and operating more efficiently. While quality control is imperative, creative approaches that look beyond traditional entry points should be sought. Nontraditional entry points, such as mission hospitals, are increasingly being used to introduce and scale up ART programs. Consideration should also be given to other delivery mechanisms, such as franchising models that have shown substantial promise in reproductive health but have been explored less frequently for their potential to provide HIV/AIDS prevention and treatment (Montague, 2002; Smith, 2002; LaVake, 2003). Indeed, the number of nonpublic Global Fund recipients is growing, and only about half of the Global Fund resources are dedicated to public-sector recipients (Schwartlander, 2004).

While private programs can provide important innovations and capacity, it will be important as well for them to coordinate with public programs and to provide assurances and evaluation data related to the quality and consistency of the care they provide. Mechanisms will be needed to address the lack of sufficient training and access to updated regimens and protocol changes among private-sector practitioners, as well as the irregular and frequent movement of patients from provider to provider and the higher cost of private-sector ARVs (Brugha, 2003).

It must be recognized that the selection of particular locations and regions for the rapid implementation of scale-up, whether based on quantitative assessments or not, has important ethical implications. In particular, it is essential to ensure that the integration of ART programs into existing efforts does not further widen the gap between those who have access to health care (e.g., those living in urban areas and having access to hospitals and clinics) and those who do not (e.g., those living in remote, rural areas). To this end, efforts must be directed simultaneously at building the necessary infrastructure and capacity in areas where they do not exist. This and other human resource and infrastructure issues surrounding the management of ART scale-up are discussed in greater detail in Chapter 5 and in Appendix E.

Finally, as important as assessing readiness may be to introducing ART programs in the manner most likely to achieve maximal ARV coverage, it is equally important that scale-up efforts be able to proceed without having every detail in place.

> **Recommendation 2-1. Antiretroviral therapy scale-up in resource-constrained settings should proceed immediately through coordinated, aggressive action by national governments, donors, international agencies, and nongovernmental organizations.** *Donors must attempt to maximize the distribution of scarce resources—human, financial, and technical—for people in need within and among all resource-constrained countries and areas. To this end, multiple HIV/AIDS prevention and treatment initiatives need to be coordinated and integrated through national leadership and entitities that best meet the needs of their populations and of all individuals.*

FISCAL SUSTAINABILITY

The promised funds and efforts of the U.S. government, WHO, the Global Fund, UNAIDS, and others represent a historic change in the global attitude and political will toward alleviating the burden of HIV/AIDS. In the absence of a cure, however, the provision of ART must be for life, and the funding for widespread ART must be sustainable in the long run and for an indefinite period of time. Moreover, all of the 40 million currently infected people will eventually require treatment, thus creating a very large, steady demand for ARVs for decades to come. Yet the global HIV/AIDS funding available today does not even meet the needs of the 6 million people currently eligible for ARVs according to WHO's clinical criteria (Royal Danish Ministry for Foreign Affairs, 2000).

Based on 2001 calculations, the estimated annual cost of HIV/AIDS prevention and care for all people living with HIV/AIDS in 135 low- and middle-income countries is US$9.2 billion by 2005 (Schwartlander et al.,

2001). This figure includes $4.8 billion for prevention and $4.4 billion for care and support (i.e., ART, palliative care, prophylaxis and treatment for opportunistic infections, and support for orphans). More recently, UNAIDS has estimated the total need for HIV/AIDS funding to be $10.7 billion for 2005 and $14.9 billion by 2007 (Henry J. Kaiser Family Foundation, 2004a). These estimates cover prevention, care, and treatment delivery, but not research or infrastructure costs. By contrast, the total estimated funding for global HIV/AIDS in 2003 was US$4.2 billion, including $852 million in bilateral U.S. assistance, $1.163 billion in bilateral assistance from other countries (e.g., Canada, the European Commission, Germany, Japan, the Netherlands, the United Kingdom), $547 million from the Global Fund, $350 million from UN agencies, $120 million from The World Bank, $200 million from NGOs and foundations, and $1 billion from affected country governments (Henry J. Kaiser Family Foundation, 2004a). As already mentioned, the actual spending for 2003 was only $3.6 billion.

Achieving 3-by-5 and ultimately providing ARVs to all people in need will require substantially strengthening and upgrading the existing health system infrastructure. Otherwise, expanded ARV coverage may lead to increasing inefficiencies in resource allocation and higher costs per person for delivering interventions. A recent economic analysis of 83 countries showed that achieving high ARV coverage by 2015 will require additional annual spending of an estimated $US6.8 to 9.2 billion, including 25 percent for infrastructure (additional annual costs for prevention and care total more than an estimated $8.5 and $5.5 billion, respectively) (Kumaranayake et al., 2002). This same study showed that without infrastructure investments, ART will be able to expand by only about 10 percent.

As an example of how limited funds can impact affected countries, medications, counseling, and testing cost an estimated US$600 per patient per year in Botswana. Over 5 years, with 20,000 new patients added each year, the cumulative total cost will be $180 million. The Gates Foundation has committed $50 million over 5 years, with Merck matching that amount in ARVs. Concerns have been raised, however, about the sustainability of the program after the funding providing by the Gates Foundation and Merck ends (Rollnick, 2002; Attawell and Mundy, 2003).

As another example, in a recent study on the cost of comprehensive HIV/AIDS treatment in Mexico, ARVs account for an estimated 72.7 to 78.3 percent of the total annual cost of treatment per patient on ART (Bautista et al., 2003). It is interesting to note that, in contrast to what has been observed in Brazil (Ministry of Health [Brazil], 2003), the use of ARVs in Mexico is not cost-saving. Even though ART leads to a decline in hospital days, the decline is nowhere near large enough to offset the increase in ARV-related costs. Even a small reduction in the price of ARVs would have a measurable impact on the overall cost of therapy and make it easier for the government to provide ARVs to the country's estimated 64,000 people with symptomatic AIDS and another 116,000 to 177,000 infected with HIV. As is the case in so many other countries, access to HIV/AIDS treatment, including ARVs, varies considerably throughout Mexico; to meet the needs of the poor, the uninsured, and other HIV-infected people who cannot afford currently priced ARVs, the Minister of Health has committed to providing ARVs to all who need them by 2006.

In Zambia, a 2003 report on the per-patient costs and human resource requirements for scaling up ART in that country concluded that, at a per-patient annual cost of US$480, the current ART budget allows for provision of therapy to only about 10,000 people (Kombe and Smith, 2003). Given the uncertain future of the Global Fund and the unclear status of the $4.9 million already awarded to Zambia for HIV/AIDS interventions, however, the fiscal sustainability of treating even these initial 10,000 people, let alone the thousands of other infected people who need or will eventually need treatment, is uncertain. There are about 850,000 HIV-infected adults living in Zambia, including 100,000 who are already clinically eligible for ART. An estimated 85,000 to 110,000 new AIDS cases will likely continue to appear each year.

In Nigeria, about 10,000 patients receive therapy through the government program (at a heavily subsidized cost of US$8 per month) and 5,000 through state or private institutions, including NGOs (at a cost of about $90 to $100 per month). But even $8 is too much for many people, particularly in rural areas (Idoko, 2004). The added cost of basic laboratory monitoring—including CD4 counts, which are recommended at least every 6 months, as well as additional toxicity assays depending on the drug regimen and clinical symptoms—is prohibitively high for many patients. Since the Global Fund insists that drugs be free, it was not clear as of January 2004 how Nigeria would deal with the fact that its public program is based on heavily subsidized—not free—drugs. The program plan currently targets only 15,000 patients, yet there are about 4 to 5 million HIV-infected Nigerians (Idoko, 2004).

Procurement Strategy of the Clinton Foundation HIV/AIDS Initiative[1]

The Clinton Foundation's established procurement agreements are with suppliers of both APIs (active pharmaceutical ingredients, which represent 60–75 percent of the cost of producing ARVs) and formulations, as well as with suppliers of diagnostic tests (including both CD4 and viral load tests). For example, under an agreement with Becton, Dickinson, and Company,

---

[1]The discussion in this section is based on Margheiro (2004).

which was announced in January 2004, CD4 tests will be made available at US$8 per test. This figure includes the cost of reagents, an operational lease for the necessary instruments (including service, training, and controls), and consumables. This represents a substantial cost savings for what would otherwise be prohibitively expensive for many programs, as the retail price of the type of high-throughput instrument required for monitoring runs upwards of $100,000 to $130,000 per instrument, plus annual service costs are usually about 10 to 20 percent of the price of the instrument. The Clinton Foundation has also negotiated price reductions for CD4 assays with Beckman Coulter and for viral load assays with Roche Diagnostics, Bayer Health Care, and bioMerieux. The latter reductions make the price up to 80 percent lower as compared with the currently available lowest-price viral tests.

To illustrate the tremendous cost savings made possible by this type of combined agreement, the expected per-person cost of ART and CD4 and viral load monitoring in South Africa has been reduced from US$800 to less than $250, representing a savings of $500 million in a single year. In the Bahamas, procurement negotiations reduced the cost of generic ARVs per patient per year from approximately $3,800 to $500, a cost savings that allowed the Ministry of Health to increase the number of patients on ART from 350 to 1,200 without additional funding. Following the conclusion of another recent agreement, this annual cost is expected to be reduced even further, to about $300.

The increased buying power made possible by this type of procurement strategy not only is immediately beneficial to countries in need and to those living with HIV/AIDS, but also may lead to near- and long-term ARV price reductions. (For details on this strategy, see Box 5-3.) Given that there are only 300,000 people worldwide on ART, the current ARV marketplace is highly fragmented, with many small orders. For the ARV supplier, this situation translates into excess capacity, the production of small batches, little leverage with API suppliers, and relatively high prices (given that the APIs account for about 60–75 percent of the cost of drug production). Larger ARV orders should improve plant utilization at many levels and increase leverage with API suppliers, both of which should lead in turn to price reductions. A predictable future demand would also increase incentives to invest in research, development, and process improvement.

Although procuring the lowest possible price for ARVs is critically important to ensuring that as many people as possible receive the drugs, equally important is the need to ensure that all drugs being distributed are safe and of high quality. The Clinton Foundation uses WHO's prequalifying Procurement Quality and Sourcing Project (WHO, 2004b) criteria as accepted by the South African Medicines Control Council (Medicines Control Council, 2004) and its own technical assistance to ensure that drug distribution systems are secure and that inventory is properly maintained. Médicins sans Frontières, another organization that has made remarkable headway in procuring affordable ARVs for use in its pilot clinics in South Africa and elsewhere, has reportedly sought and received authorization from the South African Medicines Control Council for the use of Brazilian generic ARVs (Attawell and Mundy, 2003). Issues related to drug safety and quality are discussed in detail in Chapter 5.

Need for Continuous Funding

Not only will the sustainability and success of ART scale-up depend on long-term funding, but it is vitally important that such funding from external donors be continuous while upstream issues such as debt and trade rules are being addressed in ways that could reduce the long-term dependence of developing countries on this philanthropy. In some countries, uncertainties in funding are already putting ART programs at risk of failure by interrupting the procurement and timely delivery of drugs. In Nigeria, for example, where only 5,000 of more than 1 million symptomatic HIV-infected people are currently receiving ART through a national program initiated in 2002, promised Global Fund monies have been slow to arrive: although about $12 million is expected, only $1 to 1.2 million had arrived as of the end of January 2004 (Idoko, 2004). The result has been serious procurement problems and widespread treatment interruptions.

Self-Sustainability

While philanthropy is unquestionably an essential component of ART scale-up, particularly during the emergency phase of the next 20 years or so, the long-term sustainability of these efforts will ultimately depend on addressing the complex underlying socioeconomic and political factors that drive the HIV/AIDS pandemic, as they do other infectious disease epidemics, in resource-constrained settings. Infectious diseases have and will continue to persist, emerge, and be influenced by the backdrop of rapid and profound demographic, economic, social, and ecological change (Benatar, 2002). Addressing these underlying factors will require imaginative and creative new approaches that are beyond the scope of this report.

Recommendation 2-2. Donors should commit to continuous funding of antiretroviral therapy scale-up for decades to ensure the sustainability necessary to avert the medical hazard of interruptions in the continuity of treatment. *Delays in donor funding after treatment programs are initiated will jeopardize the long-term durability of treatment regimens. Because it is estimated that 40 million people are currently infected* *with HIV, and 5 million new infections occur each year, donors should plan now for increasing support in the future. To this end, innovative mechanisms should continue to be pursued by national governments and donors in partnership with industry to ensure the continuous procurement of quality drugs, diagnostics, and other commodities at the lowest possible cost. At the same time, national governments in countries severely affected by HIV/AIDS must begin to invest in and develop priorities for prevention and treatment programs to ensure those programs' long-term sustainability and effectiveness.*

ETHICAL ISSUES

As ART programs are scaled up throughout the developing world, many difficult decisions will be necessary, and in many cases, both local and institutional/international ethical issues will be faced. The public health ethical dimension of ART scale-up is just beginning to enter the arena of bioethical debate, and there are as yet few answers to the multitude of ethical questions raised by ART scale-up.

Local Issues

One of the most pressing questions is how to determine priorities for who should receive treatment. This question is crucial given that WHO's ambitious 3-by-5 plan still targets only half of the 6 million people worldwide currently in need of life-sustaining treatment, and given that millions more infected but currently immunocompetent persons will need treatment in the future. There is no easy answer, no universally obvious single best or "right" ethical framework or theory of justice (e.g., egalitarian, utilitarian, libertarian) to apply. Even if there were agreement on a particular theory of justice, there would probably still be logistical and other practical challenges to address in translating that theory into health care rationing. Nevertheless, the question of how to select those to treat should not paralyze initiatives to provide life-sustaining ART.

Different organizations and countries are currently basing the selection of individuals for treatment on variable criteria, many of which are ethically defensible from one viewpoint or another. Although WHO and this report recommend using medical criteria, even this apparently objective measure involves certain judgments about providing the greatest good for the greatest number of individuals. An example would be recommending less-expensive regimens (in terms of both initial cost and the level of expensive laboratory monitoring) despite concern that some of these regimens appear to be considerably more susceptible to resistance in poor adherence settings, thus increasing the risk of long-term failure of scale-up. Box 2-6

BOX 2-6
Treatment Selection Criteria for ART Scale-Up Programs

• In Uganda, an argument has been put forth that people at greatest risk of transmitting infection, such as HIV-infected pregnant women, should receive treatment first.
    • Some communities have argued that every HIV-infected person deserves an equal chance, and therefore, persons receiving treatment should be selected by random lottery.
    • Some communities have argued that social worth should be used to determine who receives treatment first, and therefore, treatment selection should be based on age, level of education, vocation (e.g., health care personnel), and the like.
    • Others argue that, to ensure political stability in countries characterized by war or unrest, military personnel should receive priority (so that ARVs can be distributed).
    • In Kenya, the argument has been made that particular groups merit special consideration, such as victims of rape, people who have become infected with HIV during vaccine trials, HIV orphans, or infected pregnant women.
    • To be eligible for Médicins sans Frontières' pilot ART program in South Africa, patients must meet certain biomedical, adherence, and social criteria, including residence within a certain geographic area, number of dependents, health status, income, and level of activism in seeking improved access and care for individuals suffering from HIV/AIDS.

SOURCE: Wasunna, 2004.

---

presents some of the treatment selection criteria proposed for ART scale-up programs.

One proposed criterion is that patients be selected on the basis of provider predictions regarding who is most likely to adhere to lifetime treatment. As mentioned in Chapter 4, however, studies have shown that providers are rarely able to make such predictions accurately, and that all too often the process becomes discriminatory against poor, disadvantaged people. On the other hand, one study showed that, although screening for the selective treatment of patients more likely to adhere to their regimens may result in lower levels of resistance, it is also likely to lead to a higher incidence of drug-sensitive HIV and AIDS than would a policy of treating all HIV-infected individuals (Tchetgen et al., 2001).

In addition to patient selection, the reality that there is a limited supply of ARVs, as well as other resources needed to deliver them, raises important questions about where to begin ART scale-up. It may be necessary to start with relatively small programs in places where the capacity exists, and while these programs are running, to steadily increase the supporting infrastructure needed for larger programs. Alternatively, starting small may create greater ethical challenges by resulting in even more injustice in societies already suffering enormous disparities in health and wealth, given that ART programs would be implemented where the capacity already exists and people already have access. Meanwhile, those without access to health care would need to wait until, with donor aid, the country had built enough infrastructure to treat them. Yet delaying the provision of treatment to those who can access it now because doing so would widen existing health disparities is not necessarily any more ethical. Is it not better to save any life than none?

That there are no easy resolutions for these and similar ethical issues can lead to endless philosophical controversy and raises important questions about what, if anything, global donors can do with respect to recommending criteria or specific decision-making strategies. One proposed approach to priority setting is described in Box 2-7.

Some experts believe that, because of the enormous variation in ethical perspectives among different cultures and communities, the decision-making process on such matters should remain entirely the responsibility of

---

BOX 2-7
Accountability for Reasonableness

In the absence of a satisfactory theory of justice that can be applied in everyday practice, American scholars Daniels and Sabin have proposed a process for priority setting that they call "accountability for reasonableness." According to this framework, a fair priority-setting process meets four conditions. First, decisions must be made on the basis of the best available data by people who are fair minded and willing to make compromise good-faith decisions that are contextually relevant. Second, the rationale for how such decisions were reached must be made public. Third, allowance must be made for appeals so that decisions can be reconsidered in the light of new evidence or arguments. Fourth, there must be an enforcement process that facilitates the implementation of the previous three conditions.

This process was developed in the context of the U.S. privately funded health care system, but it has also been found to be workable and acceptable within the Canadian publicly funded system. In the latter context, researchers identified the importance of seeking multiple perspectives on the problem under review, ensuring transparency and honesty in the decision-making process, identifying potential conflicts of interest, and achieving consensus. A recent detailed qualitative study of how the framework of accountability for reasonableness can be applied to access to intensive care units for neurosurgical patients provides evidence that such a process improves the fairness of priority setting.

SOURCES: Daniels and Sabin, 1997; Martin et al., 2002, 2003.

individual countries. Others believe a minimum set of criteria for patient selection in treatment programs, based on international human rights, should be established to help countries make these very difficult decisions, and that countries should have a structured process in place for implementing context-specific decisions about the distribution and administration of treatment.

The question then arises, however, of how such a national ethical decision-making process should be created. What can countries do to ensure that the process is fair? To avoid a first-come, first-served system open to corruption and abuse, countries need some sort of legitimate process, even an imperfect one, so they can at least begin ART rollout as they simultaneously begin working toward a more fair and just system. It has been suggested that each country create its own independent, properly constituted, legally recognized, transparent decision-making body and that the decisions made by this body be subject to monitoring and evaluation just as any component of ART scale-up should be. However, the difficulties of establishing an independent ethical review process within each country cannot be underestimated. Many resource-limited countries may not have the capacity to develop ethical guidelines. Nor can the pragmatic challenges of implementing ethically sound theory and policy be overestimated. Scientific progress takes place slowly and requires much human energy and skill, as well as abundant resources. Moral progress will likewise be slow, but it can be can be made if time, energy, and resources are devoted to this end. The decision-making process described above suggests the way forward. As such processes are gradually implemented, further lessons will be learned.

What is to be done, however, about dictator-ruled countries without the political will to establish such a process? How should such countries be treated by the international community? What are the ethical issues surrounding the provision of funds and resources to countries without ethical decision-making processes in place?

As with other aspects of ART scale-up, waiting until a perfect ethical decision-making process has been designed and implemented creates its own ethical challenge, as thousands of people continue to die each day from AIDS-related causes. As critically important as the ethical components of ART scale-up may be, providing treatment in the absence of detailed guidelines has itself become an ethical imperative.

Institutional and International Issues

Although AIDS is an epidemic of unprecedented proportions, people living in resource-constrained settings also suffer from a wide range of other life-threatening ailments, most notably TB and malaria. Not only do many of these people not have access to the medical and health resources needed to treat, cure, or prevent these ailments, but they often do not have access to some of the most basic necessities of survival, such as safe drinking water. This situation is perhaps the greatest international ethical challenge (Benatar, 1998).

It is imperative that ART programs be strategically situated within existing health care systems so that funding for HIV/AIDS can contribute to building a sustainable health care infrastructure that can benefit all people in need, whether they suffer from HIV/AIDS, TB, malaria, or some other health complication. Otherwise, practical and public health considerations aside, it would be necessary to justify using ART to save the lives of HIV/AIDS patients and not the lives of those in immediate need of other life-sustaining drugs to treat malaria and other life-threatening diseases. ART scale-up must be implemented in such a way that instead of exacerbating existing inequities, it helps rectify some of those inequities by instituting programs that help meet the life-sustaining demands of all people in need.

Clearly, the ethical challenges and implications of ART scale-up are extraordinarily complex—more so, some would argue, than the medical and logistical challenges outlined in detail throughout this report. Even if WHO's 3-by-5 campaign and other efforts to accelerate the introduction of ARVs achieve the highest levels of success, insufficient drug supplies and the reality that not all infected individuals in need can receive treatment will necessitate making decisions about whom to treat. Yet this is by no means the only ethical problem that will arise. Indeed, we are living in the midst of an ethical dilemma even now as we watch patients die and children become orphaned while we struggle with valid technical questions of how to balance the risks and benefits associated with the new opportunities outlined earlier in this chapter. These and other ethical issues are described further in Appendix D.

The goal of ART scale-up should be to prolong survival while also reducing illness and the numbers of newly infected people. Therefore, success should be measured by survival, and drug regimens should be selected on the basis of providing therapy to as many people as possible. This is the case despite some concern that the use of more-expensive regimens than those currently being recommended by WHO might better serve to reduce the eventual emergence of resistance. The threat of resistance and the implications of its emergence are as yet unclear. Since the use of more-expensive regimens would reduce the number of people treated and since the goal of ART scale-up should be to reduce mortality now, the use of simpler, less-expensive regimens is recommended. As noted earlier, there are many valid ethical and cultural perspectives from which to judge whether a particular HIV/AIDS intervention or treatment program is ethical. The committee takes the perspective that the use of simple, standardized regimens that maximize not only the number of people treated but also the likelihood that

ART programs will be introduced into even the most remote, resource-constrained areas currently provides the best balance between the ethical complications of deciding who should receive treatment and the ethical imperative to act now.

REFERENCES

Alban A. 2002. Priorities of AIDS Interventions in Africa: Principles and Practice in Five Countries. Copenhagen, Denmark: EASE International.

American Enterprise Institute. 2004. *Remarks given by Ambassador Randall L. Tobias, U.S. Global HIV/AIDS Coordinator at the Department of State, in Washington, DC.* [Online]. Available: http://www.state.gov/s/gac/rl/rm/2004/29181.htm [accessed August 24, 2004].

Attawell K, Mundy J. 2003. *WHO, UK Department for International Development. Provision of Antiretroviral Therapy in Resource-Limited Settings: a Review of the Literature up to August 2003.* [Online]. Available: http://www.who.int/3by5/publications/documents/en/ARTpaper_DFID_WHO.pdf [accessed August 24, 2004].

Bautista SA, Dmytraczenko T, Kombe G, Bertozzi SM. 2003 (June). Costing of HIV/AIDS Treatment in Mexico, Technical Report No. 020. The Partners for Health Reform*plus* Project, Abt Associates Inc., Bethesda, MD.

Benatar SR. 1998. Global disparities in health and human rights. *American Journal of Public Health* 88:295–300.

Benatar SR. 2002. The HIV/AIDS pandemic: A sign of instability in a complex global system. *Journal of Medicine and Philosophy* 27:163–177.

Brugha R. 2003. Antiretroviral treatment in developing countries: The peril of neglecting private providers. *British Medical Journal* 326:1382–1384.

Daniels N, Sabin J. 1997. Limits to health care: Fair procedures, democratic deliberation and the legitimacy problem for insurers. *Philosophy & Public Affairs* 26(4):303–350.

Goosby E. 2004 (January 28). *Assessing the Readiness for ARV Program Implementation.* Presentation at the Institute of Medicine Workshop on Antiretroviral Scale-up in Resource Constrained Settings, Washington, DC. Institute of Medicine Committee on Antiretroviral Drug Use in Resource-Constrained Settings.

Henry J. Kaiser Family Foundation. 2004a. Global Funding for HIV/AIDS in Resource Poor Settings (HIV/AIDS Policy Fact Sheet #6114). *The Henry J. Kaiser Family Foundation.* [Online]. Available: http://www.kff.org [accessed August 24, 2004].

Henry J. Kaiser Family Foundation. 2004b. U.S. Government Funding for HIV/AIDS in Resource Poor Settings (HIV/AIDS Policy Fact Sheet #6115). *The Henry J. Kaiser Family Foundation.* [Online]. Available: http://www.kff.org [accessed August 24, 2004].

Hirschhorn L, Fullern A, Shaw C, Prosser W, Noguera M. 2002. *Tool to Assess Site Program Readiness for Initiating Antiretroviral Therapy (ART).* [Online]. Available: http://www.deliver.jsi.com/2002/archives/hivaids/SofR_tool/index.cfm [accessed January 7, 2004].

Idoko J. 2004 (January 27). *The 2003 WHO Guidelines for ARV use: Perspectives from a User.* Presentation at the Institute of Medicine Workshop on Antiretroviral Scale-up in Resource Constrained Settings, Washington, DC. Institute of Medicine Committee on Antiretroviral Drug Use in Resource-Constrained Settings.

Kim J. 2004 (January 27). *The Challenge of HIV in 2004 and the UNAIDS/WHO "3 by 5" Program.* Presentation at the Institute of Medicine Workshop on Antiretroviral Scale-up in Resource Constrained Settings, Washington, DC. Institute of Medicine Committee on Antiretroviral Drug Use in Resource-Constrained Settings.

Kombe G, Smith O. 2003 (October). The Costs of Anti-retroviral treatment in Zambia. The Partners for Health Reform*plus* Project, Abt Associates Inc., Bethesda, MD.

Kumaranayake L, et al. 2002. Estimating the infrastructure requirements for an expanded response to HIV/AIDS in low and middle-income countries (Abstract TuPeE5185). Presented at the 14th International AIDS Conference, Barcelona, Spain. [Online]. Available: http://www.aids2002.com/Program/ViewAbstract.asp?id=/T-CMS_Content/Abstract/200206290751023109.xml [accessed July 1, 2004].

LaVake S. 2003. Applying social franchising techniques to youth reproductive health/HIV services. *YouthNet Youth Issues Paper #2*. Family Health International. [Online]. Available: http://www.fhi.org/NR/rdonlyres/cijal2kvvmtazwuqnkoqk4hbxmdazuanzwojv55tghflkma7sj2k2gusgfv6276emct5uxnwl6iamc/YI4.pdf [accessed July 1, 2004].

Margheiro L. 2004. Paper presented at the Institute of Medicine ARV Workshop, Washington, DC. Institute of Medicine Committee on Antiretroviral Drug Use in Resource-Constrained Settings.

Martin DK, Giacomini M, Singer PA. 2002. Fairness, accountability for reasonableness, and the views of priority setting decision-makers. *Health Policy* 61:279–290.

Martin DK, Singer PA, Bernstein M. 2003. Access to ICU beds for neurosurgery patients: A qualitative case study. *Journal of Neurology, Neurosurgery and Psychiatry* 74:1299–1303.

Medicines Control Council. *Home page*. [Online]. Available: http://www.mccza.com/ [accessed March 11, 2004].

Ministry of Health (Brazil). 2003. *The Experience of the Brazilian AIDS Program*. [Online]. Available: http://www.aids.gov.br/final/biblioteca/resposta/resp_ingles.pdf [accessed July 1, 2004].

Montague D. 2002. Franchising of health services in low-income countries. *Health Policy and Planning* 17(2):121–130.

Office of Legislative Policy and Analysis. 2004. *Legislative Update, 108th Congress: United States Leadership Against Global HIV/AIDS, Tuberculosis, and Malaria Act of 2003, P.L. 108-25 (S. 250, H.R. 1298)*. [Online]. Available: http://olpa.od.nih.gov/legislation/108/publiclaws/hivtbmal.asp [accessed July 1, 2004].

Office of the United States Global AIDS Coordinator. 2003. The President's Emergency Plan for AIDS Relief. 2003. *The White House*. [Online]. Available: http://www.state.gov/s/gac/ [accessed August 24, 2004].

Quinn TC, Chaisson RE. 2004. *International Epidemiology of Human Immunodeficiency Virus in Infections Diseases*. 3rd ed. Gorbach SL, Bartlett JG, and Blacklow NR, eds. Philadelphia, PA: WB Saunders Company.

Rollnick R. 2002. Botswana's high stakes assault on AIDS. *Africa Recovery* 16(2). [Online]. Available: www.un.org/ecosocdev/geninfo/afrec/vol16no2/.

Royal Danish Ministry for Foreign Affairs. 2000. Building a global community: Globalization and the common good. Copenhagen: Royal Danish Ministry for Foreign Affairs.

Schwartlander B, Stover J, Walker N, Bollinger L, Gutierrez JP, McGreevey W, Opuni M, Forsythe S, Kumaranayake L, Watts C, Bertozzi S. 2001. AIDS. Resource needs for HIV/AIDS. *Science* 292:2434–2436.

Schwartlander B, Stover J, Walker N, Bollinger L, Gutierrez JP, McGreevey W, Opuni M, Forsythe S, Kumaranayake L, Watts C, Bertozzi S. 2004 (January 28–29). The Global Fund's Lessons Learned Regarding ARV Drug Scale-up in Resource-Constrained Settings. Paper presented at the Institute of Medicine ARV Workshop, Washington, DC. Institute of Medicine Committee on Antiretroviral Drug Use in Resource-Constrained Settings.

Smith E. 2002. *Social franchising reproductive health services: Can it work? Marie Stopes International Working Paper #5.* [Online]. Available: http://www.mariestopes.org.uk/pdf/working-paper-no5-social.pdf [accessed July 1, 2004].

South African National Treasury. 2003. Intergovernmental Fiscal Review. *South African National Treasury Table 5.6, page 79.* [Online]. Available: http://www.treasury.gov.za/documents/ifr/2003/default.htm [accessed July 1, 2004].

Tchetgen E, Kaplan EH, Friedland GH. 2001. Public health consequences of screening patients for adherence to highly active antiretroviral therapy. *Journal of Acquired Immune Deficiency Syndrome* 26:118–129.

The Foreign Press Center. 2003. *Adapted from "O'Neill, Fauci Discuss President's AIDS Initiatives," Washington, DC on May 29, 2003.* [Online]. Available: http://www.whitehouse.gov/news/releases/2003/05/print/20030529-8.html [accessed August 24, 2004].

The Global Fund. 2003a. *The Global Fund Pledges and Contributions.* [Online]. Available: http://www.theglobalfund.org/en/files/pledges&contributions.xls [accessed March 9, 2004].

The Global Fund. 2003b. Round 3 portfolio and programmatic analysis (unpublished). In: Summers T, Kates J, eds. *U.S. Government Funding for HIV/AIDS in Resource Poor Settings,* The Henry J. Kaiser Foundation.

The Global Fund. 2004a. *The Global Fund Home Page.* [Online]. Available: http://www.theglobalfund.org/en/ [accessed July 1, 2004].

The Global Fund. 2004b. *The Global Fund to Fight AIDS, Tuberculosis and Malaria Progress Report.* [Online]. Available: http://www.theglobalfund.org [accessed February 10, 2004].

The White House. 2003. *The President's Emergency Plan for AIDS Relief Fact Sheet.* [Online]. Available: http://www.state.gov/g/oes/rls/2003/22270.htm [accessed July 2, 2003].

The World Bank Group. 2001. *The US $500 Million Multi-Country HIV/AIDS Program (MAP) for Africa Progress Review Mission—FY01.* [Online]. Available: http://www.worldbank.org/afr/aids/map/prog_rpt_01.pdf.

UNAIDS (Joint United Nations Programme on HIV/AIDS). 2003. *Report on the State of HIV/AIDS Financing.* Geneva: UNAIDS.

U.S. Department of State. 2004. *The President's Emergency Plan for AIDS Relief, U.S. Five-Year Global HIV/AIDS Strategy.* Washington, DC: U.S. Department of State.

Wasunna A. 2004 (January 28). *Ethical Issues in the Scale-up of ARV Programs in Resource-Poor Settings.* Paper presented at the Institute of Medicine Workshop on Antiretroviral Scale-up in Resource Constrained Settings, Washington, DC. Institute of Medicine Committee on Antiretroviral Drug Use in Resource-Constrained Settings.

WHO (World Health Organization). 2003a. *Treating 3 Million by 2005. Making it Happen. The WHO Strategy.* Geneva: WHO. [Online]. Available: http://www.who.int/3by5/en/ [accessed July 26, 2004].

WHO. 2003b. *The World Health Report 2003: Shaping the Future.* Geneva: WHO.

WHO. 2004a. *WHO/UNAIDS Workshop on Strategic Information for Anti-Retroviral Therapy Programmes.* [Online]. Available: http://www.who.int/hiv/strategic/mt300703/en/ [accessed March 11, 2004].

WHO. 2004b. *World Health Organization Prequalification Project.* [Online]. Available: http://mednet3.who.int/prequal/hiv/hivdefault.shtml [accessed March 11, 2004].

William J. Clinton Foundation. 2004. *Foundation Programs.* [Online]. Available: http://www.clintonpresidentialcenter.com/foundation_programs.html [accessed January 5, 2004].

3

Lessons Learned

With the many policy, research, and funding initiatives now supporting and recommending antiretroviral therapy (ART) scale-up for resource-constrained settings, it will be critical to understand the experience gained by both the developed and developing worlds in treating people with HIV/AIDS. One lesson learned is that poor early treatment decisions can limit a patient's future therapeutic options and irrevocably alter the course of the disease and treatment response. One fear associated with use of ART in all settings is treatment failure as a result of the emergence of resistant virus. If widespread drug resistance were to emerge, the long-term public health impact of and financial capacity for HIV/AIDS treatment could be threatened. Preventing treatment failure—whether because of resistance or other factors—will be paramount to ensuring the long-term durability and sustainability of efforts to combat this pandemic. Thus it is essential that the many lessons learned about the causes and implications of treatment success, treatment failure, and drug resistance in the developed and developing worlds guide ART scale-up programs. While the successes achieved in more resource-constrained settings may have occurred on a small scale, they, too, can provide invaluable lessons for the scale-up of treatment to the millions in need now and in the future.

This chapter first describes the problem of drug resistance and then examines its implications for ART scale-up. The final section reviews lessons learned from early scale-up efforts around the world.

THE PROBLEM OF RESISTANCE

Highly Active Antiretroviral Therapy

During the initial years of treating the HIV/AIDS epidemic in the United States and other parts of the developed world where treatment was available, ART consisted of the use of one or two drugs, known as mono or dual therapy. By the mid-1990s, as additional drugs were developed for HIV, it became clear that other therapy regimens might be better. Highly active antiretroviral therapy (HAART), a regimen based on using at least three ARVs from a minimum of two classes in combination, was developed in the mid- to late 1990s following the introduction of additional classes of ARVs and the recognition that using more drugs in combination is more effective in restoring immune function, decreasing HIV burden, and preventing the emergence of drug resistance. The three main classes are nucleoside reverse transcriptase inhibitors (NRTIs), nonnucleoside reverse transcriptase inhibitors (NNRTIs), and protease inhibitors (PIs). (A drug from a fourth, newer class was approved in the United States in 2003 but is not yet widely used clinically and is not discussed further in this report.) HAART is now the standard treatment recommended in the United States. Appendix B provides a more thorough discussion of HAART.

Overview of Resistance

Drug resistance can render treatment ineffective for individual patients and has implications for the treatment of whole populations should they receive a high burden of transmitted drug-resistant virus. Resistance to HIV drugs arises in the presence of incomplete suppression of viral replication in the face of the selective pressure of drug treatment. The resistance-conferring mutations accumulate during rapid, error-prone HIV replication. The longer viral replication continues in the presence of inadequate ART regimens (i.e., failure of drugs to completely suppress viral replication), the more resistance will emerge. Even with low levels of virus present (i.e., between 50 and 500 copies/ml), drug resistance can develop (Fischl, 1999; Hirsch et al., 1998, 2000, 2003; Richman et al., 2004). The emergence of drug-resistant virus is one factor that can contribute to the failure of ART (Deeks, 2003). The fact that drug-resistant HIV-1 viral variants can still replicate well contributes to the rapid evolution of HIV in the face of potent drug pressure.

Although most resistance mutations confer a functional virus, the mutations can produce a virus with less replicative capacity than its wild-type relative. In theory, new mutations that emerge over time may often but not completely compensate for this defect. The lower fitness (or infectivity) of drug-resistant variants, as well as the lower viral load in partially treated patients (compared with untreated patients), may contribute to a lower rate of transmission of drug-resistant virus (Leigh Brown et al., 2003). Nevertheless, public health efforts should be focused on trying to minimize the rate of acquiring resistance (i.e., by treating drug-sensitive cases appropriately), rather than on trying to prevent the transmission of drug-resistant strains.

Thus resistance to HIV drugs can be acquired, and HIV-resistant viruses can be transmitted. And most HIV-infected individuals with drug-resistant virus are initially infected with a drug-sensitive virus that acquires resistance during ART (Deeks, 2003).

The prevalence of drug resistance among HIV strains in the United States may be as high as 50 percent, based on the results of a large cohort study of HIV-infected adults receiving HAART (Richman et al., 2004). Drug resistance has been found for each class of drugs available for ART, and resistance may be present for more than one drug or class—a phenomenon known as multidrug resistance (Richman et al., 2004).

Acquired resistance is dependent upon several factors, including patient adherence to therapy, the mutation rate of the virus, and the efficacy of the ART regimen (Blower et al., 2003a; Deeks, 2003; Leigh Brown et al., 2003; Hirsch et al., 1998, 2000, 2003) (see Box 3-1). Adherence rates of less than 90 percent and less than 80 percent have been shown to result in drug resistance and virological failure (Hirsch et al., 1998, 2000, 2003; Paterson et al., 2000; Sethi et al., 2003). As discussed above, ineffective regimens that do not completely suppress viral replication will lead to resistant virus, and the use of sequential mono or dual therapy is no longer recommended because of its now-recognized association with the development of a high rate of drug resistance (Deeks, 2003; Hirsch et al., 1998, 2000, 2003; Leigh Brown et al., 2003).

Transmitted resistance occurs when a person is infected with a virus that has previously acquired resistance. Cases of drug-resistant virus in the United States were first documented in the mid-1990s, and several recent reports have suggested that the percentage of new infections demonstrating some form of drug resistance has risen significantly since then (Grant et al., 2002; Little et al., 2002; Simon et al., 2002). If transmitted drug-resistant virus is not faced with the continuous selection pressure of ART, it can revert back to the drug-sensitive, wild type of virus (Hirsch et al., 2003). Hence, the drug-resistant virus may not be measured at a particular point in time. However, the first documented case of a resistant virus that was stably transmitted from one person to a another, who then passed it on to a third person, was reported in 2003 (Taylor et al., 2003). See Appendix B for a more-detailed discussion of resistance.

BOX 3-1
Resistance Determinants:
Factors That Affect Virological Response to Therapy

Logistics
  • Interrupted drug supply causing lapses in treatment

Medication factors
  • Inadequate drug potency
  • Interaction with other drugs

Patient factors
  • Altered drug metabolism
  • Poor drug absorption
  • Altered intracellular metabolism of drugs
  • Advanced HIV disease stage (low pretreatment CD4 count or high pretreatment viral load)
  • Anatomic compartmentalization of virus replication with limited drug exposure ("reservoirs")
  • Host genetic variability in HIV susceptibility and drug efficacy
  • Incomplete adherence to regimen (due, e.g., to side effects, pill burden, requirement for coadministration with food/water)

Virus factors
  • HIV virulence
  • Preexisting drug resistance

Provider factors
  • Incomplete counseling (e.g., on medication effects, schedules, importance of adherence)
  • Prescription of ineffective combination of drugs
  • Inadequate clinical follow-up

SOURCE: Deeks, 2003.

Resistance to Antiretroviral Drugs and Their Classes

As noted above, drug resistance has been found for all classes of drugs available for treatment of HIV/AIDS (Clavel and Hance, 2004). The NRTI drug lamivudine (3TC) and drugs within the NNRTI class are the preferential components of regimens for resource-constrained settings. The ease with which resistance can emerge to 3TC and NNRTIs when regimens containing these drugs are not used effectively underscores the critical need to focus on adherence with these programs. NNRTI-based regimens are the most frequently used first-line regimens in North America and Europe;

however, PI-based regimens are necessary for patients with either acquired or transmitted NNRTI-resistant HIV infection.

The World Health Organization (WHO) recommends that, despite their cost, PI-based regimens be considered first-line regimens in populations where the prevalence of NNRTI resistance is greater than 5 to 10 percent (Hirsch et al., 2003). In the developed world, a drug resistance test would be used to select a regimen (Hirsch et al., 2003). Other reasons for considering a PI-based regimen as a first-line regimen include the presence of viral types with known insensitivity to NNRTIs (e.g., HIV-2 or HIV-1 group O) and situations in which the patient cannot tolerate NNRTIs. Although nevirapine, for example, is a potent NNRTI with demonstrated clinical efficacy, it is also associated with rash and hepatotoxicity, both of which can be severe and life-threatening (Ena et al., 2003; Law et al., 2003; Martin-Carbonero et al., 2003). Even mild rashes can cause poor adherence and treatment failure.

Given concerns about resistance, particularly with the WHO-recommended NNRTI-based regimens, high adherence rates will be absolutely critical to the success of ART scale up. There is no known reason not to expect that, if patients adhere to currently available triple-combination drug regimens, success rates could approach 80 to 90 percent (in terms of complete viral suppression), thus minimizing the rates of emergence of drug resistance over time. Yet while studies have shown that good adherence is quite feasible in resource-constrained settings under certain circumstances (e.g., in clinical settings where the studies are conducted) (Laniece et al., 2003; Orrell et al., 2003), the replicability of these results in other circumstances has been questioned.

Questions have been raised regarding the durability of NNRTI-versus PI-based regimens for ART scale-up in resource-constrained settings and the extent to which the WHO-recommended first-line NNRTI-based regimens appropriately address concerns about resistance (Redfield, 2004). How should concerns about resistance and the need for excellent adherence be balanced with the reality that the NNRTI-based regimens are otherwise the best choice for use in resource-constrained settings (i.e., with respect to toxicity, effectiveness, side effects, pill burden, and affordability) (Barreiro et al., 2002)? Such regimens have similarly been selected as the preferred first-line regimens in developed country settings.

Nevirapine Resistance: Implications for Mother, Child, and the Pandemic

While single-dose nevirapine may be a cost-effective and simple regimen for preventing HIV transmission from mother to child in resource-constrained settings, concerns regarding nevirapine resistance have arisen and may limit the drug's future utility for this purpose (Jackson et al., 2000). In a recent study from Thailand, women with a history of limited nevirapine exposure for a single pregnancy had reduced rates of successful treatment responses subsequently with a treatment regimen containing nevirapine (Jourdain et al., 2004).

In a prior study conducted in Uganda, although 19 percent of the women and 46 percent of the infants who had received single-dose nevirapine had detectable nevirapine resistance at 6 weeks postpartum, resistance had faded from detection in all women and infants by 12 to 18 months (Eshleman et al., 2001). In this case, it is possible that drug resistance was not detected when the mother discontinued the nevirapine prophylaxis because drug-sensitive wild-type virus had reemerged in the viral population. Rather than having been eliminated, the nevirapine-resistant virus may simply have been "archived," with the potential to reappear as a therapeutic challenge in the future when infected mothers and children were placed on therapy (Ekouvi et al., 2004).

Work in Cote d'Ivoire by Chair and colleagues revealed that 21 of 74 women had a detectable nevirapine resistance mutation at 4 weeks postpartum, as did 6 (23 percent) of the offspring evaluated. As reported, follow-up plasma and DNA-(PBMC) samples collected at 3 months (1 child) and until 12 months (1 child) revealed the persistence of NVP-resistance mutations (Ekouevi et al., 2004). Other studies have also documented high rates of nevirapine-resistance mutations (Gordon et al., 2004; Loubser et al., 2004).

Another factor to consider is the consequence of the emergence of nevirapine-resistant virus among different HIV subtypes, since the pattern of nevirapine-resistance mutations varies among subtypes. One recent study showed that women with subtype D had a higher rate of nevirapine resistance than women with subtype A (Eshleman et al., 2004a,b). Interestingly, nevirapine-resistance mutations differ between babies and their mothers, suggesting that resistance is not transmitted. Rather, babies have active, ongoing viral replication at the time of intra- and/or postpartum exposure to nevirapine.

Clearly, concern is rapidly growing that the use of ARVs that readily select for resistance and have long half-lives in settings where mother-to-child transmission is common and the support of potent combinations is lacking may compromise future treatment of mothers and children. The search for less problematic alternatives to prevent mother-to-child transmission should thus be a top priority. More needs to be known about the prevalence of nevirapine and 3TC resistance at the initiation of HAART in therapy-naïve but prophylaxis-experienced women and perhaps in their partners as well.

Modeling Resistance

Mathematical models have been used to describe and predict the HIV/
AIDS pandemic. Of particular interest for scale-up of ART in resource-
constrained settings is the implication of ARV usage rates for HIV incidence and the emergence of resistance. The prevalence of resistant HIV and
the level of transmission of drug-resistant strains are a direct function of the
number of persons treated and the amount of therapy provided (Blower
and Farmer, 2003; Blower et al., 2000, 2001, 2003a,b; Velasco-Hernandez
et al., 2002). Both high usage rates (as modeled in the United States) and
low usage rates (as modeled in the developing world) have demonstrated
this relationship. Since the ARV usage rate in Africa will be low (less than
10 percent of infected persons for at least the first several years), the level of
transmitted resistance will be low.

It is true that modeling studies have shown that—as demonstrated in a
U.S. population of gay men—high rates of usage can significantly reduce
the total number of new HIV infections, but will result in increases in the
prevalence of drug resistance (Blower and Farmer, 2003; Blower et al.,
2000, 2003b). However, the low usage rates expected in Africa under even
the best of circumstances suggest that in this setting, therapy will not have
much impact on the total number of new HIV infections, and that for this
reason, other interventions that support prevention must continue to receive a strong emphasis. According to these same modeling studies, most
drug resistance is acquired, not due to transmission of resistant strains
(Blower et al., 2003a). Finally, based on modeling studies, it is expected
that the level of drug-resistant strains of HIV will first rise and then level off
and stabilize. This phenomenon is expected because of the competitive
dynamics between drug-resistant and drug-sensitive strains of HIV.

One modeling study (Blower et al., 2003a) considered the potential
impact of the rate of ARV use on (1) the future prevalence of drug-resistant
HIV, (2) the future transmission rate of drug-resistant strains of HIV, and
(3) the cumulative number of HIV infections prevented over time by widespread use of ART. If 10 percent of the infected population is treated, the
prevalence of ARV resistance can be as low as 4 percent after 10 years. If
the proportion of individuals treated increases to 50 percent, the prevalence
of ARV resistance can be as high as 53 percent after 10 years. The prevalence of drug resistance rises as risky behaviors increase, as the relative
fitness (or "infectivity") of ARV-resistant strains increases, and as the effectiveness of the ARV regimen in suppressing viral load decreases. In this
same study, assuming that 10–50 percent of the infected population receives ART (again, a level of coverage not realistic anytime soon) and that
the rate of emergence of acquired resistance varies from 20 to 70 percent,
the models indicate the likelihood of very little transmitted resistance even

after 10 years of ARV usage (median of 5.9 percent of new cases expected to be drug-resistant). However, extremely high levels of transmission (greater than 40 percent) could occur in the following scenarios: increased ARV usage, greater transmissibility (or fitness) of the virus (resistant variants generally tend to be less transmissible than their wild-type relatives), increased risky behaviors, higher levels of acquired resistance, and increased use of ineffective treatment regimens (i.e., those that do not adequately suppress viral replication). The predicted relatively small impact of anticipated levels of ART on HIV incidence at the population level is illustrated in Figure 3-1.

Even under the best possible conditions, WHO's 3-by-5 campaign aims to treat no more than 50 percent of the world's HIV-infected population currently in need of treatment and a much smaller fraction (less than 10 percent) of all those HIV-infected. Thus it is unlikely that the growth of the HIV epidemic in sub-Saharan African will be curtailed to a major degree by the use of ART (Blower and Farmer, 2003; Blower et al., 2003a, 2004).

Based on the experiences and studies cited above, it would appear that appropriate interventions to minimize resistance include ensuring that patients with failed first-line regimens are treated with effective second-line

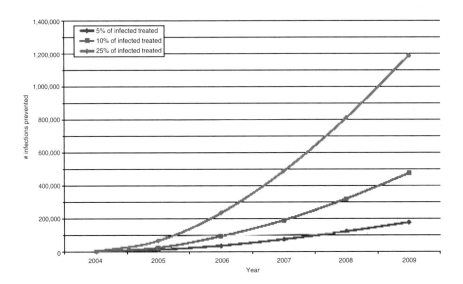

FIGURE 3-1 Potential for prevention of HIV infections by percent of HIV-infected persons under ART.
SOURCE: Sally Blower, David Geffen School of Medicine at UCLA.

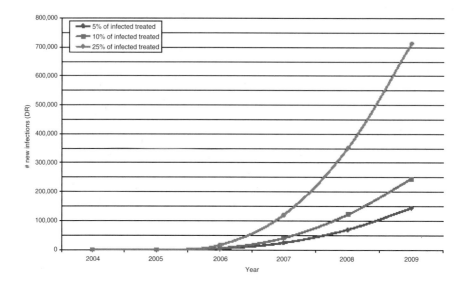

FIGURE 3-2 Drug-resistant new infections over time as a function of the percent of infected persons treated.
SOURCE: Sally Blower, David Geffen School of Medicine at UCLA.

regimens, that increases in risky behavior are prevented, and that high levels of adherence to effective regimens are maintained. Finally, because modeling studies demonstrate increased emergence of HIV resistance only with implausibly high levels of use of ART, widespread emergence of resistance may not occur during ART scale-up, when treatment rates will be relatively low (see Figure 3-2).

IMPLICATIONS OF RESISTANCE FOR SCALE-UP

While HAART has improved the lives of thousands with HIV/AIDS, HAART regimens are complex and as such have the potential for failure. As emphasized in this chapter, one reason for failure that is of particular concern as planning occurs for wide-scale introduction of ART into resource-constrained settings is the emergence of drug resistance.

The emergence of drug resistance is a concern mainly for the individual patient being treated, but also has implications for the durability of standard treatment regimens for the population as a whole. Second-line drug regimens needed once resistance to first-line regimens has developed may be unavailable or unaffordable in resource-limited settings. Moreover, resistance detection using laboratory tests will be of highly limited availability in resource-constrained settings.

While aggressive and innovative price-reduction mechanisms have lowered the cost of many ARVs, the drugs needed for a second-line ART regimen should initial treatment fail are particularly expensive. According to a November 2003 Médecins sans Frontières report, costs for second-line regimens average US$1,203 in South Africa, $1,875 in Malawi, $1,594 in Kenya, and $4,763 in Cameroon, versus $400–1,000, $288, $1,594, and $292, respectively, for first-line drugs (Médecins sans Frontières, 2003b). Not only are these second-line regimens more expensive, but their increased complexity with regard to dosing, scheduling, and monitoring requirements makes them a difficult choice for resource-constrained settings. As suggested above, moreover, resistance may go undetected in resource-constrained settings, where resistance testing may be unavailable because of costs and technical and infrastructure needs. Thus while the many lessons learned in the developed world about the causes and implications of drug resistance should guide the use of ART in resource-limited settings, the resource-intensive, laboratory-focused monitoring for drug resistance that is typical in wealthy countries may not, at this point in time, be as appropriate or necessary for more resource-constrained settings.

Although the emergence of some degree of drug resistance is inevitable, as is common with most drug-treated pathogens, widespread resistance should not be a necessary consequence of a broad treatment program. As noted earlier, despite years of (now-recognized) inadequate mono and dual ART in the United States and Europe, no cases of drug-resistant HIV transmission were recognized until the mid-1990s (Little, 2000). Thus even if ART scale-up in resource-constrained settings is conducted poorly, widespread population- or epidemic-level resistance will not likely emerge with HAART for several years. In part this is because only a small fraction of the 40 million people worldwide infected with HIV will actually be exposed to ART in the next several years; thus, HIV transmission will be largely from persons with susceptible virus. Although there are very limited data on the prevalence of resistant viral strains, even in the United States, one recent South African study showed that among 37 drug-naïve HIV-positive women screened in an antenatal clinic, none had any of 23 mutations known to be associated with ARV resistance, suggesting that even after 3 years of ART, resistance is still low to undetectable at the level of untreated patients (Pillay et al., 2002).

At the same time, the possibility that higher levels of resistance and increases in transmitted resistance could eventually emerge, although not viewed as a major issue for the near term, raises the question of when general clinical screening for drug-resistant strains should be implemented. The question also arises of what should be done now, short of laboratory-intensive resistance screening, to predict and prepare (in terms of surveillance) for the emergence of a higher level of resistance should it occur.

Certain measures can be taken now to monitor conditions that foster emergence without implementing extensive, formal, laboratory-intensive resistance surveillance systems. WHO's Global HIV Resistance Surveillance Network (HIV Resnet), a group of global experts convened to identify and implement resistance-evaluation methods, has developed a non–laboratory-based early warning system. This system is based on the use of "indicators," most of which consist of various data being collected for other purposes that can provide indirect but helpful indications of situations in which resistance is likely to emerge. For example, given that the use of substandard treatment regimens (e.g., monotherapy) has been associated with resistance, data on the use of such regimens, such as prescription records from pharmacies, could be used to alert program managers of conditions that foster resistance. The relative yield of different laboratory and nonlaboratory markers for identifying an emerging problem with drug resistance should be considered an important topic for operations research.

Meanwhile, few studies have measured population-level resistance at a large scale in areas where ART has already been available for many years, even in the United States. Most studies involve insufficient sample sizes to allow accurate estimation of the prevalence of resistant virus within the larger HIV-infected population. Moreover, the proportions of risk groups in most study samples do not represent the actual proportions in the HIV population at large. For example, among the widely cited population-level studies of transmitted resistance, the overwhelming majority of subjects within the study samples are white men who have sex with men (Boden et al., 1999; Grant et al., 2002; Little et al., 2002; Simon et al., 2002). Yet male-to-male sexual contact now accounts for only about 40 percent of new HIV diagnoses in the United States, while fewer than 30 percent of newly diagnosed individuals in the United States are white (CDC, 2004). Large, representative cohort studies are needed to derive more accurate estimates of the prevalence of HIV drug resistance and achieve a better understanding of population factors that impact such prevalence.

Recommendation 3-1. For individual patients about to embark on therapy, general clinical screening for resistance to antiretroviral drugs is not recommended at this time for two reasons: because the prevalence of resistance in HIV-infected individuals not previously exposed to antiretroviral therapy is expected to be undetectable or low, and because the proportion of total persons with HIV who are receiving therapy in a given country will also be relatively small in the short term. Coordinated, systematic testing for resistance to antiretroviral drugs should, however, be conducted among a subset of patients failing treatment. *These latter results will be critical in evaluating ART programs and in determining whether and when routine population-based resistance testing might eventually prove effective. Sentinel surveillance of treatment-naïve HIV-positive persons may also be indicated in the future.*

LEARNING BY DOING:
SCALE-UP AROUND THE WORLD

This section reviews lessons learned from ART scale-up in five countries: Brazil, Haiti, South Africa, Nigeria, and Uganda.

Brazil

Brazil, with a per capita income of about US$3,000, is much less resource-constrained than most of sub-Saharan Africa, the Caribbean, and other countries being targeted for current ART scale-up programs, and its national HIV prevalence rate is much lower. Nontheless, the success of that country's ART program—considered the most advanced such national program in the developing world—serves as an important example of how sound policy can profoundly improve treatment and prevention efforts, save lives and money, and halt the expansion of an epidemic.

In 1996, the Brazilian public health system began widespread and free provision of ARVs for all citizens. Late in 1996, the Brazilian president signed a law establishing this free distribution. By 2001, public and private laboratories were manufacturing 63 percent (43 percent of expenditures) of the ARVs available to Brazilians (Galvão, 2002). Seven of the 13 ARVs being used to treat Brazilians are domestically produced; others have been procured by the government on the international market through aggressive negotiation of prices. As one example, the threat to break patent law for efavirenz resulted in Merck, the drug's producer, reducing its price by 60 percent (Galvão, 2002). Overall, Brazil saw the median cost of ART drop 67 percent from 1997 to 2002 (Schechter, 2004). In part because of Brazil's leadership in addressing patent law, in 2001 the UN Human Rights Commission announced that access to medical drugs during pandemics is a human right.

The ARVs in Brazil are distributed by 486 centers located in public health hospitals or health centers. A structural component integral to the distribution effort is the Unified Health System, established in 1988. This system provides free comprehensive care to the entire population of Brazil.

An estimated 35,900 Brazilians with HIV/AIDS received medication in 1997, 1 year after program initiation. In 2003, with 280,000 cases of AIDS and 600,000 cases of HIV infection, Brazil provided 128,000 people with medication (Lima, 2004). (It is predicted that 148,500 persons with HIV/

AIDS will receive therapy in 2004.) In addition, because of free access to effective therapy, more Brazilians have been tested for HIV, and epidemiologic surveillance of the disease has improved. As an example, in 1996 there was a 40 percent increase in the number of AIDS cases reported. From 2000 to 2002, epidemiologic surveillance revealed a decline in HIV incidence from 17,504 to 7,361 cases (Boletin Epidemiologico, 2004).

There are many reasons for Brazil's success in addressing its HIV/AIDS epidemic. Community advocacy and the government's leadership are particularly noteworthy (Levi and Vitória, 2002). Especially active in the process have been religious organizations, sexual minorities, and organizations representing persons living with HIV/AIDS. The Brazilian government acknowledged the problem, and citizens participated in committees designing the country's response. Following passage of the law guaranteeing free, universal ART in 1996, an independent advisory committee established national treatment guidelines and criteria, and the treatment program was integrated into the existing health care infrastructure.

Early on in program implementation, prevention and treatment initiatives were integrated. In the 1990s, it was predicted that there would be over 1 million cases of HIV/AIDS in Brazil by 2000. The actual number of cases in 2000 was only about half that figure, largely as a result of wide-scale prevention efforts (Schechter, 2004). One successful prevention initiative was a significant increase in the use of condoms, as demonstrated by minimal use in the early 1980s and a rate of use at first intercourse of over 70 percent by the late 1990s (Schechter, 2004).

A unique feature of the Brazilian program that has contributed to its success is the use of information technology for program management (Lima, 2004). Two computerized systems were developed to assist in monitoring patient care (see the discussion in Chapter 5).

Government spending for ART and HIV/AIDS care in Brazil increased from US$34 million in 1996 to $232 million in 2001. Because of a substan-

---

The Brazilian Experience: Summary of Lessons Learned

- Early government commitment and response and active civil society participation are necessary for success.
- Scale-up must be integrated with prevention.
- The establishment of national treatment criteria that have the force of the law is important.
- Integrating the treatment program into existing health infrastructure is indispensable.
- Targeted development and national coordination of information technology and computerized systems have proven essential.

tial reduction in opportunistic infections and hospital admissions, this increased spending has been cost-effective. The Brazilian Ministry of Health estimates cost savings of over US$1 billion (Galvão, 2002).

Haiti

Haiti is one of the world's poorest countries, with an annual per capita income of around US$440 (World Bank, 2004). The estimated prevalence of HIV among adults in Haiti is 6 percent (Fitzgerald, 2004; WHO, 2003a). About 60 percent of HIV-infected people live in Port-au-Prince and surrounding urban areas, while the other 40 percent live in the rural countryside.

Pre-HAART cohort studies in Haiti showed that the estimated survival time from HIV infection to death was $7 \frac{1}{2}$ years for adults and less than 1 year for newborns—both of these rates being dramatically accelerated compared with people living with HIV/AIDS in the pre-HAART era in the United States and Europe (Fitzgerald, 2004). Despite these alarming statistics, however, the HIV epidemic in Haiti has not doubled in size, as was predicted in the mid-1990s. Indeed, seroprevalence data indicate that the epidemic is contracting rather than expanding (Fitzgerald, 2004; UNAIDS, 2002).

Two noteworthy initiatives have been established in Haiti to help address the epidemic. In urban Haiti, the Haitian Study Group on Kaposi's Sarcoma and Opportunistic Infections, commonly known as GHESKIO, was established in 1982 with the support of the Cornell University Medical College (GHESKIO, 2004). In rural Haiti, the HIV Equity Initiative was established in 1998 with assistance from the Boston-based Partners in Health, which is affiliated with Harvard Medical School (WHO, 2003a).

Urban Haiti: GHESKIO

The GHESKIO Center operates in a central slum district in Port-au-Prince. Patients visit the clinic each month. Some patients are counseled more aggressively and are visited at home. Patients are followed by a physician every 3 months and by a nurse every month. Therapy is monitored by clinical signs and symptoms, as well as routine CD4 counts at baseline and every 6 months. Adherence is ensured through a team approach that includes pharmacists, community health workers, and a growing number of patients who are employed as social workers and peer educators (Fitzgerald, 2004). The GHESKIO program provides comprehensive care. One component of the program is an evaluation of patients' nutritional needs and the provision of nutritional support when necessary. Although physicians take a very active role during the first 3 months of ART, the frequency of contact is reduced as treatment progresses. The ownership in this program with respect to care belongs to nurses, social workers, pharmacists, and community health workers.

As of January 2004, 972 patients were on ART under the program (Fitzgerald, 2004). The first-line regimen comprises zidovudine, lamivudine, and efavirenz. Pregnant women are given nevirapine instead of efavirenz. Fully 75 percent of all patients had clinical AIDS at the start of therapy, and the median CD4 count was 114. Approximately 10 percent of patients have required a regimen change because of drug toxicity (anemia and rash are the most common complications). During a 1-year follow-up examination, mortality was found to be 6 percent; many of these deaths were among patients with advanced disease at the time therapy was initiated (Fitzgerald, 2004).

Rural Haiti: The HIV Equity Initiative

Partners in Health's HIV Equity Initiative is frequently cited as a remarkable success story in the introduction and implementation of ART in a resource-constrained setting (WHO, 2003a; Farmer et al., 2001a,b). Its mission was to provide integrated preventive and comprehensive treatment services to those living with HIV/AIDS, using the already successful directly observed therapy (DOT) model for tuberculosis. The aim was to deliver HAART to those people in the direst need of therapy—the sickest and closest to death from AIDS. The clinical facility in Cange, Clinique Bon Sauveur, was set up in a province with no electricity and limited road access, and began to offer HAART in 1999. Within the first 2 years of the program's establishment, the availability of HAART contributed to a more than 300 percent increase in use of HIV counseling and testing services (Farmer et al., 2001b; Walton et al., 2004).

The HIV Equity Initiative in Haiti harnessed the capacity of human infrastructure and trained a cadre of community health workers in the administration and follow-up of ART. These workers, called *accompagnateurs*, provided HAART and served as an essential link between those with HIV/AIDS in the community and the resources of the Clinique Bon Sauveur, which is more than 5 hours away by foot for some of those served. Building on the success of the directly observed therapy short course (DOTS) for tuberculosis, HAART was provided by directly observed interventions.

Prior to 2002, initiation of therapy was based on clinical status. Patients were selected for DOT-HAART if they met the following criteria (WHO, 2003a):

• Absence of active tuberculosis

- Recurrent opportunistic infections that were difficult to manage with antibacterial or antifungal agents
  - Chronic enteropathy with wasting
  - Otherwise unexplained significant weight loss
  - Severe nervous system complications attributable to HIV disease
  - Severe leucopenia, anemia, or thrombocytopenia

Laboratory determination of HIV serology, hematocrit, and white blood cell count was prerequisite to beginning HAART. Of note, a CD4 determination was not necessary. If symptoms of gastrointestinal side effects, anemia, or thrombocytopenia developed, a liver function test or complete blood count was ordered as appropriate. To monitor response to therapy, again a CD4 determination was not the tool. Rather, the patient's weight, a studied predictor of survival and disease progression, was used.

Patients enrolled in the HIV Equity Initiative received a three-drug regimen consisting of stavudine, lamivudine, and nevirapine.[1] Approximately 10 percent of patients initiated on this regimen switched regimens because of toxicity (Fitzgerald, 2004). In their three-drug regimens, pregnant women received zidovudine instead of stavudine, and patients with tuberculosis received efavirenz instead of nevirapine.

While two physicians assessed persons with HIV/AIDS, it was the accompagnateurs who provided the care. For those on HAART, an accompagnateur would visit daily and observe the patients taking their medications. In some cases, a second daily visit would occur to observe subsequent taking of medication. While visiting patients, the accompagnateurs would provide educational and emotional support. They also were trained in recognizing complications of the disease and its therapies; as complications arose, patients would be referred back to the Clinique Bon Sauveur for a more skilled evaluation. Routinely, however, patients treated through the HIV Equity Initiative were followed up in clinic on a monthly basis. In addition to daily visits by accompagnateurs, efforts to improve adherence to HAART included assessments of the patients' living quarters, social support system, and financial system. Monthly meetings involving people living with HIV/AIDS also were held to facilitate information exchange and provide support.

The program has been lauded for reducing AIDS-associated stigma and for achieving success in reducing mortality from HIV/AIDS in a rural area without electricity and paved roads at low cost. All services provided

---

[1]Second line regimens were zidovudine/didanosine/PI or stavudine/didanosine/PI. The PI options were indinavir, nelfinavir, or lopinavir boosted by ritonavir.

through the HIV Equity Initiative (e.g., laboratory monitoring, home visits, medical consultations) were provided free of charge.

The Partners in Health program currently provides ART to about 700 patients living with HIV/AIDS. The majority of these patients now have undetectable viral loads (86 percent of a small subset of 65 patients whose viral loads were measured with at least 3 months of follow-up) and are able to live normal, active lives. One-year mortality is about 5 percent, with almost all of this mortality associated with very advanced disease (i.e., severe wasting and low CD4 counts) at the initiation of ART (Fitzgerald, 2004).

With the international and multilateral financial support that has been provided and is forthcoming, the Partners in Health program hopes to provide comprehensive care for HIV and tuberculosis on a much larger scale in Haiti. Several strategies are being employed to make the scale-up feasible. ART as a fraction of program costs has decreased from 80 percent to below 15 percent because of three endeavors: purchase of drugs from WHO-prequalified manufacturers, concessional pricing agreements with pharmaceutical companies, and collaboration with a wholesale distributor of essential medicines based in the Netherlands (WHO, 2003a). Also, in anticipation of further scale-up of treatment, Partners in Health has established a logistical monitoring system that includes web-based medical records, an application allowing for off-line data entry, and a system to monitor drug inventory.

Summary

GHESKIO and the HIV Equity Initiative provide ART to over 1,600 people living in resource-constrained settings and serve as helpful examples for ART scale-up. As the result of two national conferences attended by representatives from the Haitian Ministry of Health, U.S. and European

---

The Haitian Experience: Summary of Lessons Learned

- Early government response and private–public partnership are important.
- The provision of free care and ARVs is an essential element of program success.
- Strengthening the primary care infrastructure is critical.
- It is important to develop local, field-tested solutions to monitor adherence.
- An uninterrupted drug supply and coordination among multiple donors are essential.

universities, and people living with HIV/AIDS, Haitian national guidelines based on the WHO-recommended regimens have been established. Appropriate modifications for strengthening adherence have been made in accordance with lessons learned in both Port-au-Prince and rural Haiti.

South Africa

Khayelitsha, South Africa, is a resource-poor, periurban township just outside of Cape Town. It has a population of approximately 500,000, 50,000 of whom are estimated to be HIV-infected (WHO, 2003b). The majority of people in the township live in informal housing such as shacks built from corrugated iron, and many live without electricity and running water. With the help of Médecins sans Frontières (see Box 3-2), HIV/AIDS

**BOX 3-2
At a Glance: Médecins sans Frontières**

Médecins sans Frontières (MSF) is an international, independent medical humanitarian organization founded in 1971. With the help of 2,500 international volunteers per year and 15,000 national staff, it currently has 400 relief projects ongoing in 80 countries. Because of its efforts worldwide, MSF received the Nobel Peace Prize in 1999.

One activity in which MSF is engaged is the provision of ART and HIV/AIDS care to countries in need. All of MSF's ART programs, the first of which was initiated in 2001, are pilot projects designed to demonstrate the efficacy and feasibility of ART in resource-poor settings. Currently there are 42 ART programs in 19 countries throughout Africa, Asia, Latin America, and the former Soviet Union serving some 11,000 people on ART. Key components of MSF-sponsored programs for HIV/AIDS are as follows:

- The sickest patients are served first.
- All treatment is provided free.
- Treatment is education based (as opposed to directly observed).
- Prior attendance in programs is considered as an indicator of the ability to adhere.
- Eligibility committees are established for determining treatment initiation.
- Community involvement is emphasized.
- Affordable, quality medicines are selected, most of which are generic drugs.
- Comprehensive HIV/AIDS care includes:
  - opportunistic infection prophylaxis
  - nutritional support
  - adherence support
  - home visits

SOURCE: Cohen, 2004.

clinics were set up within community health centers in Khayelitsha in 2000, and in 2001, ART began to be provided at these clinics to patients in advanced stages of the disease. The clinics provide comprehensive care for patients with HIV/AIDS and were initially staffed in each case by one physician, one nurse, and one lay counselor. Additional staff members have since been added, and the clinics are now more heavily nurse based. They currently serve more than 1,800 patients per month among three clinics (WHO, 2003b).

Eligibility for ART is based on both clinical and social indicators; ability to adhere to therapy is also a factor. To be clinically eligible, patients must have CD4 cell counts of less than 200/mm^3 and Stage III or IV disease based on WHO criteria. (See Appendix C for the WHO guidelines.) A clinic staff member visits each patient's home to assess the social support network. Potential ability to adhere to therapy is based on an assessment of adherence to cotrimoxazole prophylaxis and tuberculosis treatment, as well as regular attendance at HIV clinics in the period leading up to the beginning of treatment (WHO, 2003b; Médecins sans Frontières, 2003a). The first-line treatment regimen is stavudine, lamivudine, and either efavirenz or nevirapine. In the case of the latter two drugs, the decision on which to use takes into account whether a patient is also being treated for tuberculosis, has indications of abnormal liver function, or is pregnant. Patients receive clinical assessments either weekly or biweekly for the first 2 months of treatment, after which they are evaluated on a monthly basis.

By the end of 2003, 776 individuals had been started on ART. A full analysis of the 287 treatment-naïve adult patients who initiated therapy during the first year and a half of the program has been performed (Médecins sans Frontières, 2003a). Among these 287, HIV RNA levels were reduced to undetectable in 89.2 percent of patients at 6 months and remained undetectable in 84.2 percent of patients at 12 months, 75.0 percent at 18 months, and 69.7 percent at 24 months (Coetzee et al., 2004). Patients showed a median weight gain of 5.0 kg and 9.0 kg at 6 and 12 months, respectively, as well as a median gain in CD4 cell count of 288 cells/mm^3 after 24 months. The survival rate at 24 months was 86.3 percent for all patients and 91.4 percent for patients who began treatment with a CD4 count greater than 50 cells/mm^3 (Coetzee et al., 2004). Nearly three-fourths of patient deaths occurred in the first 3 months after treatment initiation.

The Khayelitsha program has also witnessed encouraging rates of both patient retention and adherence to therapy. Of the patient cohort just described, only one individual was entirely lost to follow-up by July 2003, while a dozen more either moved to a different province or stopped therapy for other reasons. Separately, a prospective study of self-reported adherence to ART regimens found that 87.5 percent of patients reported "high" levels of adherence (having taken at least 95 percent of their drug doses in a 4-day recall period) at 1 month, 89.0 percent at 3 months, and 87.7 percent at 12 months (Médecins sans Frontières, 2003a). To achieve these levels of adherence, Médecins sans Frontières has promoted a dual strategy of simple, standardized pill regimens and a robust patient education program combining several elements (Médecins sans Frontières, 2003a; WHO, 2003b):

• **Individual support**—Patients are required to identify another individual close to them (such as a friend or other household member) who will act as a treatment assistant, accompanying them during the enrollment process and learning basic ART principles. Lay counselors are also provided to assist with individual adherence plans.
• **Peer support**—Clinics host regular meetings for individuals on ART, where participants can discuss adherence barriers, adverse events, and community and psychosocial issues, such as disclosing their condition to others.
• **Material support**—Individuals receiving ART are provided with educational materials and supplies, including pillboxes, schedules, drug-related information charts, and educational materials such as pamphlets and newsletters on the risks and benefits of ART.

The success of the program in Khayelitsha has been the result of a number of efforts. Médecins sans Frontières played a pivotal role in guiding the program and procuring affordable ARVs, and the Treatment Action Campaign, a grassroots advocacy group, was instrumental in mobilizing the community to be aware of HIV as a political issue and pressuring the government to address it. The latter group has also established education programs to combat the stigma and discrimination associated with the disease and to promote its prevention and treatment.

Nigeria

As of 2001, there were an estimated 3.5 million HIV-infected Nigerians, including an estimated 1.2 million with symptomatic AIDS. In 2002, the government of Nigeria initiated a nationwide ART program with the goal of treating 10,000 adults and 5,000 children with HIV (Idoko, 2004). Because there had been no pilot initiatives on which to base programmatic policies and guidelines, the program was based largely on the WHO recommendations. Decisions on exceptions to those recommendations were made by a committee. Treatment eligibility, for example, was based on a CD4 count below 350 cells/mm^3, given that many patients with CD4 counts above 200 still suffer significant immunological damage. The priority is to treat symptomatic patients.

The first-line regimen is a WHO-recommended combination of generic forms of lamivudine, stavudine, and nevirapine. Thus far, this regimen has proven potent, while its pill burden has proven acceptable. Within 12 months following the initiation of therapy, patients were gaining weight; CD4 cell counts were increasing; and, based on viral load testing at one center, about 80 percent of patients had fully suppressed viral loads (Idoko, 2004). Major adverse events that occurred with this treatment regimen included hepatotoxicity (reported as most likely from nevirapine) and a case of severe Stevens-Johnson syndrome. Other concerns with the use of this treatment regimen in Nigeria include the following:

- The risk of resistance to nevirapine, which is also used for prevention of mother-to-child transmission
- Tuberculosis coinfection (about 50 percent) and drug–drug interactions with the first-line regimen—particularly nevirapine, which can cause hepatotoxicity
- Hepatitis B coinfection
- Hepatitis C coinfection
- Price differentials between public and private purchasers

Despite these concerns, scale-up of ART has proceeded. The greatest challenges faced by Nigeria have been the establishment of a regular, continuous drug supply and the delayed procurement of second-line drugs due to delays in receipt of donor monies.

Uganda

Over the past decade and a half, Uganda has witnessed remarkable declines in HIV prevalence among its population. Surveillance data from antenatal clinics in many cases show prevalence rates as high as 20 to 30 percent in 1991 declining to 10 percent or lower just 10 years later (Uganda AIDS Commission, 2003). Despite declining rates of new infections, however, the country continues to face serious challenges, including a total number of HIV-infected individuals estimated at 600,000, many of whom are progressing to AIDS (WHO, 2003c). In an effort to improve access to ART in resource-constrained settings, UNAIDS launched a pilot project—the HIV Drug Access Initiative—to introduce structured therapy programs in four countries: Uganda, Cote d'Ivoire, Chile, and Vietnam (Katzenstein et al., 2003).

When the Uganda initiative began in June 1998, five health care facilities were accredited to provide ART, all of them located in or around Kampala. As the program has expanded in recent years, more facilities have been accredited so that by 2003, a total of 23 facilities, including six regional hospitals, were providing ART (WHO, 2003c).

In the program's initial stages, only four NRTIs and one PI were available, but by February 2000, the number of available treatments had grown to six NRTIs, four PIs, and three NNRTIs (Weidle et al., 2002). These drugs were initially employed in one of two alternative approaches. The first targeted complete suppression of viral replication and used three-drug combination therapy regimens, including two NRTIs and either a PI or an NNRTI. The second approach, which is no longer recommended, targeted partial viral suppression and focused on the use of two NRTIs, with the option of adding hydroxyurea. Given that many people could not afford the triple-drug combination, the partially suppressive therapy was felt to be justified in Uganda at the program's outset and was recommended on the grounds that partial viral suppression was better than none (WHO, 2003c). As a result of significant decreases in the cost of ART, however, more individuals have been treated with triple-drug regimens since 2000.

There are two primary suppliers of ARVs in Uganda: the Joint Clinical Research Centre and Medical Access Uganda Limited. The latter organization was established under the UNAIDS Drug Access Initiative as a not-for-profit company that would procure drugs at reduced cost from participating pharmaceutical companies and then sell these drugs to treatment centers accredited by Uganda's National Advisory Board (WHO, 2003c). Four multinational pharmaceutical groups have contributed to the company's operating costs: Glaxo-Wellcome, Bristol Myers Squibb, Roche Products Ltd., and Merck Sharpe and Dohme. In this manner, Medical Access Limited has become Uganda's principal supplier of ARVs from the pharmaceutical industry. By comparison, the Joint Clinical Research Centre is now the country's principal supplier of generic ARVs. It was first established through collaborative efforts between Uganda's Ministry of Health, Makerere University, and the Ministry of Defence and began importing generic ARVs in 2000 (WHO, 2003c).

In 1997, prior to the beginning of the Drug Access Initiative, 450 people were enrolled in ART programs in Uganda. With the initiative's assistance, this figure rose to 900 by 2000, when the UNAIDS pilot project came to an end. Early clinical assessments of patients treated through the Uganda initiative have quantified the project's efficacy and illustrated the extent to which well-organized drug procurement and distribution programs can have an impact even in such resource-constrained settings (Weidle et al., 2002, 2003; Katzenstein et al., 2003). After the project's end, further developments, including substantial reductions in drug prices and governmental efforts to train more staff and accredit additional clinical centers, helped raise the number of treated individuals to 3,000 by the end of 2001

(WHO, 2003c). This rapid escalation has continued, with an estimated 17,000 Ugandans receiving ART by the end of 2003 (Kamya, 2003).

The U.S. Experience: Summary of Lessons Learned

- Widespread use of sequential mono and dual therapy is associated with a high rate of drug resistance and is not recommended for any scale-up programs.
- Long-term HAART failure is associated with the development of resistant virus with low replicability and "fitness," particularly when a protease inhibitor is used in the triple therapy.
- Second-line regimens are more expensive than first-line treatments and require more-complex and more-intense treatment management.
- In the HAART era, 10 percent of new HIV infections are due to resistant virus strains.

REFERENCES

Barreiro P, Garcia-Benayas T, Soriano V, Gallant J. 2002. Simplification of antiretroviral treatment: How to sustain success, reduce toxicity and ensure adherence avoiding PI use. *AIDS Review* 4:233–241.

Blower SM, Farmer P. 2003. Predicting the public health impact of antiretrovirals: Prevention in developing countries. *AIDS Science* 3(11).

Blower SM, Gershengorn HB, Grant RM. 2000. A tale of two futures: HIV and antiretroviral therapy in San Francisco. *Science* 287:650–654.

Blower SM, Aschenbach AN, Gershengorn HB, Kahn JO. 2001. Predicting the unpredictable: Transmission of drug-resistant HIV. *Nature Medicine* 7:1016–1020.

Blower SM, Ma L, Farmer P, Koenig S. 2003a. Predicting the impact of antiretrovirals in resource poor settings: Preventing HIV infections whilst controlling drug resistance. *Current Drug Targets-Infectious Disorders* 3:345–353.

Blower SM, Schwartz EJ, Mills J. 2003b. Forecasting the future of HIV epidemics: The impact of antiretroviral therapies and imperfect vaccines. *AIDS Review* 5:113–125.

Blower SM, Bodine E, Kahn J, McFarland W. 2004. The impact of the antiretroviral rollout on drug resistant HIV in Africa: Insights from empirical data and theoretical models. *AIDS* (in press).

Boden D, Hurley A, Zhang L, Cao Y, Guo Y, Jones E, Tsay J, Ip J, Farthing C, Limoli K, Parkin N, Markowitz, M. 1999. HIV-1 drug resistance in newly infected individuals. *Journal of the American Medical Association* 282(12):1135–1141.

Boletin Epidemiologico. 2004. *AIDS*. [Online]. Available: http://www.aids.gov.br/ [accessed August 24, 2004].

CDC (Centers for Disease Control and Prevention). 2004. *HIV-AIDS Surveillance: General Epidemiology*. [Online]. Available: http://www.cdc.gov/hiv/graphics/surveill.htm [accessed August 2, 2004].

Clavel F, Hance A. 2004. HIV drug resistance. *New England Journal of Medicine* 350(10): 1023–1035.

Coetzee D, Hildebrand K, Boulle A, Maartens G, Louis F, Labatala V, Reuter H, Ntwana N, Goemaere E. 2004. Outcomes after two years of providing antiretroviral treatment in Khayelitsha, South Africa. *AIDS* 18(6):887–895.

Cohen R. 2004. *Positive Replication: The MSF Experience Providing HAART in Developing Countries.* Paper presented at the Institute of Medicine Workshop on Antiretroviral Use in Resource Constrained Settings, Washington, DC. Institute of Medicine Committee on Antiretroviral Drug Use in Resource-Constrained Settings.

Deeks S. 2003. Treatment of antiretroviral-drug-resistant HIV-1 infection. *Lancet* 362:2002–2011.

Ekouevi DK, Peyatvin G, Rouet F, Bequet L, Montcho C, Viho I, Fassinou P, Leroy V, Dabis F, Rouzioux C, Ditrame Plus Tsudy Grou. 2004. Persistence of nevirapine-resistant virus and pharmacokinetic analysis in women who received intrapertum NVP associated to a short course of zidovudine (ZDV) to prevent HIV-1 transmission: The Ditrame Plus ANRS 1201/02 Study, Abidjan, Cote d'Ivoire. Abstract 160. *Antiviral Therapy* 9:S176.

Ena J, Amador C, Benito C, Fenoll V, Pasquau F. 2003. Risk and determinants of developing severe liver toxicity during therapy with nevirapine-and efavirenz-containing regimens in HIV-infected patients. *International Journal of STD & AIDS* 14(11):776–781.

Eshleman SH, Mracha M, Guay LA, Deseyve M, Cunningham S, Mirochnick M, Musoke P, Fleming T, Glenn Fowler M, Mofenson LM, Mmiro F, Jackson JB. 2001. Selection and fading of resistance mutations in women and infants receiving nevirapine to prevent HIV-1 vertical transmission (HIVNET 012). *AIDS* 15:1951–1957.

Eshleman SH, Wang J, Guay LA, Cunningham SP, Mwatha A, Brown ER, Musoke P, Mmiro F, Jackson JB. 2004a. Distinct patterns of selection and fading of K103N and Y181C are seen in women with subtype A vs D HIV-1 after single dose nevirapine: HOVNET 012. Abstract 50. *Antiviral Therapy* 9:S59.

Eshleman SH, Guay LA, Mwatha A, Brown ER, Cunningham SP, Musoke P, Mmiro F, Jackson JB. 2004b. Characterization of nevirapine resistance mutations in women with subtype A vs. D HIV-1 6–8 weeks after single-dose nevirapine. *HIV Journal of Acquired Immune Deficiency Syndromes* 35(2):126–130.

Farmer P, Léandre F, Mukherjee J, Claude M, Nevil P, Smith-Fawzi M, Koenig S, Castro A, Becerra M, Sachs J, Attaran A, Kim JY. 2001a. Community-based approaches to HIV treatment in resource-poor settings. *Lancet* 358:404–409.

Farmer P, Léandre F, Mukherjee J, Gupta R, Tarter L, Kim JY. 2001b. Community-based treatment of advanced HIV disease: Introducing DOT-HAART (directly observed therapy with highly active antiretroviral therapy). *Bulletin of the World Health Organization* 79(12):1145–1151.

Fischl MA. 1999. Antiretroviral therapy in 1999 for antiretroviral-naïve individuals with HIV infection. *AIDS* 13(Supplement 1):s49–s59.

Fitzgerald D. 2004 (January 27). *Lessons Learned from the Use of ARVs in Very Low-Resource Settings: The Haiti Experience.* Paper presented at the Institute of Medicine Workshop on Antiretroviral Scale-up in Resource Constrained Settings, Washington, DC. Institute of Medicine Committee on Antiretroviral Drug Use in Resource-Constrained Settings.

Galvão J. 2002. Access to antiretroviral drugs in Brazil. *Lancet* 360(9348):1862–1865.

GHESKIO (Haitian Study Group on Kaposi's Sarcoma and Opportunistic Infections). 2004. *Homepage.* [Online]. Available: http://www.haitimedical.com/gheskio/ [accessed July 1, 2004].

Gordon M, Graham N, Bland R, Rollins N, De Oliveira T, Monosi B, Van Laethem K, Vandamme A, Cassol S. 2004. Surveillance of resistance in KZN South Africa, including mother-infant pairs 6 weeks after single-dose NVP. Abstract 71. *Antiviral Therapy* 9:S80.

Grant RM, Hecht FM, Warmerdram M, Liu L, Liegler T, Petropoulos CJ, Hellmann NS, Chesney M, Busch MP, Kahn JO. 2002. Time trends in primary HIV-1 drug resistance among recently infected persons. *Journal of the American Medical Association* 288(2): 181–188.

Hirsch MS, Conway B, D'Aquila RT, Johnson VA, Brun-Vezinet F, Clotet B, Demeter LM, Hammer SM, Jacobsen DM, Kuritzkes DR, Loveday C, Mellors JW, Vella S, Richman DD. 1998. Antiretroviral drug resistance testing in adults with HIV infection. *Journal of the American Medical Association* 279:1984–1991.

Hirsch MS, Brun-Vezinet F, D'Aquila RT, Hammer SM, Johnson VA, Kuritzkes DR, Loveday C, Mellors JW, Clotet B, Conway B, Demeter LM, Vella S, Jacobsen DM, Richman DD. 2000. Antiretroviral drug resistance testing in adult HIV-1 infection. *Journal of the American Medical Association* 283:2417–2426.

Hirsch MS, Brun-Vezinet F, Clotet B, Conway B, Kuritzkes DR, D'Aquila RT, Demeter LM, Hammer SM, Johnson VA, Loveday C, Mellors JW, Jacobsen DM, Richman DD. 2003. Antiretroviral drug resistance testing in adults infected with human immunodeficiency virus type 1: 2003 recommendations of an International AIDS Society-USA panel. *Clinical Infectious Diseases: An Official Publication of the Infectious Diseases Society of America* 37:113–128.

Idoko J. 2004. *The 2003 WHO Guidelines for ARV Use: Perspectives from a User.* Paper presented at the Institute of Medicine Workshop on Antiretroviral Scale-up in Resource Constrained Settings, Washington, DC. Institute of Medicine Committee on Antiretroviral Drug Use in Resource-Constrained Settings.

Jackson JB, Becker-Pergola G, Guay LA, Musoke P, Mracna M, Fowler MG, Mofenson LM, Mirochnick M, Mmiro F, Eshleman SH. 2000. Identification of the K103N mutation in Ugandan women receiving nevirapine to prevent HIV-1 vertical transmission. *AIDS* 14:FT111–FT115.

Jourdain G, Ngo-Giang-Huong N, Tungyai P, Kummee A, Bowonwatanwong C, Kantipong P, Lechanachai P, Hammer S, Lallemant M; Perinatal HIV Prevention Trial Group. 2004 (February 8–11). *Exposure to Intrapartum Single-Dose Nevirapine and Subsequent Maternal 6-Month Response to NNRTI-Based Regimens.* Paper presented at the 11th Conference on Retroviruses and Opportunistic Infections, San Francisco, CA.

Kamya M. 2003. *The National Strategic Framework for HIV/AIDS Activities in Uganda: 2000/1-2005/6. Mid-Term Review Report—Theme 2: Care and Treatment Technical Working Group.* [Online]. Available: http://www.aidsuganda.org/pdf/Annex_2_TWG_2_Report.pdf [accessed August 6, 2004].

Katzenstein D, Laga M, Moatti JP. 2003. The evaluation of the HIV/AIDS drug access initiatives in Côte d'Ivoire, Senegal and Uganda: How access to antiretroviral treatment can become feasible in Africa. *AIDS* 17(Supplement 3):S1–S4.

Laniece I, Ciss M, Desclaux A, Diop K, Mbodj F, Ndiaye B, Sylla O, Delaporte G, Ndoye I. 2003. Adherence to HAART and its principal determinants in a cohort of Senegalese adults. *AIDS* 17:S103-S108.

Law W, Dore G, Duncombe C, Mahanontharit A, Boyd M, Ruxrungtham K, Lange J, Phanuphak P, Cooper D. 2003. Risk of severe hepatotoxicity associated with antiretroviral therapy in the HIVNAT cohort, Thailand, 1996–2001. *AIDS* 17(15):2191–2199.

Leigh Brown AJ, Frost SDW, Mathews WC, Dawson K, Hellmann NS, Daar ES, Richman DD, Little SJ. 2003. Transmission fitness of drug-resistant human immunodeficiency virus and the prevalence of resistance in the antiretroviral-treated population. *Journal of Infectious Diseases* 187:683–686.

Levi G, Vitória M. 2002. Fighting against AIDS: The Brazilian experience. *AIDS* 16:2373–2383.

Lima R. 2004. *Information Management and Technology Considerations for ARV Programs in Resource-Constrained Settings*. Paper presented at the Institute of Medicine Workshop on Antiretroviral Scale-up in Resource Constrained Settings, Washington, DC. Institute of Medicine Committee on Antiretroviral Drug Use in Resource-Constrained Settings.

Little SJ. 2000. Transmission and prevalence of HIV resistance among treatment-naïve subjects. *Antiviral Therapy* 5(1)33–40.

Little SJ, Holte S, Routy JP, Daar ES, Markowitz M, Collier AC, Koup RA, Mellors JW, Connick E, Conway B, Kilby M, Wang L, Whitcomb JM, Hellmann NS, Richman DD. 2002. Antiretroviral-drug resistance among patients recently infected with HIV. *New England Journal of Medicine* 347:385–394.

Loubser S, Sherman G, Chezzi C, Jones S, Cohen S, Puren S, Morris L. 2004. Characterization of nevirapine resistance mutations using RT-PCR and DNA sequencing methods in a mother-infant cohort following single dose nevirapine. Abstract 131. *Antiviral Therapy* 9:S145.

Martin-Carbonero L, Nunez M, Gonzalez-Lahoz J, Soriano V. 2003. Incidence of liver injury after beginning antiretroviral therapy with efavirenz or nevirapine. *HIV Clinical Trials* 4(2):115–120.

Médecins sans Frontières. 2003a. *Providing HIV Services Including Antiretroviral Therapy at Primary Health Care Clinics in Resource-Poor Settings: The Experience from Khayelitsha*. [Online]. Available: http://www.msf.org/source/countries/africa/southafrica/2004/1000/khayelitsha1000.pdf [accessed August 5, 2004].

Médecins sans Frontières. 2003b. *Surmounting Challenges: Procurement of Antiretroviral Medicines in Low-and Middle-Income Countries*. [Online]. Available: http://www.accessmed-msf.org/documents/procurementreport.pdf [accessed July 1, 2004].

Orrell C, Bangsberg DR, Badri M, Wood R. 2003. Adherence is not a barrier to successful antiretroviral therapy in South Africa *AIDS* 17(9):1369–1375.

Paterson DL, Swindells S, Mohr J, Brester M, Vergis EN, Squier C, Wagener MM, Singh N. 2000. Adherence to protease inhibitor therapy and outcomes in patients with HIV infection. *Annals of Internal Medicine* 136(3):253.

Pillay C, Bredell H, McIntyre J, Gray G, Morris L. 2002. HIV-1 subtype C reverse transcriptase sequences from drug-naive pregnant women in South Africa. *AIDS Research and Human Retroviruses* 18(8):605–610.

Redfield R. 2004 (January 27). *Durability of ARV Therapy: U.S. Experience and its Implications for Resource-Constrained Settings*. Paper presented at the Institute of Medicine Workshop on Antiretroviral Scale-up in Resource Constrained Settings, Washington, DC. Institute of Medicine Committee on Antiretroviral Drug Use in Resource-Constrained Settings.

Richman D, Morton S, Wrin T, Hellmann N, Berry S, Shapiro M, Bozzette S. 2004. The prevalence of antiretroviral drug resistance in the United States. *AIDS* 18:1–7.

Schechter M. 2004 (January 27). *Lessons Learned from the Scale-up of Antiretroviral Treatment in Brazil*. Paper presented at the Institute of Medicine Workshop on Antiretroviral Scale-up in Resource Constrained Settings, Washington, DC. Institute of Medicine Committee on Antiretroviral Drug Use in Resource-Constrained Settings.

Sethi A, Celentano D, Gange S, Moore R, Gallant J. 2003. Association between adherence to antiretroviral therapy and human immunodeficiency virus drug resistance. *Clinical Infectious Diseases: An Official Publication of the Infectious Diseases Society of America* 37:1112–1118.

Simon V, Vanderhoeven J, Hurley A, Ramratnam B, Louie M, Dawson K, Parkin N, Boden D, Markowitz M. 2002. Evolving patterns of HIV-1 resistance to antiretroviral agents in newly infected individuals. *AIDS* 16:1511–1519.

Taylor S, Cane P, Hue S, Xu L, Wrin T, Lie Y, Hellmann N, Petropoulos C, Workman J, Ratcliffe D, Choudhury B, Pillay D. 2003. Identification of a transmission chain of HIV type 1 containing drug resistance-associated mutations. *AIDS Research and Human Retroviruses* 19:353–361.

Uganda AIDS Commission. 2003. *Follow-up to the Declaration of Commitment on HIV/ AIDS (UNGASS): Uganda Country Report, January–December 2002.* [Online]. Available: http://www.unaids.org/html/pub/topics/ungass2003/sub-saharan-africa/uganda_ ungassreport_2003_en_pdf.pdf [accessed August 6, 2004].

UNAIDS (Joint United Nations Programme on HIV/AIDS). 2002. *HIV/AIDS and Sexually Transmitted Infections: Haiti. 2002 Update.* [Online]. Available: http://www.unaids.org/ [accessed August 4, 2004].

Velasco-Hernandez JX, Gershengorn HB, Blower SM. 2002. Could widespread use of combination antiretroviral therapy eradicate HIV epidemics? *Lancet Infectious Diseases* 2:487–493.

Walton D, Farmer P, Lambert W, Léandre F, Koenig S, Mukherjee J. 2004. Integrated HIV prevention and care strengthens primary health care: Lessons from rural Haiti. *The Journal of Public Health Policy* 25(2):137–158.

Weidle PJ, Malamba S, Mwebaze R, Sozi C, Rukundo G, Downing R, Hanson D, Ochola D, Mugyenyi P, Mermin J, Samb B, Lackritz E. 2002. Assessment of a pilot antiretroviral drug therapy programme in Uganda: Patients' response, survival, and drug resistance. *Lancet* 360(9326):34–40.

Weidle P, Downing R, Sozi C, Mwebaze R, Rukundo G, Malamba S, Despess R, Hertogs K, Larder B, Ochola D, Mermin J, Samb B, Lackritz E. 2003. Development of phenotypic and genotypic resistance to antiretroviral therapy in the UNAIDS HIV Drug Access Initiative—Uganda. *AIDS* 17(Supplement 3):S39–S48.

WHO (World Health Organization). 2003a. *Access to Antiretroviral Treatment and Care: The Experience of the HIV Equity Initiative, Cange, Haiti.* [Online]. Available: http:// www.who.int/hiv/pub/prev_care/en/Haiti_E.pdf [accessed July 1, 2004].

WHO. 2003b. *Antiretroviral Therapy in Primary Health Care: Experience of the Khayelitsha Programme in South Africa.* [Online]. Available: http://www.who.int/hiv/pub/prev_care/ en/South_Africa_E.pdf [accessed July 1, 2004].

WHO. 2003c. *Scaling up Antiretroviral Therapy: Experience in Uganda.* [Online]. Available: http://www.who.int/hiv/pub/prev_care/en/Uganda_E.pdf [accessed July 1, 2004].

World Bank. 2004. *World Development Report 2004: Making Services Work for Poor People.* Washington, DC: World Bank.

4

Principles of Scale-up

Much has been learned from both developed and developing nations that have accomplished large-scale antitretroviral therapy (ART), and it is now clear that effective scale-up is a realistic objective in many settings. Before this can happen, however, the stigma and discrimination that can hamper efforts to curb the global HIV/AIDS pandemic must be addressed. To initiate the scale-up process, countries will have to identify those needing treatment, as well as the various possible points of entry into treatment programs. Once persons in need have been identified, scale-up efforts should be guided by a core set of principles. The many lessons learned from previous country efforts (see Chapter 3) have allowed the World Health Organization (WHO) to formulate a set of such guidelines that countries may wish to use as a template for beginning scale-up. These guidelines include strategies for diagnosing HIV and AIDS, deciding when to initiate therapy, determining which regimen to use given the characteristics of the population needing treatment, and deciding when and how to monitor therapy.

While these strategies can serve as a useful guide, however, treatment providers must remain cognizant of the limitations associated with their particular setting. Resource-constrained settings are beset by other health problems, such as tuberculosis (TB) and malnutrition—both of which will affect the opportunities and challenges faced during scale-up. Additionally, the success of any ART program will depend upon many factors, crucial among which is adherence to therapy. The many lessons learned about adherence from past experience with ART (see Chapter 3) can be applied during the initiation and implementation of treatment programs in resource-constrained settings. Finally, the integration of prevention and treatment is essential, as is palliative care for AIDS patients in developing countries.

REDUCING STIGMA AND DISCRIMINATION

Stigma and discrimination, often driven by fear, can undermine efforts to treat and care for persons with HIV/AIDS. With HIV/AIDS, fear of illness, contagion, and death can affect not only patients themselves, but also those living with and caring for them, such as family members, co-workers, and health care workers. In addition to the stigma associated with the infection and the disease itself, persons with HIV/AIDS may face the stigma associated with belonging to a specific group, such as homosexuals, prostitutes, injection drug users, or persons engaging in "casual" sex. Stigma can result in silence, denial, ostracism, and violence.

Clearly, these reactions can impact interest in and ability to seek diagnosis and care for HIV/AIDS. Stigma and discrimination can discourage people from finding out about and revealing their HIV status, which in turn can affect prevention and treatment efforts. In Africa, 90 percent of HIV-infected people still do not know of their status (Harries et al., 2002); fear of stigma could be one reason for this. Stigma also can affect the quality of care received by people diagnosed with HIV/AIDS. A survey of 1,000 Nigerian physicians, nurses, and midwives, for example, assessed the prevalence of stigma and discrimination (UNAIDS, 2003a). Fully 10 percent of providers admitted to having refused care or denied admission to a hospital for a patient with HIV/AIDS. Almost 40 percent of those interviewed believed that a person's appearance revealed his or her HIV-positive status, while 20 percent believed that people with HIV/AIDS had behaved immorally and deserved their fate. Factors contributing to these attitudes and behaviors included a lack of knowledge about the virus; a lack of protective equipment, prompting fear among health care providers of acquiring the infection from patients; and frustration at not having medications to treat HIV/AIDS patients, who therefore were "doomed" to die.

Strategies to reduce stigma may include providing information, counseling, imparting coping skills, and promoting social interaction with persons living with HIV/AIDS. It is possible that providing treatment for HIV/AIDS may decrease stigma by restoring health, which in turn will allow those infected to live symptom-free and engage in work and community activities, and by reducing fear of contagion and death. By providing hope to people living with HIV/AIDS, the widespread availability of ART may reduce the stigma associated with seeking testing and treatment.

Unfortunately, the literature documenting effective methods for reducing the stigma associated with HIV/AIDS in resource-poor settings needs to be strengthened considerably. Referring to health-related stigma in developing countries in general, the Fogarty International Center of the National Institutes of Health (NIH) has written: "Little is known about the pervasiveness of stigma in the developing world and how healthcare systems can tackle its negative consequences. Effective action has been slow in coming, in part because of the continuing gaps in knowledge" (NIH, 2003). In recognition of this lack of knowledge, in 2002 NIH launched a Stigma and Global Health Research Program. The first 19 awards under the program were announced in October 2003; expected 5-year funding for the program is approximately $16.5 million (NIH, 2003). The NIH grant recipients will establish a global network of researchers to "develop the field of stigma and global health research by testing hypotheses and generating data on the etiology of stigma and effective interventions for its negative effects on health" (NIH, 2003). The network will help identify best practices, opportunities, and obstacles in research on stigma related to global health. Through the studies conducted by this network and others, culture-specific interventions to reduce stigma, perhaps tailored to different demographic groups, should be tried and evaluated.

In June 2001, the United Nations General Assembly Special Session on HIV/AIDS issued a Declaration on Commitment on HIV/AIDS. This declaration included a provision for UN Member States to "develop strategies to combat stigma and social exclusion connected with the epidemic" and "enact, strengthen or enforce, as appropriate, legislation, regulations and other measures to eliminate all forms of discrimination against . . . people living with HIV/AIDS..." (UNAIDS, 2003a). According to a UNAIDS report in 2003, almost half of all African countries had adopted no legislation to prevent discrimination against people living with HIV/AIDS (UNAIDS, 2003b).

> **Recommendation 4-1.** Governmental and community leaders at all levels of civic life should spearhead an effort to create a culture of openness and support in order to eliminate stigma and ensure the successful continuance of antiretroviral treatment and HIV prevention programs.

IDENTIFYING POINTS OF ENTRY

Identifying persons in immediate need of treatment provides one challenge for the efficient and effective scale-up of ART. As noted earlier, there are multiple possible points of entry for treatment programs, each of which may target different sectors of the population and initially identify infected persons at different stages of the disease.

Early detection and counseling to prevent subsequent transmission, with regular follow-up, are desirable even though patients initially entering care at a later stage of infection are more likely to be immediately clinically eligible to begin ART under the WHO guidelines endorsed by the committee. The former patients also may be more likely to remain in care. At the same time, the challenges of beginning care and treatment for those in the latest stages of disease include reconstituting a highly suppressed immune system and the necessity of treating opportunistic infections, such as TB. For these and other reasons, mortality may be higher for patients entering care at later disease stages, as was the case for patients enrolled in treatment programs in Haiti (Fitzgerald, 2004) (see Chapter 3).

Existing health care facilities—already providing services for other health needs—may take on HIV/AIDS testing and treatment as scale-up unrolls. The screening of military personnel and other occupational groups can also serve as entry points for ART. Three additional points of entry may be considered during scale-up: voluntary counseling and testing centers, mother-to-child transmission prevention programs, and TB treatment and control programs.

Voluntary Counseling and Testing Programs

Only 5–7 percent of people in most developing countries know their HIV status (WHO, 2003a). Clearly then, counseling and testing must precede ART and HIV/AIDS care. At the same time, voluntary counseling and testing (VCT) centers established to provide these services offer the opportunity to address a comprehensive range of measures for HIV/AIDS prevention, treatment, and care. Though the majority of apparently healthy persons seeking to know their status can be diagnosed most effectively in VCT programs, some asymptomatic persons will be found HIV-positive through other mechanisms, such as blood bank screening. Such patients should still be referred to VCT programs to ensure that preventive counseling is provided in conjunction with entry into ART programs. Requiring that capable HIV-positive patients obtain VCT clinic counseling prior to receipt of ARVs may encourage disclosure and foster the linkage of treatment, prevention, and care.

Counseling and testing involve risk evaluation, facilitated decision making following testing, and education about preventive measures for those found to be HIV-negative or -positive. UNAIDS has identified several critical elements of counseling and testing programs: testing should be voluntary; results should be kept confidential; counseling should focus on the individual client's needs; HIV-positive and -negative persons should be referred for ongoing support; and stigma-reducing activities should be incorporated into the services provided (CDC, 2004; UNAIDS, 2000). Centers offering VCT services can serve as an important link to medical and support programs that provide treatment and care for those eligible to receive ART. Same-day testing sites can facilitate this linkage.

Mother-to-Child Transmission Prevention Programs

Pregnancy can provide an opportune point of entry for women who might not otherwise seek health care for themselves. In addition, antenatal clinics are used to collect data for HIV prevalence estimates (UNAIDS, 2003a).

In the history of treating and caring for those with HIV/AIDS, special attention has focused on preventing transmission of the virus from mother to child. Mother-to-child-transmission (MTCT) prevention programs have been established to provide specialized services to women during their pregnancy and then to the children they bear during the immediate postpartum period. While MTCT prevention programs can provide an opportunity for women to enter health care, in some regions of resource-poor settings only 1 percent of women have access to these services. Moreover, partner opposition can reduce the likelihood of participating in these programs.

Building on the success of these programs, the Maternal-to-Child-Transmission-Plus (MTCT-Plus) Initiative was established in 2002 (Columbia University Mailman School of Public Health, 2004). The goal of this initiative is to provide specialized care, including ART, to HIV-infected women during and following pregnancy, to their children, and to their partners. The program's comprehensive reach provides an opportunity for family members to enter a system of care and for mothers to receive continued care following childbirth.

The MTCT-Plus Initiative is coordinated by the Mailman School of Public Health at Columbia University and is funded by private foundations and the U.S. Agency for International Development (USAID). The programs operate in 12 sites ranging from rural clinics to teaching hospitals—11 in sub-Saharan Africa and 1 in Thailand. The comprehensive HIV/AIDS care provided includes ART, therapy for the prevention and treatment of opportunistic infections, TB prevention services, nutrition support, family planning, and supportive services. Recognizing that HIV/AIDS has psychosocial as well as clinical dimensions, the programs use multidisciplinary teams of providers and supporters that include nurses, counselors, and pediatric and adult physicians.

As of November 2003, 2,000 people had been enrolled in MTCT-Plus programs. Women can enroll in the programs either during or following pregnancy; currently, 40 percent are enrolled antepartum and 60 percent postpartum. In recognition of the fact that HIV/AIDS affects families, not just individuals at risk for or with HIV/AIDS, and that family-based endeavors may improve overall treatment and care, enrollment is offered to other members of the household as well. Of the 2,000 people enrolled as of November 2003, one-third were children, and one-fifth were partners of the (index) women.

The programs target people at the earlier stages of disease. The mean CD4 count of patients beginning treatment is 379. The index women are at a less advanced stage of disease than their partners who become enrolled. Most of the infants enrolled in the program are of indeterminate status; they are followed clinically as an effort to provide comprehensive family care.

Each MTCT-Plus site uses standardized protocols with respect to treatment eligibility criteria, treatment monitoring, toxicity management, drug regimens, and pediatric dosing. An attempt is made to harmonize these protocols with both country-specific and WHO guidelines. The antiretrovirals (ARVs) used in these programs are procured by UNICEF; approximately half are generic products.

CLINICAL PRINCIPLES

Because of the complexity of HIV and AIDS, WHO established clinical guidelines in 2003 as part of its 3-by-5 campaign (see Chapter 2) to assist programs in scale-up of ART (WHO, 2003b). These guidelines take into account experience gained in the clinical management of HIV/AIDS in the developed world and lessons learned from treating the disease in the developing world. Data from clinical trials and observational studies underlie the guidelines.

In recognition of the limitations faced by resource-constrained settings, such as cost and availability of drugs and diagnostics, the WHO guidelines offer suggestions specific to these settings. The guidelines provide a framework that can be used to standardize and simplify treatment for this complex disease and encompasses the point at which to start therapy; first- and second-line combination regimens; considerations involved in treating subgroups of patients, such as those coinfected with TB, pregnant women, and children; means of monitoring therapy; and indicators for changing regimens. As noted earlier, these recommendations are based on scientific and clinical experience and evidence, drug availability and cost, the requirement to refrigerate some ARVs, the need for and availability of laboratory monitoring, drug toxicity profiles, and the risk of drug interactions. The guidelines acknowledge limitations in areas in urgent need of research, such as the treatment of pregnant women and individuals coinfected with TB. Nonetheless, they provide a critically important starting point by outlining simple criteria and steps that can be used in even the most resource-poor settings.

The WHO guidelines can be used by providers with a range of experience in diagnosing and treating people with HIV/AIDS. The simplified, standardized guidance they offer can be indispensable given that many ART scale-up programs in resource-limited settings need to rely on community involvement and the recruitment of unskilled workers or health care professionals with little or no experience in managing such programs. At the same time, however, HIV/AIDS experts warn that these guidelines should not be considered a substitute for local program manuals. Nor should they be used to underestimate the complex nature of ART, the need for context-specific individualized care, and the reality that early treatment decisions can profoundly alter the course of disease and limit a patient's response to future therapy in the case of first-line failure.

> **Recommendation 4-2. Before countries develop their own directives, the World Health Organization's 2003 guidelines for the treatment of adults, children, and pregnant women should serve as an initial template for the design of antiretroviral therapy programs with respect to when to start therapy, which regimens to use, how to monitor the progress of therapy, and when to switch drugs or terminate therapy.** *As new evidence becomes available, through the efforts of international, national, and local research, the WHO guidelines, particularly with regard to pregnant women and those coinfected with tuberculosis, may require refinement or modification.*

One clinical principle that deserves mention is that because therapy for HIV/AIDS is an ongoing process, an adequate longitudinal medical record is an essential tool in patient management. In many developing countries, medical records systems will need significant improvement, especially where those records are currently held by the patient or where documentation is organized around discrete visits rather than continuity of care. Relevant training in longitudinal medical record keeping and changes in patient flow through the clinic should be considered, where needed, to facilitate this process.

The remainder of this section reviews in turn considerations involved in using the laboratory to diagnose, initiate, and monitor ART; selecting a treatment regimen; treating dual epidemics of HIV and TB; treating women; treating pregnant women; treating children; and addressing the role of nutrition in HIV/AIDS and its treatment.

Using the Laboratory to Diagnose, Initiate, and Monitor ART

In the developed world, laboratory and clinical criteria weigh heavily in the initiation and monitoring of ART. Cost and infrastructure needs may limit the ability of resource-constrained settings to use such a laboratory-intensive approach for treating patients with HIV/AIDS.

In the developed world, standard tests administered prior to beginning therapy include a test to detect HIV, followed by a confirmatory test; a test to determine CD4 T cell count—a marker of immune function and disease stage; and a test to determine the amount of virus present in the blood (viral RNA or viral load)—a marker of disease burden. The WHO guidelines do recommend baseline HIV testing and, when possible, CD4 T cell count (or the surrogate marker, total lymphocyte count [TLC]) prior to initiation of therapy (see Appendix B, Table A). While a confirmatory test to diagnose HIV is preferable, if a second test (e.g., rapid antibody test, Western Blot) is not available, therapy should proceed based on clinical criteria defining AIDS stage (see Appendixes B and E).

In the developed world, CD4 T cell count and viral RNA load are assessed throughout therapy to monitor progress and determine the success of the therapeutic regimen. When laboratory tests such as CD4 T cell count and viral load are not available, the WHO guidelines recommend the use of clinical criteria for symptomatic appraisals to ensure that therapy can be monitored in settings without sophisticated laboratory capacity or personnel.

Finally, because of potential side effects and toxicities of ARVs—and the progression of HIV infection—additional baseline laboratory tests obtained in less resource-constrained countries include determinations of red blood cell count, renal function, liver enzymes and function, and lipid status (U.S. Department of Health and Human Services, 2003). WHO recommends additional tests such as these when infrastructure allows (see Appendix B, Table E).

Laboratory testing can be costly and require sophisticated laboratory infrastructure and trained technicians. A CD4 T cell count is typically determined using a flow cytometer for measurement and is costly. Of note, there are no data indicating what degree of CD4 or viral load testing translates into cost-effective clinical or public health benefits. For example, in the United States, no trial has been conducted to compare clinical endpoints between patients who received viral load testing and those who did not.

Less-expensive technologies and surrogate laboratory markers are available and have been used in the developing world to monitor therapy. While a flow cytometer is commonly used to quantify CD4 T cell count and assess disease stage and progression, some countries have used alternative technologies to garner this information. A West African study, for example, demonstrated the utility of Dynabeads, a low-cost alternative to the flow cytometer based on epifluorescent microscopy (Diagbouga et al., 2003). The cost of an epifluorescent microscope is approximately half that of the least-expensive flow cytometry equipment, and the reagent cost per assay is only 12 percent of the cost of the assay for a CD4 T cell count (Diagbouga et al., 2003). Another technology, the Cytosphere bead assay, is reportedly easier to use but more expensive (US$8/test, compared with $3–5/ Dynabead test, as of December 2002). Even these alternative technologies, however, are limited by the need for trained technicians, an element of subjective interpretation, the need for refrigeration and a reliable power source, and fatigue associated with the manual nature of the technology. Because of these concerns and limited formal evaluation, WHO has recommended that both methods be evaluated in a multicenter study before being officially recommended to laboratories in the developing world.

As noted, TLC has been suggested as a surrogate for CD4 T cell count; indeed, it is recommended by WHO. Since the CD4 T cell is one type of lymphocyte, CD4 T cell count correlates with TLC. A number of reports have shown TLC to be a useful predictor of significant immunosuppression, as measured by a CD4 cell count of less than 200/μL in HIV-infected persons. If TLC were used to determine who was eligible to start therapy, a lower level would increase specificity (by increasing the likelihood that people with high CD4 counts would not be incorrectly targeted for therapy) but decrease sensitivity (by increasing the likelihood that people with low CD4 counts would not be identified).

The cost of laboratory tests is only one of many costs associated with laboratory monitoring of HIV/AIDS patients. The procurement and proper use of assays and reagents depend on an enormous amount of infrastructure, which may include data management programs; laboratory equipment and supplies (e.g., refrigerators, freezers, centrifuges, thermocyclers, and pipettes); proficiency testing programs; laboratory accrediting agencies, and skilled technicians. At an even more basic level, effective laboratory monitoring relies on a range of nonlaboratory resources that are taken for granted in resource-rich countries, such as reagent-grade water, electrical power, and theft prevention measures. Securing infrastructure and resources can be very costly and is particularly important given that theft is a large problem in many resource-constrained settings. It may be particularly challenging to obtain and maintain these resources in rural areas of resource-constrained settings, where infrastructure may be even weaker.

Recognizing the infrastructure costs and limitations in resource-constrained settings, WHO has set forth guidelines for conducting laboratory testing prior to initiating therapy, for monitoring therapy, and for defining treatment failure (see Box 4-1). The WHO recommendations are tiered for primary health centers, district hospitals, and regional referral hospitals.

Recommendation 4-3. Donors and program managers should plan and budget for laboratory activities that will foster more accurate and effective HIV diagnosis and management, using the World Health Organization's 2003 guidelines as the initial template. *Incorporating*

98 SCALING UP TREATMENT

BOX 4-1
WHO Guidelines for the Initiation of Antiretroviral Therapy in Adults and Adolescents

1. If CD4 Testing Is Available:
   i)   For persons with WHO Stage IV disease, therapy should begin regardless of CD4 count.
   ii) For persons with WHO Stage III disease, therapy should begin with consideration of using CD4 cell count < 350 /mm^3.
   iii) For persons with WHO Stage I or II disease, therapy should begin with CD4 cell counts ≤ 200/mm^3.
2. If CD4 Testing Is Not Available:
   i)   For persons with WHO Stage IV disease, therapy should begin regardless of total lymphocyte count.
   ii) For persons with WHO Stage III disease, therapy should begin regardless of total lymphocyte count.
   iii) For persons with WHO Stage II disease, therapy should begin with a total lymphocyte count ≤ 1200/mm^3.*

   * A total lymphocyte count = 1200/mm^3 can be substituted for the CD4 count when the latter is unavailable and HIV-related symptoms (Stage II and III) exist. It is not useful in the asymptomatic patient. Thus, in the absence of CD4 cell testing, asymptomatic HIV-infected patients (Stage I) should not be treated because there is currently no other reliable marker available in severely resource-constrained settings.

   SOURCE: WHO, 2003b.

---

emerging evidence and resources into their decision-making process, countries should consider developing population-specific guidelines reflective of the best possible practices in their particular circumstances. In those localities where it is possible to go beyond the WHO guidelines, treatment failure should be defined through viral RNA determination; otherwise, it should be defined by means of clinical or other laboratory markers consistent with the guidelines.

Recommendation 4-4. Under the leadership of their ministries of health and national reference laboratory experts, all countries should develop hierarchical laboratory networks that integrate the local, district, and referral hospital levels through tiered quality assurance programs and provide referral support for increasingly complex laboratory assays. Full development of these networks is not required before the initiation of scaled-up antiretroviral therapy programs, however. *National reference laboratories should promulgate tier-specific quality assurance protocols, and donors supporting ART programs should provide the means*

*to properly ensure acceptable technical performance by these labora-
tory networks. Dedicated funds, training, and other resources to ensure
the maintenance of laboratory equipment employed in these networks
should be provided. To better facilitate the diagnosis and treatment of
HIV infection in infants less than 18 months of age, the laboratory
networks should put in place a capacity for the direct detection of HIV,
such as HIV DNA, HIV RNA, or HIV p24 antigen.*

Clinical criteria for monitoring treatment progress have been used in
developing countries. While there are many reasons during both health and
disease for weight gain or loss, patient weight has been one clinical marker
used in developing countries to judge the success of ART. In the event that
clinical criteria are used for treatment monitoring, however, it must be
recognized that such criteria do not always provide an accurate assessment
of viral suppression, and even patients who appear to be doing well may fail
in their regimen if viral suppression is not above a certain threshold. Initial
treatment regimens should be selected based on this awareness. The degree
to which laboratory services for toxicity monitoring are used also requires
special consideration in resource-constrained settings with limited infrastructure. The necessity for laboratory monitoring may be tailored to the
use of certain ARVs. For example, when nevirapine is used in combination
with other drugs, hepatoxicity testing may be important, whereas when
zidovudine is used, a hemoglobin determination for anemia might be considered.

Selecting a Treatment Regimen

In the developed world, regimen selection is quite intricate because of
the availability of numerous drugs and the infrastructure needed to deliver
and monitor therapy, the affordability of drugs (through third-party payers
in some cases), and the ability to tailor regimens to virus susceptibility.
Because resource-constrained settings may not have these advantages, WHO
has recommended four first-line regimens for HIV/AIDS treatment. These
regimens, summarized in Table 4-1, take into account toxicities, appropri-
ateness for use in TB-coinfected patients and in pregnant women, availability as a fixed-dose combination (FDC) (see Box 4-2), cost, and laboratory
monitoring requirements. Regimen design also must take into account the
population being treated with respect to age, gender, pregnancy status, and
comorbid infections.

According to the WHO guidelines, ARV regimens that have been shown
scientifically to be ineffective or less effective than other available regimens
should not be used. Specifically, mono- or dual-therapy regimens and
nucleoside-only regimens should be avoided. According to a recent

TABLE 4-1 WHO-Recommended Antiretroviral Therapy Regimens for Persons in Resource-Constrained Settings

Regimen	Major Potential Toxicities	Used for Women of Childbearing Age During Pregnancy	Used for Those with TB Coinfection	Fixed-Dose Combination Available	Laboratory Monitoring Requirements
d4T/3TC/NVP	d4T-related neuropathy, pancreatitis, and lipoatrophy; NVP-related hepatotoxicity and severe rash	Yes	Yes, in rifampicin-free continuation phase of TB treatment; used with caution in rifampicin-based regimens	Yes	No
ZDV/3TC/NVP	ZDV-related gastrointestinal intolerance, anemia, and neutropenia; NVP-related hepatotoxicity and severe rash	Yes	Yes, in rifampicin-free continuation phase of TB treatment; used with caution in rifampicin-based regimens	Yes	Yes, because of ZDV-associated bone marrow suppression
d4T/3TC/EFV	d4T-related neuropathy, pancreatitis, and lipoatrophy; EFV-related central nervous system toxicity and potential for teratogenicity	No	Yes, but EFV should not be given to pregnant women or women with childbearing potential unless effective contraception can be ensured	No (d4T/3TC available in FDC)	No
ZDV/3TC/EFV	ZDV-related gastrointestinal intolerance, anemia, and neutropenia; EFV-related central nervous system toxicity and potential for teratogenicity	No	Yes, but EFV should not be given to pregnant women or women with childbearing potential unless effective contraception can be ensured	No (ZDV/3TC available in FDC)	Yes, because of ZDV-associated bone marrow suppression

NOTE: 3TC = lamivudine; d4T = stavydube1; EFV = efavure bz1; FDC = fixed-dose combination; NVP = nevirapine; TB = tuberculosis; ZDV = zidovudine.
SOURCE: Adapted from WHO, 2003:Table B.

BOX 4-2
At a Glance: Fixed-Dose Combination Therapy

Fixed-dose combinations (FDCs) are pills that contain more than one drug per tablet. FDCs are available for a variety of disease conditions, including HIV and AIDS.

The World Health Organization has recommended using FDCs, when available, for the treatment of HIV/AIDS, provided their quality and bioequivalence to individual drug therapy have been proven, and they would be advantageous to individual programs delivering ART.

FDCs have a number of potential advantages:

• Adherence effect: fewer tablets per day need to be taken.
• Adherence effect: assists providers in complying with treatment standards.
• Resistance deterrent: limits likelihood of taking only one or two of the three drugs needed for effective highly active antiretroviral therapy (HAART).
• Supply management assistance: fewer drugs need to be stored.

At the same time, FDCs pose several challenges:

• Allergies to one or more components
• Different pharmokinetic or pharmodynamic profiles
• Dose titration

SOURCES: MSF Briefing Note, 2004; WHO, 2003b.

Cochrane review of randomized controlled trials comparing the effects of three- or four-drug ARV regimens versus two-drug regimens, the latter were associated with higher levels of failure of viral suppression and resistance (Rutherford et al., 2004) (see also Chapter 3). Although it may be desirable in some cases to reduce the number of drugs for adherence or toxicity reasons, ART with at least three drugs should be the standard.

> **Recommendation 4-5. Antiretroviral therapy programs should be designed to optimize the balance between individual efficacy and population effectiveness while minimizing toxicity and resistance.** *ART regimens or programs shown to be significantly less effective or ineffective—such as mono- or dual-therapy and nucleoside-only regimens—must be avoided. Because resources and population and patient needs will vary considerably among different countries and regions, countries should develop population-specific guidelines.*

An initial template guiding regimen selection may prove especially useful to programs that have not yet developed their own treatment guidelines.

The need for such a template is illustrated by the case of Harare, Zimbabwe, where national guidelines were not available to the practitioners and pharmacists who prescribed and stocked ARVs. The treatment and management of HIV/AIDS patients in that setting have been described as "therapeutic anarchy," with at least 17 percent of 92 patients receiving AZT monotherapy, a regimen not recommended by HIV/AIDS experts (Nyazema et al., 2000; U.S. DHHS, 2003).

Treating Dual Epidemics of HIV and TB

The TB and HIV/AIDS epidemics exist in parallel in many resource-constrained settings (see Box 4-3). Of the 42 million people worldwide infected with HIV, an estimated 11 million are coinfected with TB (WHO, 2003c) (see Figure 4-1). While ART programs may be new for many countries, these same countries may have experience with TB control and treat-

---

BOX 4-3
At a Glance: Tuberculosis and HIV/AIDS—
An Intersection of Epidemics

Tuberculosis (TB) is one of the leading causes of AIDS-related death; together, TB and HIV/AIDS represent the two greatest infectious disease killers in the world. Worldwide, 42 million people are infected with HIV, and 2 billion are infected with TB. Of the 42 million people with HIV, nearly one-third are coinfected with TB. In sub-Saharan Africa, TB is the leading cause of death in coinfected persons (Ridzon and Mayanja-Kizza, 2002).

Primary TB infection occurs when a person inhales a threshold amount of *Mycobacterium tuberculosis* bacilli. In most persons, no signs or symptoms are present, and the infection is contained. This then becomes "latent" TB infection. If the immune system is sufficiently compromised—which occurs in a variety of non-infectious diseases—latent TB can progress to active TB, which can be pulmonary, or extrapulmonary or disseminated. Most active TB results in pulmonary disease. With advanced immune compromise, such as when a person has AIDS (CD4 cell count < 200 /mm^3), extrapulmonary or disseminated disease is more likely. Examples of extrapulmonary TB infection include brain abscesses, meningitis, pericarditis, gastric TB, scrotal TB, and bone marrow infection.

While the risk of developing active disease from latent TB infection is 10 percent during the lifetime of an immunocompetent person, the risk in a person with HIV/AIDS is 4–10 percent *yearly* (Corbett et al., 2003; Fennelly and Ellner, 2004). Additionally, having TB accelerates the progression of HIV/AIDS (Ridzon and Mayanja-Kizza, 2002). TB is the most common opportunistic infection in HIV-infected patients. Additionally, TB is the only opportunistic infection that can be transmitted to persons without HIV. Of note, though, is that HIV-infected persons

ment programs. As the rate of coinfection is high, the latter programs may, as noted earlier, be a useful point of entry for HIV/AIDS diagnosis and care. Indeed, it is estimated that 500,000 people with HIV/AIDS could be reached through existing TB programs (Kim, 2004). WHO recognizes this opportunity to detect HIV/AIDS cases and recommends that in countries with an HIV prevalence exceeding 5 percent, HIV testing and counseling be offered to everyone with TB (WHO, 2003a).

In 1998, the World Health Initiative began its ProTEST initiative to provide collaborative services for both HIV and TB (London School of Hygiene and Tropical Medicine, 2002; Elzinga and Nunn, 2002; Gorkom, 2003). The project was begun in South Africa, Malawi, and Zambia and later expanded to additional African countries. VCT is used as the entry point for prevention and care services. Clients are screened for sexually transmitted infections, including HIV, and HIV-infected persons are

---

with TB are no more infectious than HIV-negative persons with TB (Ridzon and Mayanja-Kizza, 2002). Latent TB is noninfectious.

TB can be difficult to diagnose in immunocompromised people; if diagnosed, however, it is easily treatable. Treatment reduces morbidity and mortality in TB–HIV coinfected persons. Even treatment of latent TB infection can be successful.

Using isoniazid for latent TB infection and highly active antiretroviral therapy (HAART) for HIV can reduce the risk of conversion from latent to active TB infection. With one exception, treatment for active TB is the same for HIV-infected and HIV-negative persons and requires the administration of multiple drugs in combination. The one exception is the rifamycin component of therapy, which requires a particular type of administration for HIV-infected persons who simultaneously are on HAART. With respect to the treatment of HIV and of TB, because of drug–drug interactions, pill burden, and potentially additive toxicities of regimens, the decision to start therapy for each condition and when to do so requires careful consideration and additional research. The 2003 WHO guidelines for the treatment of HIV-infected persons in resource-limited settings provide some initial guidance for beginning treatment for HIV in the coinfected (WHO, 2003b). (For further information, refer to Appendix B, Table A. and Section VIII C.)

Directly observed therapy for TB has been shown to be effective in both the developed and developing worlds and may be considered, when feasible, for improving adherence and treatment outcomes.

Finally, the emergence of multidrug-resistant tuberculosis (MDR-TB) in the setting of HIV treatment should be noted. TB in HIV clinics in general, and MDR-TB specifically, constitutes an important nosocomial threat that should be addressed proactively through appropriate infection control initiatives.

SOURCES: Fennelly and Ellner, 2004; WHO, 2003c,d.

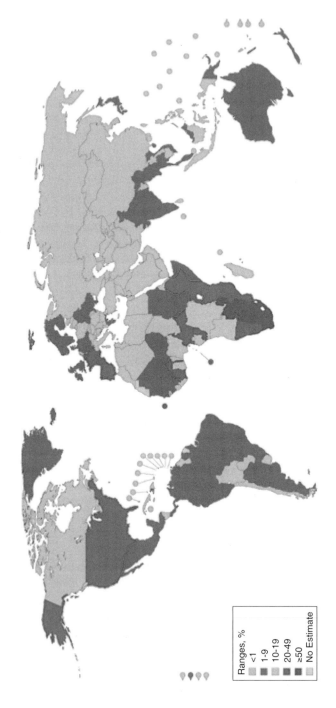

FIGURE 4-1 Proportions of adult tuberculosis cases attributable to human immunodeficiency virus by country in 2000.
SOURCE: Corbett et al., 2003.

screened for TB. Those diagnosed with infections are then referred for further support and treatment.

The immune deficiency created by HIV infection increases the risk of developing active TB, while TB increases the mortality of those with HIV (Havlir and Barnes, 1999). Indeed, TB is the leading cause of death in HIV-positive patients in the developing world (Corbett et al., 2003; Harries et al., 2002). Specifically, individuals latently infected with TB who are HIV-negative have a 10 percent lifetime risk of developing active TB after infection, while those who are HIV-positive may have nearly a 10 percent annual risk of developing active disease (Corbett et al., 2003). The coexistence of the two diseases in populations thus has implications for disease progression and prevention, as well as treatment priorities.

> **Recommendation 4-6. Program managers, international donors, and national policy makers should ensure that strong tuberculosis control programs continue in parallel with antiretroviral treatment scale-up programs, given that nearly one-third of HIV-infected persons in the world are coinfected with tuberculosis.** *Because dual infection with HIV and tuberculosis poses a life-threatening diagnostic and therapeutic dilemma, strong HIV care programs must include capabilities for diagnosis, treatment, and prophylaxis of tuberculosis. Tuberculosis treatment programs should be supported as an important point of entry for HIV testing and consideration for ART. It is critical to overall treatment success that these coexisting epidemics be addressed in parallel.*

Case finding and treatment for each of these epidemics in parallel can have profound effects on morbidity and mortality. The experience in Brazil highlights some of these successes. As in the United States, when ART was made more widely accessible in Brazil, the number of cases of pulmonary TB declined (Schechter, 2004); the incidence of TB fell by 80 percent when highly active antiretroviral therapy (HAART) was introduced. Furthermore, when TB prophylaxis was prescribed for HIV-infected patients, TB mortality decreased by 80 percent in just 4 years (Levi and Vitória, 2002). In South Africa, similar success was seen. In an observational study, patients receiving HAART had a significantly lower incidence of TB than those not receiving HAART, with an overall risk reduction of 81 percent.

Isoniazid has proven effective in reducing the incidence of active TB in HIV-positive patients and has been used effectively in some resource-constrained settings, such as those in Africa (Harries et al., 2002). In a review of randomized controlled trials comparing TB preventive therapy with placebo for HIV-positive individuals, it was found that preventive therapy reduced the rate of active TB by 50 percent over an average follow-up period of 15 to 33 months. This review included trials conducted in resource-poor settings, such as Haiti and sub-Saharan Africa (Wilkinson et al., 1998).

The WHO-sponsored ProTEST projects, previously discussed as a point of entry for case finding, combine comprehensive services for the HIV/AIDS and TB epidemics. The goal is to reduce disease burden more efficiently than would be possible if care and treatment programs for each were run separately (Elzinga and Nunn, 2002).

Treating each disease in a coinfected person is complicated by treatment costs, drug interactions, pill burden, and patient acceptance of both diagnoses. WHO has suggested initial guidelines but recognizes that data are limited on which to base specific treatment recommendations for this special population. In cases in which HIV disease stage cannot be determined by CD4 T cell count, WHO recommends ART for all HIV-positive patients with TB. Additionally, WHO recommends that the treatment for TB remain a central priority and not be compromised by ART. The timing of treatment for both infections poses a challenge. WHO recommends beginning ART 2 weeks to 2 months after the patient has been stabilized on TB treatment. While ART may be lifesaving for those with TB and advanced HIV, consideration of pill burden, drug interactions, and toxicity must help guide decisions to treat both infections.

The ART regimen selected for coinfection reflects the risk of rifampicin drug interactions with nonnucleoside reverse transcriptase inhibitors (NNRTIs) and protease inhibitors (PIs); the first-line regimen for patients with coinfection is (zidovudine or stavudine) + lamivudine + efavirenz. Using abacavir instead of efavirenz offers, among other advantages, lower pill burden and no interaction with rifampicins. Of note, however, abacavir is associated with hypersensitivity syndrome and decreased viral potency; for these reasons, it was removed from the first-line regimen options for persons with HIV. Using nevirapine instead of efavirenz also is possible but must be done with caution while using rifampicin because of effects on immunological response and toxicity.

As the two epidemics have similar characteristics, including the need for long-term treatment, the possibility of drug resistance, and multidrug therapy with strict adherence requirements, TB control programs could provide a model for delivery of ART for HIV (Gupta et al., 2004; Harries et al., 2002). In particular, directly observed therapy programs for TB have been used as models for the treatment of HIV/AIDS (see Chapter 3).

Beyond the threat of TB in general as an opportunistic infection, there is the additional concern of the emergence of multidrug-resistant tuberculosis (MDR-TB) in HIV patients and its nosocomial spread. In Lima, Peru, Campos and colleagues (2003) found that the prevalence of MDR-TB was 43 percent in HIV-infected persons with TB versus 2–3 percent in non–

HIV-infected persons with TB. This finding may be attributable to concentration of HIV care in hospital-based clinics where MDR-TB patients also were obtaining care. During the scale-up of clinics for ART, it will be essential that rigorous attention be paid to environmental, personal protective, and administrative measures to ensure effective infection control. As these measures can be costly and necessitate infrastructural work, proactive planning and budgeting are important. Overcrowded, poorly ventilated clinics that bring together large numbers of HIV-infected persons, some with active TB, will be a recipe for disaster.

As important as TB is among the opportunistic infections in HIV/AIDS patients, it is only one of several for which an intervention may be beneficial. Table 4-2 summarizes recommendations for prophylaxis and immuni-

TABLE 4-2 U.S. Recommendations for Opportunistic Infection Prophylaxis and for Vaccinations in Persons with HIV/AIDS

CD4 Count Risk Factor	Infectious Agent	Prophylaxis Recommended	First Line Prophylaxis
< 200	*Pneumocystis carinii*	Yes	trimethoprim-sulfamethoxazole
< 100	*Toxoplasma gondii*	Yes	trimethoprim-sulfamethoxazole
	fungal infections	No	
< 50	*Mycobacterium avium* complex	Yes	azithromycin (or clarithromycin)
	cytomegalovirus	No	
Any	*Mycobacterium tuberculosis*	Yes if PPD[a] > 5 mm	isoniazid, pyridoxine, rifampin, pyrazinamide[b]
Any	*Pneumococcus*	Yes	pneumococcal vaccine
Any	influenza	Yes	influenza vaccine
Any	hepatitis B	Yes	hepatitis vaccine
Any	hepatitis A	Yes if history of hepatitis B or C and seronegative for hepatitis A	hepatitis vaccine

[a]Positive tuberculin skin test.

[b]A combination of these drugs is required, and regimen selection should be based upon MTB resistance epidemiology.

zation for opportunistic infections in the United States. While all of these recommendations may not be indicated in highly resource-constrained countries, prophylaxis with cotrimoxazole does provide significant benefit (Grimwade and Swingler, 2004) in settings with susceptible organisms. Specifically, a Cochrane Review meta-analysis of three African trials indicated that cotrimoxazole was associated with a reduction in death (relative risk 0.69 [95 percent confidence interval 0.55 to 0.87]), morbid events (0.76 [0.64 to 0.9]), and hospitalization (0.66 [0.48 to 0.92]).

Treating Women

Globally, women make up 50 percent of those afflicted by the AIDS pandemic. In sub-Saharan Africa, more woman than men are infected with HIV. In this region, teenage girls are infected at rates up to four to seven times those of their teenage male counterparts (Fleischman, 2004; UNAIDS/ WHO, 2003). There are biological, economic, and sociocultural reasons for this disparity (Fleischman, 2003). Biologically, women are more susceptible to HIV for several reasons, including the efficiency with which male-to-female sexual transmission occurs through the large mucosal surfaces of the female genital tract. Moreover, economic dependence upon men may create an inequitable power relationship that can have far-reaching consequences for women's health. From a sociocultural perspective, women may have limited power to negotiate when and with whom they have sex, as well as whether to use safer sex practices, and they also may have limited access to information about HIV prevention.

Women may be less likely to get tested or to seek and receive treatment because of gender-based inequalities. In a Kampala hospital, only 10 percent of women had disclosed their HIV status to their partners, with fear of abandonment and discriminination being the most common reasons cited (Phillips, 2004). Fear of violence also affects women's decision to seek testing and care. Globally, from 10 to 50 percent of women report being physically abused by intimate male partners at some point during their lifetime, and this abuse can be accompanied by sexual violence (Heise et al., 1999; UNAIDS, 2004). At a VCT center in Tanzania, 37 percent of women reported a history of one or more physically abusive partners, and HIV-positive women were more than twice as likely as HIV-negative women to report that their current partner was physically or sexually abusive (Maman et al., 2002). A recent study in South Africa also found that women in controlling or violent relationships were at higher risk of contracting HIV infection (Dunkle et al., 2004). Other factors that could influence access to and use of ART by women include household and childrearing responsibilities affecting the priority accorded to obtaining health care; lack of control over finances in the household; and a focus on treatment of other members of the family, including the unborn children of women when pregnant (e.g., in programs for prevention of MTCT).

Treating Pregnant Women

Much research has been conducted on the treatment of pregnant women with HIV/AIDS in both the developed and developing worlds, and reduction of MTCT of HIV in developed countries is considered one of the greatest success stories of the HIV/AIDS pandemic. Despite what has been learned, however, success has not been widespread. In sub-Saharan Africa, where it is common for more than 10 percent of pregnant women to be infected with HIV, only 1 percent of pregnant women in some countries have access to services aimed at preventing MTCT (WHO, 2003a).

In the early 1990s in the United States, prior to the availability of ARV prophylaxis for MTCT, approximately 1,600 HIV-infected babies were born to about 6,000 HIV-infected mothers—a transmission rate of about 25 percent (Mofenson, 2003a). Following a seminal study of zidovudine prophylaxis given to mothers ante- and intrapartum and to newborns postpartum, this rate of transmission dropped to 8 percent (Mofenson, 2003b). This study, the Pediatric AIDS Clinical Trial Group (PACTG) protocol 076, used a complex three-part zidovudine regimen administered to HIV-infected women beginning at 14 to 34 weeks gestation, then intravenously during labor, and finally to the newborn for 6 weeks (Mofenson, 2003b).

The rate of transmission in the developed world has now decreased to less than 2 percent with the use of HAART, cesarean delivery, and avoidance of breastfeeding (Mofenson, 2003a,b). As a result of these interventions, the number of infants born with HIV each year has been reduced to 400 (Mofenson, 2003a). European countries have reported similar successes (European Collaborative Study, 2001; The Italian Register for Human Immunodeficiency Virus Infection in Children, 2002). The mechanisms by which the three-part zidovudine regimen afforded such protection in PACTG 076 were (1) a modest decrease in the mother's viral load, thereby exposing the baby to less virus transplacentally; (2) preexposure prophylaxis of the baby through transplacental passage of the drug; and (3) postexposure prophylaxis of the baby after the baby had passed through the birth canal.

Despite its potency, a three-part zidovudine regimen is too complex and expensive for use in severely resource-constrained settings. Accordingly over the past 10 years, other effective and less-expensive ARV interventions for prevention of MTCT have been identified. Single-dose nevirapine is one such intervention. Not only does nevirapine prophylaxis work, but nevirapine-based programs are feasible and cost-effective for resource-limited settings. In a recent 12-month study conducted in Lusaka, Zambia,

1,654 mothers and 1,157 infants were administered nevirapine. It is estimated, based on expected transmission rates in the absence of the intervention, that at least 190 infants participating in this study were spared HIV
infection (Stringer et al., 2003). Start-up costs aside, estimated expenditures
were US$9.34 per patient counseled (17,263 pregnant women were volun-
tarily counseled), $12.96 per patient tested (12,438 women were tested),
$55.12 per seropositive woman identified (2,924 women), and $848.26 per
infection averted.

Single-dose nevirapine has been compared with other regimens. Results
from the South African Intrapartum Nevirapine Trial demonstrated the
similar efficacy and safety of two intrapartum/postpartum prevention regimens in breastfeeding women: multiple-dose zidovudine/lamivudine and
single-dose nevirapine (Moodley et al., 2003). Both regimens can be implemented in settings where women may have only limited antenatal care or
where a woman's first visit to a clinic or hospital is during labor.

Because of the described advantages of cost, availability, simplicity,
and efficacy, nevirapine has been used as the cornerstone of MTCT prevention in resource-constrained settings. In these settings, its use has decreased
MTCT from about 30 percent to 15 percent (Stephenson, 2004).

Unfortunately, as discussed more fully in Chapter 3, recent data have
raised concerns about the emergence of nevirapine resistance and its implications both for programs to prevent MTCT and for future use of the drug
in an ART regimen for mothers after childbirth. A recent study from Thailand found that women with a history of limited nevirapine exposure for a
single pregnancy had reduced rates of successful treatment response with a
nevirapine-containing treatment regimen (Jourdain et al., 2004).

Recognizing what was known about the advantages and disadvantages
of nevirapine for prevention of MTCT, WHO found that the established
benefit of single-dose nevirapine in preventing MTCT outweighed the then-
perceived potential risks. WHO currently recommends nevirapine alone or
in more-potent combinations with another medication(s) (e.g., zidovudine),
depending on local circumstances (WHO, 2004a). However, the ongoing
accumulation of data on the emergence of nevirapine resistance after single-
dose therapy and possible "archiving" of resistant strains suggests that
current policies regarding single-dose use should be reassessed and less-
problematic alternatives vigorously explored. Reflecting these concerns
about nevirapine resistance and its implications for future therapeutic options for both mother and child, WHO's 3-by-5 guidelines suggest that
determining whether single-dose nevirapine prophylaxis compromises subsequent NNRTI-based HAART is "the most pressing operational research
question facing the field." Women who have received previous single-dose
nevirapine for prevention of MTCT should be considered eligible for future
NNRTI-based regimens, but with the awareness that their treatment re-

sponses may be compromised. Recognizing that heavily planned, protocol-driven treatment systems often change slowly, efforts addressing reassessment of treatment guidelines should encompass not only identifying the mechanisms necessary to ensure that the guidelines are timely, but also for rapidly implementing any new guidelines generated.

Even with ART prophylaxis, a major obstacle to preventing MTCT is preventing transmission that occurs through breastfeeding. In resource-limited settings, where the majority of HIV-infected mothers breastfeed, the risk of MTCT with no intervention is about 30–45 percent at 24 months after delivery (DeCock et al., 2000). Evidence suggests that most of the transmission that results from breastfeeding occurs early on. One study, conducted in Nairobi, Kenya, showed that 75 percent of transmission through breastmilk had occurred by the time the infant was 6 months old (Nduati et al., 2000). In this study, the only randomized controlled trial of formula feeding versus breastfeeding, 42 percent of HIV transmission to the infant was attributable to breastfeeding.

Another study, from Malawi, followed 672 infants (HIV-negative at birth) born to HIV-infected women. Forty-seven children became HIV-infected while breastfeeding but none after weaning. Incidence per month was 0.7 percent during ages 1 to 5 months, 0.6 percent during ages 6 to 11 months, and 0.3 percent during ages 12 to 17 months ($p = 0.01$ for trend) (Miotti et al., 1999).

In the South African Intrapartum Nevirapine Trial, which included both formula-fed and breastfed infants, all of whom received effective prophylaxis against intrapartum HIV transmission, breastfeeding was identified as the most significant risk factor for MTCT. During the first 4 weeks of life, breastfed infants were 2.2 times more likely to be HIV-infected, and breastfed infants between the ages of 4 and 8 weeks were 7.9 times more likely to be infected than their non-breastfed counterparts. In the absence of HAART, breastfeeding may also impair the health of the HIV-infected mother: the mortality rate of women randomized to breastfeed their infants was three times that of women randomized to formula-feed their infants (Mbori-Ngacha, 2001).

Nonetheless, the health benefits of breastfeeding for the infant create a significant dilemma for programs designed to prevent MTCT for women in resource-constrained settings. In such settings, clean water and affordable commercial infant formula often are not widely available, and poor hygiene and sanitation conditions increase the risk and transmission of the types of diarrheal and respiratory infections for which breastfeeding provides protection. In those resource-poor settings where there is a lack of safe, affordable, and sustainable alternatives to breastfeeding, WHO recommends that HIV-infected women exclusively breastfeed their infants during the first 6 months of life. It is this early period of breastfeeding that is believed to provide the maximum health benefits to the infant in terms of nutrition and protection against diarrheal and respiratory infections (WHO Collaborative Study Team on the Role of Breastfeeding on the Prevention of Infant Mortality, 2000).

A number of ongoing and planned clinical trials are addressing whether short-course ART, including HAART, given to the mother and/or infant during the lactation period can reduce transmission through breastfeeding (Gaillard et al., 2004). Recent data show that women with advanced HIV disease (i.e., with higher viral loads in their breastmilk) are more likely to transmit the virus through breastmilk, suggesting that treatment with HAART may reduce the risk of MTCT (Rousseau et al., 2003). In a study conducted among pregnant women in the United States, Europe, Brazil, and the Bahamas, single-dose nevirapine did not further reduce MTCT transmission in women who were receiving standard HAART (Dorenbaum et al., 2002). As mentioned in the 2003 WHO treatment guidelines, several countries are considering using short-course triple-combination therapy for prevention of MTCT even in women who would not yet need HAART for their own HIV infection. While HAART may not only reduce perinatal HIV transmission to the infant but also minimize the emergence of nevirapine or 3TC resistance, which is a critical problem, the potential toxicity of such intense drug exposure in both mother and fetus may preclude this approach. Further study of these issues is needed before a recommendation can be made.

As part of a recently published Institute of Medicine report entitled *Improving Birth Outcomes: Meeting the Challenge in the Developing World*, a variety of nonretroviral strategies for reducing MTCT, including cesarean section, are discussed (IOM, 2003). The report notes that while in North American and European studies, elective cesarean section reduced the risk of perinatal HIV transmission by more than 50 percent, independent of treatment with zidovudine, its use can be associated with higher complication rates in HIV-infected women. Especially problematic is use of caesarean section in developing countries, where poor medical facilities and inappropriate staffing may further foster an increased rate of maternal complications.

While research has progressed, and rates of MTCT in the developed world are declining, UNAIDS notes that prevention of MTCT is virtually nonexistent in some of the hardest-hit countries of sub-Saharan Africa, where more than 70 percent of countries report having no such programs (UNAIDS, 2003a). Even with recent drug price cuts, most resource-constrained settings cannot support the mother–child health care infrastructure required for the implementation of MTCT prophylaxis. The problem is compounded by the social stigma of HIV infection discussed earlier and by societal or individual perceptions that treatment is not available or too complicated—all factors that may discourage women from using available health care or counseling services.

Treating Children

The vast majority of the 3.2 million children living with HIV acquired the infection through MTCT, and 90 percent of these perinatal infections occurred in resource-limited settings (Mofenson, 2003a). As discussed above, the MTCT routes of transmission are transplacentally during pregnancy, during labor and delivery when the infant's skin and mucus membranes are exposed to HIV in the mother's genital tract, and postnatally through breastfeeding.

Children account for 14 percent of all new HIV infections and 16 percent of all AIDS-related deaths (UNAIDS, 2003a). Yet children are one of the most neglected populations living with HIV/AIDS for numerous reasons, including limited or challenging pediatric ART formulations (e.g., tablets too big to swallow), a belief that therapy in children may not be effective, and a lack of pediatricians and social workers specializing in the care and treatment of this population. Despite these potential limitations, pediatric ART programs in Romania and Botswana have demonstrated success in treating HIV/AIDS (Baylor International Pediatric AIDS Initiative, 2004). Moreover, it has been learned that addressing the needs of children can serve as an important point of entry to HIV/AIDS care for the entire family.

Challenges to pediatric HIV/AIDS treatment remain, however. They include the following:

- Biological and behavioral constraints imposed by the size and age of the patient
- Problems associated with infant diagnosis
- Differences in drug disposition in children
- Changes in drug disposition during development from infant to toddler to child to adolescent
- Developmental changes that affect the way a child is counseled regarding adherence
- Limited pediatric formulations and the need to break adult tablets into halves or quarters for use in children
- Poor palatability of many pediatric formulations
- The generally low priority assigned to pediatric HIV/AIDS care (children can rarely advocate for themselves)
- Lack of experience among health professionals in the treatment and monitoring of pediatric HIV/AIDS

Among the pediatric issues that should receive priority is the need for liquid formulations and appropriate FDCs to supplement the ongoing use of single drugs where a more customized regimen is needed. The need to refrigerate some pediatric formulations is a complicating factor.

The question has been raised as to whether pediatric HIV/AIDS cases should be treated separately during ART scale-up or integrated into an adult–pediatric care system. Although integrating the two might maximize the utilization of minimal resources, there is concern that children will become lost in the effort, especially since, as noted, most children do not or cannot advocate for themselves. Thus there may be advantages to establishing a dedicated team within each ART program to focus on the specific needs of children. Ideally, as the Baylor International Pediatric AIDS Initiative has shown, this would be done within the context of treating the whole family. Relevant here is the importance of recognizing, for example, the vulnerability of children to the spread of TB from contagious family members. Hence, as part of family-centered care, household contacts should be evaluated for active TB. The fact that it is often very difficult to separate children from family members with whom they live makes a "one-stop" treatment program attractive. This strategy has been so successful for the Baylor initiative that its challenge now is accepting the overwhelming number of families that wish to enroll (Kline, 2004).

The 2003 WHO guidelines for scale-up of ART provide further specific guidance on initiating treatment in both infants and children (WHO, 2003b). A particular issue awaiting better resolution is the case of the HIV-positive infant less than 18 months of age in a circumstance in which neither a CD4 percent nor a virological assay can be obtained. Current WHO guidelines indicate that asymptomatic infants less than 18 months of age (WHO Stage I) should not be placed on therapy unless a CD4 count is obtained and found to be <20 percent.

Addressing the Role of Nutrition in HIV/AIDS and Its Treatment

Malnutrition affects one in every three people worldwide. Fully 20 percent of people in the developing world are affected, and the HIV/AIDS epidemic is occurring largely in these populations. Many of the complications of HIV infection and the associated opportunistic infections can result in micro- and macronutrient deficiencies and weight loss (Nerad et al., 2003; Kotler, 2000). (Micronutrients comprise vitamins and minerals; they have a role in immune function. Macronutrients are carbohydrates, proteins, fat, and fiber; they have a role in energy balance and in preventing wasting.) The infection-related complications that lead to malnutrition include anorexia; oral and esophageal symptoms, such as pain, that limit food intake; malabsorption; and diarrhea. The resulting malnourished state in persons with HIV/AIDS further impairs immune function and can accelerate disease progression (Kiure et al., 2002).

ART can lead to improved nutritional status. However, the use of ART requires an understanding of the interactions between diet and drugs and the adverse effects than can compromise nutritional status, as well as recognition of the metabolic complications of drugs (Castleman et al., 2003). ARVs may require certain foods for absorption and efficacy, and their absorption can be influenced by the presence of food in the gastrointestinal tract. For example, a high-fat meal enhances the absorption of tenofovir (a nucleoside reverse transcriptase inhibitor [NRTI]) and inhibits the absorption of indinavir (a PI). Excess or inadequate absorption of drugs can result in clinical toxicity or the development of resistance, respectively. Of note, the five drugs recommended by WHO for first-line therapy combinations in resource-limited settings have no food requirements (U.S. DHHS, 2003). However, efavirenz, one of these five drugs, will have increased blood levels if taken with high-fat/high-calorie meals; thus it is recommended that this drug be taken on an empty stomach (U.S. DHHS, 2003).

Side effects of ART may affect nutritional status by leading to a loss of micro- and macronutrients or to decreased food consumption. For example, zidovudine (an NRTI) may cause anorexia, nausea, or vomiting. Didanosine (an NNRTI) may cause diarrhea. These adverse effects clearly could result in direct loss of nutrients in the body (e.g., from vomiting or diarrhea) or inhibition of nutrient intake (e.g., from anorexia or nausea).

Finally, the metabolic complications of therapy can affect short- and long-term morbidity and mortality. For example, the PI class of ARVs can cause changes in the metabolism of lipids and result in hypercholesterolemia and hypertriglyceridemia. This class of drugs can also result in insulin resistance, which can lead to diabetes mellitus.

As many of the clinical trials and prospective studies of ARVs and their effects have occurred in the developed world, the extent to which the relationships among disease, drugs, and nutrition are a factor of the developed world's diet and nutritional status is unclear. At this time, it is also unclear what effect malnutrition will have on the success of ART scale-up on a large scale. It is clear that many people living with HIV/AIDS in the developing world lack access to sufficient quantity and quality of nutritious foods. In a May 2003 report entitled *Nutrient Requirements for People Living with HIV/AIDS*, WHO recognizes the limited research done in this area—specifically in resource-constrained settings—and poses research questions viewed as crucial for gaining a better understanding in this area (WHO, 2003d; see also Chapter 6). It is known, however, that micro- and macronutrients affect the progression of HIV disease and the bioavailability and efficacy of particular drugs. Indeed, a recent study has suggested that supplementation with vitamin B complex, vitamin C, and vitamin E can significantly delay the progression of AIDS and associated disease complications among HIV-infected women (Fawzi et al., 2004). Clearly, then, food and nutrition assistance programs should be a resource available to those using ART.

THE IMPORTANCE OF ADHERENCE

As noted, ART for HIV/AIDS involves taking a complex regimen of drugs with, at times, unforgiving requirements, such as dosage timing and coadministration with food. Following this regimen scrupulously is central to durable and effective HIV therapeutic responses. A first step in successful adherence, however, is agreement on all the dimensions that this term should encompass. Numerous possible interpretations of adherence fall short of the recognition that to be adherent, patients must access properly stored ARVs and then take all prescribed drugs at the prescribed frequency and intervals and when called for with alimentation. Wider-than-recommended intervals can lead to intermittently suboptimal drug concentrations and a heightened risk of resistance emergence (see Chapter 3). The complexity of the task of assessing adherence defies the use of a single simple measurement. Indicative of the challenge is that investigators have pursued multiple approaches to ascertain different aspects of compliance, including the following:

- Percentage of doses taken—total doses taken/number of prescribed doses
- Proportion of days correct doses taken—number of days correct doses were taken/number of days of follow-up
- Mean doses per day—number of doses taken/number of days cap was opened
- Mean interdose interval—sum of all intervals between doses/number of doses taken
- Drug holidays—count of intervals that were more than 3 days
- Proportion of days with no doses taken—number of days with no recorded dose/number of days of follow-up
- Dose difference—mean difference between the time each dose was taken and the "correct time" as projected from the first dose
- Proportion of doses in dosing periods—two periods defined around the prescribed interval (either 4-hour or ±25 percent interval length)

The problem of poor adherence, however measured, to prescribed, self-administered medications generally is well documented, particularly for chronic and asymptomatic conditions (WHO, 2003e). As noted, however, one concern associated with poor adherence that is specific to ART is the risk of emergence of drug-resistant virus. It has been shown that even short-term poor adherence (e.g., for as little as a week) can result in rapid rebound of plasma viremia and treatment failure, progression to AIDS, the development of multidrug resistance, and death. At the population level, poor adherence leading to the emergence of resistance could compromise the long-term sustainability of ART scale-up initiatives. Resistant infections are more expensive and challenging to treat. Considering the limitations of poor countries, these challenges may effectively eliminate practical options for the second-line therapies that are used in better-resourced settings. Thus there is an urgent need to standardize the definition of adherence and the measures required to document it, to assess reasons for poor adherence, and to address the problem through culturally appropriate strategies. This need is addressed in Chapter 6 as a topic for operations research.

> **Recommendation 4-7. Antiretroviral therapy program managers, international donors, and national planners should take the necessary measures and provide resources to ensure the strict adherence to therapy that is fundamental to program success. Such measures should include timely and adequate provision of drugs and health care, knowledgeable and available providers, and appropriate patient education.** *ART programs should encourage community involvement in the development of adherence interventions. This involvement should include people living with HIV/AIDS, family members, and community and religious leaders. Additionally, in special populations—such as migrant workers, trucking and transportation workers, and the military—multisite and transnational program links may need to be established.*

Poor adherence is common. Several U.S. studies have assessed adherence rates and their implications for HIV/AIDS. In a U.S. study of rural patients receiving ART, only 50 percent of the patients reported consistent adherence within the previous week (Heckman et al., 2004). In another U.S. study, nearly 33 percent of patients reported having missed a medication dose in the past 5 days, and 18 percent had missed doses weekly over the past 3 months; the frequency of missed doses correlated with detectable viral loads (Catz et al., 2000). In another U.S. study involving 185 patients at the Johns Hopkins Outpatient Center, cumulative adherence was only 70 to 89 percent; the missing of a single scheduled clinic visit in the previous month was associated with increased viral rebound and clinically significant resistance (Sethi et al., 2003). In yet another prospective cohort study of 140 HIV-infected individuals at a county hospital HIV clinic, subjects took 71 percent of prescribed doses over a 48-week period, with more than 95 percent of patients achieving suboptimal adherence (i.e., less than 95 percent) (Golin et al., 2002).

Many factors contribute to poor adherence (see Box 4-4). In a recent

WHO report on adherence to long-term therapies, the simplicity of the dosage regimen (e.g., using FDCs) and drug side effects were identified as the two most important therapy-related factors influencing adherence (WHO, 2003e).

About 25–33 percent of patients experience either short- or long-term side effects while using ART. These side effects include diarrhea, nausea, stomach pains, fatigue, lipodystrophy, and neuropathies. Results of a number of studies indicate that the existence of side effects per se is not as important in affecting adherence as the patient's capacity to tolerate them. Patients may be able to tolerate very uncomfortable side effects if they have sufficient support and motivation.

Financial constraints can affect adherence as well. In a study of HIV/AIDS patients in Botswana, the cost of therapy was found to be the most significant barrier to adherence; 44 percent of patients self-reported that the cost of the treatment directly interfered with their ability to comply with the regimen (Weiser et al., 2003).

Another factor affecting adherence is the patient's readiness to begin and maintain treatment (Tuldra and Wu, 2002). Since daily ART is a reminder of HIV/AIDS and potential death, many patients do not want to be on therapy at all. "Battle fatigue" can arise from the continuous need to struggle to be adherent and behave according to instruction. These observations emphasize the need to enlist patients as partners in their care and to ask them whether they feel ready to begin therapy for HIV/AIDS.

Patient education and continued support during therapy can also affect adherence. Education and support can be provided by a number of people on a health care team. One study showed that pharmacist-led interventions, which included educational counseling and telephone support, significantly improved adherence. Reminders offered by health care providers or technological devices can improve adherence. The use of alarmed medical vials and handheld devices to remind patients to take their medication have improved adherence in resource-rich settings (Simoni et al., 2003).

Direct supervision of medication intake can improve adherence. In Haiti, community health workers visit patients with HIV/AIDS in their homes daily to assist them with ART and provide support and referral when questions or complications arise (see Chapter 3 for a discussion of this program) (WHO, 2003f). The program has been found to reduce mortality, to lessen AIDS-related stigma, and to be effective in terms of clinical and virological criteria (Farmer et al., 2001). It is possible, however, that these successful outcomes are not attributable solely to the program, but may be due in part to intensive community support for these people living with HIV/AIDS (Liechty and Bangsberg, 2003). Another factor to consider before embarking on such a program is patient confidentiality. Given the

---

BOX 4-4
At a Glance: Factors That May Affect
Adherence to Medical Therapy

Patient variables
- Education level
- Economic situation
- Mental health (e.g., depression)
- Substance abuse
- Fear of stigma and discrimination

Treatment regimen
- Continuous supply of medications
- Cost burden to patient
- Number of pills
- Number of times during the day that therapy is required
- Side effects
- Toxicity
- Food restrictions or requirements

Disease characteristics
- Degree of symptoms
- Illness severity

Patient–provider relationship
- Patient's perception of provider's competence
- Trust
- Open communication
- Willingness to include patient in treatment decisions
- Common language shared between patient and provider

Clinical setting
- Clinic distance from home
- Access to transportation
- Access to child care
- Convenience in scheduling appointments
- Assurance of confidentiality
- Participation in a clinical trial
- Involvement of community support, such as other people living with HIV/AIDS

SOURCES: Ickovics and Meade, 2002; Lanlece et al., 2003; Orrell et al., 2003; Weiser et al., 2003.

---

stigma and discrimination that have been associated with HIV/AIDS, as discussed earlier in this chapter, patients may not want their status disclosed to a community health worker observing them (Liechty and Bangsberg, 2003).

Studies have shown that good adherence is feasible in resource-constrained settings under certain circumstances. Adherence in some such settings exceeds that often observed in the United States. In a 48-week South African study of adherence among 289 indigent HIV-infected patients, mean adherence was 93.5 percent; there was no association between level of adherence and socioeconomic status, sex, or HIV stage (Orrell et al., 2003). And in a 2-year Senegalese study of adherence in 158 patients, patients had taken 91 percent of each monthly dose, on average, and all patients reported having taken the full monthly dose during two-thirds of the months studied (Laniece et al., 2003).

Improved adherence with FDCs was found in a retrospective study from Spain (Ibarra et al., 2003). In this study of 76 patients, mean adherence improved from 93.7 to 96.1 percent ($p < 0.01$). Similarly, a 16-week study comparing a combination tablet of lamivudine and zidovudine administered with a PI and a regimen with all three of these drugs administered separately found that patients in the former group were less likely to miss doses at week 8 ($p = 0.007$) and week 16 ($p = 0.046$) (Eron et al., 2000). The two regimens studied had similar clinical outcome with respect to treatment failure.

FDCs can improve adherence for two reasons. First, they reduce pill burden. This has the clinical benefit of preventing a patient from using only mono or dual therapy, which, as noted previously, has been shown to cause treatment failure and drug resistance. In a meta-analysis of 23 clinical trials involving 31 independent treatment groups, higher pill burden was associated with fewer patients with plasma HIV RNA levels ≤ 50 copies/ml at 48 weeks ($p < 0.01$) (Bartlett et al., 2001). This result suggests that, while different drug combinations may provide comparable activity in terms of pharmacokinetics, differences in daily pill burden can significantly affect treatment outcomes. Second, FDCs eliminate the need to purchase more than one drug, which may reduce costs and, in turn, improve adherence to a prescribed regimen. Additionally, FDCs can simplify supply management since fewer pills need to be accounted for, ordered, and distributed.

Recognizing the benefit of FDCs, WHO recommends their use in ART scale-up programs when the formulations are available and of assured quality with proven bioequivalence. Of note, not all of the FDCs listed by WHO in its recommendations for scale-up have been prequalified as of this writing. More studies are needed to compare FDCs, blister packaging of the single formulations, and "loose" single formulations.

INTEGRATION OF PREVENTION AND TREATMENT

With 40 million people currently infected with HIV, 6 million in need of immediate treatment, and funding and resources to meet only a fraction of this need, it will be important for extensive prevention activities to be conducted while ART scale-up proceeds. Indeed, prevention and treatment need not be regarded as mutually exclusive efforts (Blower and Farmer, 2003); they can and should work in parallel and even synergistically. Though details regarding prevention are largely beyond the scope of this report, prevention activities should include general HIV health communication and education; counseling and testing; efforts to delay sexual activity for youth; encouragement of correct and consistent condom use with casual partners and in other circumstances associated with risk; and targeted prevention initiatives for high-risk transmitters, such as female sex workers, long-distance truckers, and military populations. Prevention messages must be sensitive to local cultural interpretations. For example, in some settings, "faithfulness" or "fidelity" may not be understood as monogamy. Some believe one can be "faithful" to a small number of regular partners. The existence of regular sexual networks can challenge the interpretation of the word "casual." Conceptualizations such as "zero grazing" may be better understood.

The introduction of ART on the scale proposed by WHO, UNAIDS, and the President's Emergency Plan for AIDS Relief (PEPFAR) could have a direct secondary beneficial effect on HIV prevention, but the major impact could be indirect through the increased public attention paid to HIV, widespread testing and counseling, and stigma reduction that could accompany such programs. HIV/AIDS treatment will have the primary impact of decreasing morbidity and mortality; if accompanied by prevention counseling, it should also reduce transmission from persons under treatment by altering behavior and theoretically by reducing viral load and infectivity (Blower and Farmer, 2003; Blower et al., 2000, 2003a). Additionally, as noted earlier, the availability of ART may increase the use of VTC, which serves as a cornerstone of prevention activities by providing hope to those currently discouraged from being tested and treated.

Recommendation 4-8. National and international program planners should coordinate and integrate stronger and more effective HIV/AIDS prevention initiatives concurrently with the scale-up of antiretroviral therapy programs. *Prevention initiatives should focus on those at risk for acquiring or transmitting HIV infection, in addition to those receiving treatment. To be optimally successful, voluntary counseling and testing programs and programs to prevent mother-to-child transmission should encompass both preventive and therapeutic dimensions.*

National and community leaders should be strong advocates for effective HIV prevention efforts and engage government agencies and community groups in sectors beyond health, including education and public relations, as well as legislative leaders (to prevent discrimination).

In 2003, the U.S. Centers for Disease Control and Prevention and other U.S. health, research, and policy-making organizations developed recommendations for incorporating HIV prevention initiatives into HIV treatment plans in the United States (CDC, 2003). The three main components recommended were (1) screening for HIV transmission risk behaviors, for sexually transmitted diseases (whose presence is often an indication of potential risk for acquiring HIV), and for pregnancy; (2) providing brief behavioral risk-reduction interventions in an office setting (e.g., offering simple, straightforward messages about the use of condoms and clarifying misconceptions about infectiousness while on ART) and referring selected patients for additional interventions; and (3) facilitating notification and counseling of sexual and needle-sharing partners of infected persons. It is as yet unclear how to apply some of these recommendations most effectively in the cultural milieu of different resource-constrained settings. Operations research can help identify the best alternatives. One potential concern in particular resource-constrained settings relates to the third of these recommendations: in cultures where HIV/AIDS is clouded by stigma and discrimination, partner notification under a "forced" disclosure policy could result in abuse and violence. This concern, however, should not be an excuse for inaction or timidity in addressing an important need, but rather a stimulus for exploring new approaches to involving male partners.

The 1996 National Research Council report *Preventing and Mitigating AIDS in Sub-Saharan Africa: Research and Data Priorities for the Social and Behavioral Sciences* reviews 26 AIDS prevention programs in Africa. These include a variety of community-, population-, and institution-based intervention programs. The report documents changes resulting from these programs, including more condom usage, reductions in teenage sexual activity and in numbers of sexual partners, improvements in fidelity and treatment and control of sexually transmitted diseases, and reductions in HIV seroconversion (National Research Council, 1996). More-recent African studies involving community and family approaches likewise document the potential of preventive interventions (Roth et al., 2001). It is worth noting, however, that some of this work has also highlighted underreporting of unprotected sex by study participants (Allen et al., 2003).

As noted above, placing infected persons on ART can impact the prevention of some new cases through prevention counseling and decreases in viral load. Quinn and colleagues (2000) report from a community-based study of more than 15,000 persons in Uganda that the mean serum HIV-1

RNA viral load level was significantly higher among HIV-1–positive subjects whose partners had seroconverted than among those whose partners had not seroconverted (90,254 copies per milliliter vs. 38,029 copies per milliliter, p = 0.01). Reflecting the population benefits of suppressed viral replication, no instances of transmission were noted from the 51 HIV-infected partners with less than 1,500 copies per milliliter. Overall in this community, however, transmission was substantial, with 90 of 415 initially seronegative partners seroconverting (11.8 per 100 person-years) (Quinn et al., 2000). Modeling studies also suggest that suppression of viral load in a high proportion of infected people can significantly reduce transmission in a population (Blower et al., 2000, 2003a, 2004).

While treatment for HIV/AIDS could positively impact the prevention of new cases by decreasing viral load and reducing the infectiousness of those already afflicted with the disease, past experience with the introduction of treatment in the developed world has highlighted the potential for an increase in behaviors linked to HIV/AIDS transmission (Blower and Farmer, 2003; Blower et al., 2000, 2001). Substantial decreases in HIV mortality in the United States and other developed countries have been accompanied by a resurgence of HIV infection rates among some communities of gay men in these countries (Katz et al., 2002; Miller et al., 2000).

An observational study of adults—mainly homosexual men—with AIDS in the era of HAART found an increase in sexually transmitted infections over a 4-year period in the late 1990s. A survey of 54 homosexual men found that 26 percent felt "less concerned about becoming HIV-positive" with the availability of ART. This increase in risky behavior following receipt of ART in the developed world has not been documented for other risk groups (e.g., intravenous drug abusers, heterosexuals). Factors that could contribute to this increase in risk behaviors, also called "disinhibition," include a greater sense of security from knowing that therapy is available and improved health, leading to more or resumption of higher-risk sexual activities. Another concern is that the increase in life expectancy that can be brought about by ART affords a greater opportunity for HIV-positive persons to infect others (although as noted, treated patients should have decreased HIV viral load burdens and thus be less infectious).

Modeling has been used to predict the interactions between use of ART and risk behaviors and the subsequent effect on HIV prevalence. Given otherwise optimal ART scale-up conditions (i.e., use of potent regimens that completely suppress viral replication, near-perfect adherence, and widespread use), but absent efforts to prevent increased risk behaviors, the potential benefits of increased ARV usage could be masked by increased transmission resulting from such behaviors, as was seen in the gay community in the United States (Blower and Farmer, 2003; Blower et al., 2000, 2003a,b, 2004; Velasco-Hernandez et al., 2002). Evidence from both empirical and modeling studies, then, demonstrates that HIV prevention activities must be strengthened and integrated into ART scale-up programs if success in combating the pandemic is to be achieved.

PALLIATIVE CARE FOR AIDS PATIENTS IN DEVELOPING COUNTRIES

Despite advances in the treatment of AIDS patients and the potential for adding even decades of additional quality life to what might have been the case without ARVs, many of these persons will eventually face death due to the infection. Thus a humane approach to this disease includes steadfast care not only while the patient is responsive to ARVs, but also when all that can be offered is palliative care. Comprehensive national programs to care for patients with HIV/AIDS should address the needs of those who are in the terminal stage of AIDS.

WHO defines palliative care as care that:

- Provides relief from pain and other distressing symptoms.
- Affirms life and regards dying as a normal process.
- Intends neither to hasten nor to postpone death.
- Integrates the psychological and spiritual aspects of patient care.
- Offers a support system to help patients live as actively as possible until death.
- Offers a support system to help the family cope during the patient's illness and in its own bereavement.
- Uses a team approach to address the needs of patients and its families, including bereavement counseling, if indicated.
- Enhances quality of life and may also positively influence the course of illness.
- Is applicable early in the course of illness in conjunction with other therapies intended to prolong life, such as chemotherapy or radiation therapy, and includes those investigations needed to better understand and manage distressing clinical complications.

There are particular challenges to palliative care in developing countries. Palliative care of terminal AIDS patients often centers on pain management. A Ugandan study found that more than half of terminally ill patients cited pain as their chief problem (Kikule, 2003). Morphine and other analgesic opioids are inexpensive, though tight regulations hinder their availability in developing countries (Carlisle, 2003). Table 4-3, based on 2001 figures for per capita morphine consumption in African countries heavily affected by HIV/AIDS, highlights this problem. According to David Joranson of the Pain and Policy Studies Group, University of Wisconsin/

TABLE 4-3 Per Capita Consumption of Morphine, 2001

Country	Per Capita Consumption (mg)
Global mean	5.9
Africa regional mean	0.5
South Africa	3.7
Namibia	2.5
Botswana	1.7
Uganda	0.1
Tanzania	0.09
Zambia	0.03
Rwanda	0.01
Mozambique	0.01
Kenya	0.003
Cote d'Ivoire	0.002
Ethiopia	0.0002
Nigeria, Haiti, and Guyana	NA[a]

[a]NA = not available. These countries did not report for 2001.
NOTE: 2001 consumption is estimated with 2000 United Nations Population Data.
SOURCE: David Joranson, Pain and Policy Studies Group, University of Wisconsin/WHO Collaborating Center, using 2003 International Narcotics Control Board and United Nations *Demographic Yearbook*, 2000.

WHO Collaborating Center, the 14 countries originally selected for PEPFAR accounted for only 0.8 percent of the world's morphine consumption in 2001 (personal communication to Hellen Gelband). Joranson further notes:

All of the 14 governments are parties to the United Nation's Single Convention on Narcotic Drugs, 1961, but it is clear from the consumption statistics that there has been little effort aimed at ensuring the availability of opioids which is a treaty obligation. This may be due to many reasons, or barriers, involving pain relief being a low healthcare priority in cancer and AIDS, lack of infrastructure to deliver medical care and pain relief, lack of medical demand (prescriptions) for opioids, inadequate education of physicians, general misunderstanding and fear of morphine, and lack of governmental action.

It has been reported that patients in India have significant difficulty receiving morphine because of government fears of its diversion for nonmedical use (Ghooi and Ghooi, 2003). Culture-specific palliative guidelines are rare, though some research has been done. A recent study to determine the palliative needs of Ugandans concluded that a "good death" occurs when patients are at home, free from pain, and without stigma, and do not feel dependent on others for their basic needs (Kikule, 2003).

WHO's Program on Cancer Control and Departments of Care for HIV-AIDS are currently enganged in an intitiative to enhance palliative care in southern Africa. The principal objectives are as follows (WHO, 2004b):
- To develop/reinforce palliative care programs with a public health approach in response to the needs and gaps identified, considering:
  — A holistic approach to palliative care, giving special emphasis to pain relief.
  — A systemic approach to program implementation that considers policy development, provision of care, drug availability, training, and education in the context of HIV/AIDS and cancer health problems.
  — Integration with the existing health system at all levels of care, with special emphasis on home-based care.
  — A team approach at the organizational and care levels.
  — The elements of good quality performance, including improving access, acceptability, efficiency, and effectiveness.
- To advocate for drug availability and policy development among the governments of the participating countries.
- To develop a network among the participating countries that will:
  — Promote the exchange of information and collaboration.
  — Advocate for the integration of such programs into national strategic plans for health and social services.

WHO Staging System for HIV Infection and Disease in Adults and Adolescents[1]

Stage I
- Asymptomatic
- Generalized lymphadenopathy
Performance scale 1: asymptomatic, normal activity

Stage II
- Weight loss, < 10% of body weight
- Minor mucocutaneous manifestations (seborrheic dermatitis, prurigo, fungal nail infections, recurrent oral ulcerations, angular cheilitis)
- Herpes zoster within the last 5 years
- Recurrent upper respiratory tract infections (e.g., bacterial sinusitis)
And/or performance scale 2: symptomatic, normal activity

Stage III
- Weight loss, > 10% of body weight
- Unexplained chronic diarrhea, > 1 month
- Unexplained prolonged fever (intermittent or constant) > 1 month
- Oral candidiasis
- Oral hairy leucoplakia
- Pulmonary tuberculosis
- Severe bacterial infections (i.e., pneumonia, pyomyositis)

And/or performance scale 3: bedridden < 50% of the day during the last month

Stage IV
- HIV wasting syndrome
- *Pneumocystis carinii* pneumonia
- Toxoplasmosis of the brain
- Cryptosporidiosis with diarrhea > 1 month
- Cryptococcosis, extrapulmonary
- Cytomegalovirus disease of an organ other than liver, spleen, or lymph nodes (i.e., retinitis)
- Herpes simplex virus infection, mucocutaneous (> 1 month) or visceral
- Progressive multifocal leucoencephalopathy
- Any disseminated endemic mycosis
- Candidiasis of esophagus, trachea, bronchi
- Atypical mycobacterioris, disseminated or lungs
- Nontyphoid salmonella septicemia
- Extrapulmonary tuberculosis
- Lymphoma
- Kaposi's sarcoma
- HIV encephalopathy

And/or performance scale 4: bedridden > 50% of the day during the last month

[1]Appendix B. WHO Staging System for HIV Infection and Disease in Adults and Adolescents. Scaling up antiretroviral therapy in resource-limited settings: Treatment guidelines for a public health approach. 2003 Revision. World Health Organization 2003.

REFERENCES

Allen S, Meinzen-Derr J, Kautzman M, Zulu I, Trask S, Fideli U, Musonda R, Kasolo F, Gau F, Haworth A. 2003. Sexual behavior of HIV discordant couples after HIV counseling and testing. *AIDS* 17(5):733–740.

Bartlett JA, DeMasi R, Quinn J, Moxham C, Rouseau F. 2001. Overview of the effectiveness of triple combination therapy in antiretroviral-naive HIV-1 infected adults. *AIDS* 15:1369–1377.

Baylor International Pediatric AIDS Initiative. 2004. *Baylor International Pediatric AIDS Initiative Homepage*. [Online]. Available: http://bayloraids.org/ [accessed February 19, 2004].

Blower SM, Farmer P. 2003. Predicting the public health impact of antiretrovirals: Preventing HIV in developing countries. *AIDScience* 3(11).

Blower SM, Gershengorn HB, Grant RM. 2000. A tale of two futures: HIV and antiretroviral therapy in San Francisco. *Science* 287:650–654.

Blower SM, Aschenbach AN, Gershengorn HB, Kahn JO. 2001. Predicting the unpredictable: Transmission of drug-resistant HIV. *Nature Medicine* 7(9):1016–1020.

Blower SM, Ma L, Farmer P, Koenig S. 2003a. Predicting the impact of antiretrovirals in resource poor settings: Preventing HIV infections whilst controlling drug resistance. *Current Drug Targets-Infectious Disorders* 3:345–353.

Blower SM, Schwartz EJ, Mills J. 2003b. Forcasting the future of HIV epidemics: The impact of antiretroviral therapies and imperfect vaccines. *AIDS Reviews* 5(2):113–125.

Blower SM, Bodine EJ, Kahn J, McFarland W. 2004. The impact of the antiretroviral rollout on drug resistant HIV in Africa: Insights from empirical data & theoretical models. *AIDS* [in press].

Campos PE, Suarez PG, Swanchez J, Zavala D, Arevalo J, Ticona E, Nolan CM, Hooton TM, Holmes KK. 2003. Multidrug resistant *Mycobacterium tuberculosis* in HIV-infected persons in Peru: Prevalence and risk factors. *Emerging Infectious Diseases* 9:1571–1578.

Carlisle D. 2003. Africans are dying of AIDS without pain relief. *British Medical Journal* 327:1069.

Castleman T, Suemo-Fosso E, Cogill B. 2003. *Food and Nutrition Implications of Antiretroviral Therapy in Resource Limited Settings. Food and Nutrition Technical Assistance Project. Academy for Educational Development*. [Online]. Available: http://www.fantaproject.org/downloads/pdfs/tn7_ARVs.pdf [accessed July 29, 2004].

Catz SL, Kelly JA, Bogart LM, Benotsch EG, McAuliffe TL. 2000. Patterns, correlates, and barriers to medication adherence among persons prescribed new treatment for HIV disease. *Health Psychology* 19:124–133.

CDC (Centers for Disease Control and Prevention). 2003. *Incorporating HIV Prevention into the Medical Care of Persons Living with HIV: Recommendations of CDC, the Health Resources and Services Administration, the National Institutes of Health, and the HIV Medicine Association of the Infectious Diseases Society of America*. [Online]. Available: www.cdc.gov/mmwr/PDF/rr/rr5212.pdf [accessed February 21, 2004].

CDC. 2004. *Global Aids Program: Strategies. 2.1 Voluntary Counseling and Testing (VCT)*. [Online]. Available: http://www.cdc.gov/nchstp/od/gap/Strategies/2_1_vct.htm [accessed July 29, 2004].

Columbia University Mailman School of Public Health. 2004. *MTCT-Plus: Saving Mothers, Saving Families*. [Online]. Available: http://www.mtctplus.org/index.html [accessed July 29, 2004].

Corbett E, Watt C, Walker N, Maher D, Williams B, Raviglione M, Dye C. 2003. The growing burden of tuberculosis. *Archives of Internal Medicine* 163(9):1009–1021.

DeCock KM, Fowler MG, Mercier E, de Vincenzi I, Saba J, Hoff E, Alnwick DJ, Rogers M, Shaffer N. 2000. Prevention of mother-to-child HIV transmission in resource-poor countries: Translating research into policy and practice. *Journal of the American Medical Association* 283:1175–1182.

Diagbouga S, Chazallon C, Kazatchkine MD, van dePerre P, Inwoley A, M'boup S, David MP, Tenin AT, Soudre R, Aboulker JP, Weiss L. 2003. Successful implementation of a low-cost method for enumerating CD4+ T lymphocytes in resource-limited settings: The ANRS 12-26 study. *AIDS* 17:2201–2208.

Dorenbaum A, Cunnungham CK, Gelber RD, Culnane M, Mofenson L, Britto P, Rekacewicz C, Newell ML, Delfraissy JF, Cunningham-Schrader B, Mirochnick M, Sullivan JL, International PACT G 316 Team. 2002. Two-dose intrapartum/newborn nevirapine and standard antiretroviral therapy to reduce perinatal HIV-1 transmission: A randomized trial. *Journal of the American Medical Association* 288:189–198.

Dunkle K, Jewkes R, Brown H, Gray G, McIntryre J, Harlow S. 2004. Gender-based violence, relationship power, and risk of HIV infection in women attending antenatal clinics in South Africa. *Lancet* 363(9419):1415–1421.

Elzinga G, Nunn P. 2002. TB and HIV: Joint problems, joint solutions? *Bulletin of the World Health Organization* 80(6):469–470.

Eron JJ, Yetzer ES, Ruane PJ, Becker S, Sawyer GA, Fisher RL, Tolson JM, Schaefer MS. 2000. Efficacy, safety, and adherence with a twice-daily combination lamivudine/zidovudine tablet formulation, plus a protease inhibitor, in HIV infection. *AIDS* 14:671–681.

European Collaborative Study. 2001. HIV-infected pregnant women and vertical transmission in Europe since 1986. *AIDS* 15(6):761–770.

Farmer P, Leandre F, Mukherjee J, Gupta R, Tarter L, Kim JY. 2001. Community-based treatment of advanced HIV disease: Introducing DOT-HAART (directly observed therapy with highly active antiretroviral therapy). *Bulletin of the World Health Organization* 79(12):1145–1151.

Fawzi W, Msamanga G, Spiegelman D, Wei R, Kapiga S, Villamor E, Mwakagile D, Mugusi F, Hertzmakr E, Essex M, Hunter D. 2004. A randomized trial of multivitamin supplements and HIV disease progression and mortality. *New England Journal of Medicine* 351(1):23–32.

Fennelly K, Ellner J. 2004. Tuberculosis. In: Gorbach, Bartlett, Blacklow, eds. *Infectious Diseases*, 3rd Edition. Philadelphia, PA: Lippincott, Williams & Wilkins.

Fitzgerald, D. 2004 (January 27). *Lessons Learned from the Use of ARVs in Very Low-Resource Settings: The Haiti Experience.* Paper presented at the Institute of Medicine Workshop on Antiretroviral Scale-up in Resource Constrained Settings. Washington, DC. Institute of Medicine Committee on Antiretroviral Drugs in Resource-Constrained Settings.

Fleischman J. 2003. *Fatal Vulnerabilities: Reducing the Acute Risk of HIV/AIDS among Women and Girls. Center for Strategic and International Studies Task Force on HIV/AIDS.* [Online]. Available: http://www.csis.org/africa/0302_fatalvulnerabilities.pdf [accessed July 29, 2004].

Fleischman J. 2004. *Breaking the Cycle: Ensuring Equitable Access to HIV Treatment for Women and Girls. Center for Strategic and International Studies Task Force on HIV/AIDS.* [Online]. Available: http://www.csis.org/africa/0402_breakingcycle.pdf [accessed July 29, 2004].

Gaillard P, Fowler MG, Dabis F, Coovadia H, Van der Horst C, Van Rompay K, Ruff A, Taha T, Thomas T, DeVincenzi I, Newell ML, Ghent IAS Working Group on HIV in Women and Children. 2004. Use of antiretroviral drugs to prevent HIV-1 transmission through breastfeeding. From animal studies to randomized clinical trials. *Journal of Acquired Immune Deficiency Syndrome* 35:178–187.

Ghooi RB, Ghooi SR. 2003. Freedom from pain: A mirage or a possibility? Experience in attempts to change laws and practices in India. *Journal of Pain & Palliative Care Pharmacotherapy* 17:3–4.

Golin CE Liu H, Hays RD, Miller LG, Beck CK, Ickovics J, Kaplan AH, Wenger NS. 2002. A prospective study of predictors of adherence to combination antiretroviral medication. *Journal of General Internal Medicine* 17:756–765.

Gorkom J. 2003 (February 3–6). *TB/HIV Lessons Learned: ProTEST Meeting.* Paper presented at the ProTEST Lessons Learned Workshop, Durban, South Africa.

Grimwade K, Swingler G. 2004. Cotrimoxazole prophylaxis for opportunistic infections in adults with HIV (Cochrane Review). In: *The Cochrane Library,* Issue 2. Chichester, UK: John Wiley & Sons.

Gupta R, Irwin A, Raviglione M, Kim J. 2004. Scaling up treatment for HIV/AIDS: Lessons learned from multi-drug resistant tuberculosis. *Lancet* 363:320–324.

Harries A, Hargreaves N, Chimzizi R, Salaniponi. 2002. Highly active antiretroviral therapy and tuberculosis control in Africa: Synergies and potential. *Bulletin of the World Health Organization* 80(6):464–469.

Havlir D, Barnes P. 1999. Tuberculosis in patients with human immunodeficiency virus infection. *New England Journal of Medicine* 340(5):367–373.

Heckman BD, Anderson ES, Sikkema KJ, Kochman A, Kalichman SC, Anderson T. 2004. Adherence to antiretroviral therapy in rural persons living with HIV disease in the United States. *AIDS Care* 16:219–230.

Heise L, Ellsberg M, Gottemoeller M. 1999. Ending violence against women. *Population Reports, Series L,* no. 11. Baltimore, MD: Johns Hopkins University School of Public Health, Population Information Program. [Online]. Available: http://www.infoforhealth. org/pr/l11/violence.pdf [accessed July 29, 2004].

Ibarra I, Martin-Bengoechea MJ, Peral J, Santos A, Illaro A, Lertxundi U. 2003. Assessing adherence in a treatment simplification. 2nd IAS Conference on HIV Pathogenesis and Treatment, Paris.

Ickovics JR, Meade CS. 2002. Adherence to antiretroviral therapy among patients with HIV: A critical link between behavioral and biomedical sciences. *Journal of Acquired Immune Deficiency Syndrome* 31:98–102.

IOM (Institute of Medicine). 2003. *Improving Birth Outcomes: Meeting the Challenge in the Developing World.* Washington, DC: The National Academies Press.

Jourdain G, Ngo-Giang-Huong N, Tungyai P, Kummee A, Bowonwatanwong C, Kantipong P, Lechanachai P, Hammer S, Lallemant M; Perinatal HIV Prevention Trial Group. 2004 (February 8–11). *Exposure to Intrapartum Single-Dose Nevirapine and Subsequent Maternal 6-Month Response to NNRTI-Based Regimens.* Paper presented at the 11th Conference on Retroviruses and Opportunistic Infections, San Francisco, CA.

Katz MH, Schwarz SK, Kellogg TA, Klausner JD, Dilley JW, Gibson S, McFarland W. 2002. Impact of highly active antiretroviral treatment on HIV seroincidence among men who have sex with men: San Francisco. *American Journal of Public Health* 92:388–394.

Kikule E. 2003. A good death in Uganda: Survey of needs for palliative care for terminally ill people in urban areas. *British Medical Journal* 327:192–194.

Kim J. 2004 (January 27). *The Challenge of HIV in 2004 and the UNAIDS/WHO "3 by 5" Program.* Paper presented at the Institute of Medicine Workshop on Antiretroviral Drug Use in Resource Constrained Settings, Washington, DC. Institute of Medicine Board on Global Health.

Kiure A, Msamanga G, Fawzi W. 2002. Nutrition and HIV infection. In: Essex M, Mboup S, Kanki P, Marlink R, Tlou S, eds. *AIDS in Africa.* 2nd Edition. Boston, MA: Plenum Publishers.

Kline M. 2004 (January 27). *Pediatric Considerations for ARV Programs in Resource-Constrained Settings.* Paper presented at the Institute of Medicine Workshop on Antiretroviral Scale-up in Resource Constrained Settings, Washington, DC. Institute of Medicine Committee on Antiretroviral Drug Use in Resource-Constrained Settings.

Kotler D. 2000. Nutritional Alterations Associated with HIV Infection. *Journal of AIDS Research* 25(Supplement 1):s81–s87.

Laniece I, Ciss M, Desclaux A, Diop K, Mbodj F, Ndiaye B, Sylla O, Delaporte E, Ndoye I. 2003. Adherence to HAART and its principle determinants in a cohort of Senegalese adults. *AIDS* 17:S103–S108.

Levi GC, Vitória MA. 2002. Fighting against AIDS: The Brazilian experience. *AIDS* 16:2373–2383.

Liechty C, Bangsberg D. 2003. Doubts about DOT: Antiretroviral therapy in resource-poor countries. *AIDS* 17:1383–1387.

London School of Hygiene and Tropical Medicine. 2002. *Issue No. 000004: The Cost Effectiveness of the Zambian ProTEST Project.* [Online]. Available: http://www.lshtm.ac.uk/dfid/tb/Briefing%20Note%205.htm [accessed March 31, 2004].

Maman S, Mbwambo J, Hogan N, Kilonzo G, Campbell J, Weiss E, Sweat M. 2002. HIV-positive women report more lifetime partner violence: Findings from a voluntary counseling and testing clinic in Dar es Salaam, Tanzania. *American Journal of Public Health* 92(8):1331–1337.

Mbori-Ngacha D. 2001. Morbidity and mortality in breastfed and formula-fed infants of HIV-1-infected women: A randomized clinical trial. *Journal of the American Medical Association* 286(19):2413–2420.

Miller M, Meyer L, Boufassa F, Persoz A, Sarr A, Robain M, Spira A. 2000. Sexual behavior changes and protease inhibitor therapy. *AIDS* 14:F33–F39.

Miotti PG, Taha TE, Kumwenda NI, Broadhead R, Mtimavalye LA, Van der Hoeven L, Chiphangwi JD, Liomba G, Biggar RJ. 1999. HIV transmission through breastfeeding: A study in Malawi. *Journal of the American Medical Association* 282(8):744–749

Mofenson L. 2003a. Tale of two epidemics: The continuing challenge of preventing mother-to-child transmission of human immunodeficiency virus. *The Journal of Infectious Diseases* 187:721–724.

Mofenson L. 2003b. Advances in the prevention of HIV vertical transmission. *Seminars in Pediatric Infectious Diseases* 14(4):295–308.

Moodley D, Moodley J, Coovadia H, Gray G, McIntyre J, Hofmyer J, Nikodem C, Hall D, Gigliotti M, Robinson P, Boshoff L, Sullivan JL, South African Intrapartum Nevirapine Trial (SAINT) Investigators. 2003. A multicenter randomized controlled trial of nevirapine versus a combination of zidovudine and lamivudine to reduce intrapartum and early postpartum mother-to-child transmission of HIV-1. *Journal of Infectious Diseases* 187:725–735.

MSF Briefing Note. 2004 (February). *Two Pills a Day Saving Lives: Fixed-Dose Combinations (FDCs) of Antiretroviral Drugs.* Geneva: Medécins sans Frontières.

National Research Council. 1996. Preventing and Mitigating AIDS in sub-Saharan Africa: Research and Data Priorities for the Social and Behavioral Sciences. Washington, DC: National Academy Press.

Nduati R, Mbori-Ngacha D, Richardson B, Overbaugh J, Mwatha A, Ndinya-Achola J, Bwayo J, Onyango FE, Hughes J, Kreiss J. 2000. Effect of breastfeeding and formula feeding on transmission of HIV-1: A randomized clinical trial. *Journal of the American Medical Association* 283:1167–1174.

Nerad J, Romcyn M, Silverman E, Allen-Reid J, Dieterich D, Merchant J, A Pelletier V, Tinnerello D, Fenton M. 2003. General nutrition management in patients infected with human immunodeficiency virus. *Clinical Infectious Diseases* 36(Supplement 2).

NIH (National Institutes of Health). 2003. *Fogarty International Center Announces First Awards for Research Program in Stigma and Global Health.* [Online]. Available: http://www.nih.gov/news/pr/oct2003/fic-27.htm [accessed August 24, 2004].

Nyazema NZ, Khoza S, Landman I, Sibanda E, Gael K. 2000. Antiretroviral (ARV) drug utilisation in Harare. *Central African Journal of Medicine* 46(4):89–93.

Orrell C, Bangsberg DR, Badri M, Wood R. 2003. Adherence is not a barrier to successful antiretroviral therapy in South Africa. *AIDS* 17:1369–1375.

Phillips D. 2004. *Making Women Central to Family Care: Global Health Council.* [Online]. Available: http://www.globalhealth.org/reports/report.php3?id=139 [accessed July 29, 2004].

Quinn TC, Wawer MJ, Sewankambo N, Serwadda D, Li C, Wabwire-Mangen F, Meehan MO, Lutalo T, Gray RH. 2000. Viral load and heterosexual transmission of human immunodeficiency virus type 1. *New England Journal of Medicine* 342(13):921–929.

Ridzon R, Mayanja-Kizza H. 2002. Tuberculosis. In: Essex, M, Mboup S, Kanki P, Marlink R, Tlou S, eds. *AIDS in Africa.* 2nd Edition. Boston, MA: Plenum Publishers.

Roth DL, Stewart KE, Clay OJ, van der Straten A, Karita E, Allen S. 2001. Sexual practices of HIV discordant and concordant couples in Rwanda: Effects of a testing and counseling programme for men. *International Journal of Sexually Transmitted Diseases and AIDS* 12(3):181–188.

Rousseau CM, Nduati RW, Richardson BA, Steele MS, John-Stewart GC, Mbori-Ngacha DA, Kreiss JK, Overbaugh J. 2003. Longitudinal analysis of human immunodeficiency virus type 1 RNA in breast milk and of its relationship to infant infection and maternal disease. *Journal of Infectious Diseases* 187:741–747.

Rutherford GW, Sangani PR, Kennedy GE. 2004. Three- or four- versus two-drug anti-retroviral maintenance regimens for HIV infection (Cochrane Review). In: *The Cochrane Library,* Issue 1. Chichester, UK: John Wiley & Sons.

Schechter, M. 2004 (January 27). *Lessons Learned from the Scale-up of Antiretroviral Treatment in Brazil.* Paper presented at the Institute of Medicine Workshop on Antiretroviral Drug Use in Resource-Constrained Settings, Washington, DC. Institute of Medicine Board on Global Health.

Sethi AK, Celentano DD, Gange SJ, Moore RD, Gallant JE. 2003. Association between adherence to antiretroviral therapy and human immunodeficiency virus drug resistance. *Clinical Infectious Diseases* 37:1112–1118.

Simoni JM, Frick PA, Pantalone DW, Turner BJ. 2003. Antiretroviral adherence interventions: A review of current literature and ongoing studies. *Topics in HIV Medicine* 11:185–198.

Stephenson J. 2004. Researchers report findings on HIV drug resistance, new infections. *Journal of the American Medical Association* 291(12):1431–1433.

Stringer EM, Sinkala M, Stringer JS, Mzyece E, Makula I, Goldenberg RL, Kwape P, Chilufya M, Vermund SH. 2003. Prevention of mother-to-child transmission of HIV in Africa: Successes and challenges in scaling-up a nevirapine-based program in Lusaka, Africa. *AIDS* 17:1377–1382.

The Italian Register for Human Immunodeficiency Virus Infection in Children. 2002. Determinants of mother-to-infant human immunodeficiency virus 1 transmission before and after the introduction of zidovudine prophylaxis. *Archives of Pediatric and Adolescent Medicine* 156(9):915–921.

Tuldra A, Wu AW. 2002. Interventions to improve adherence to antiretroviral therapy. *Journal of Acquired Immune Deficiency Syndrome* 31:S154–S157.

UNAIDS (Joint United Nations Programme on HIV/AIDS). 2000. *Voluntary Counseling and Testing (VCT): UNAIDS Technical Update 2000.* [Online]. Available: http://www.unaids.org [accessed August 24, 2004].

UNAIDS. 2003a. *AIDS Epidemic Update.* [Online]. Available: http://www.unaids.org [accessed August 24, 2004].

UNAIDS. 2003b. *Combating Stigma and Discrimination Is Vital to Improving Access to AIDS Care.* [Online]. Available: http://www.unaids.org [accessed May 28, 2004].

UNAIDS. 2004. *Violence against Women and AIDS*. [Online]. Available: http://www.unaids. org/html/pub/una-docs/gcwa_violence_02feb04_en_pdf.pdf [accessed July 29, 2004].

UNAIDS/WHO (Joint United Nations Programme on HIV/AIDS and World Health Organization). 2003. *AIDS Epidemic Update: December 2003*. [Online]. Available: http:// www.unaids.org/html/pub/publications/irc-pub06/jc943-epiupdate2003_en_pdf.pdf [accessed July 29, 2004].

U.S. DHHS (United States Department of Health and Human Services). 2003. *Guidelines for the Use of Antiretroviral Agents in HIV-1-Infected Adults and Adolescents*. [Online]. Available: http://AIDSinfo.nih.gov [accessed August 24, 2004].

Velasco-Hernandez JX, Gershengorn HG, Blower SM. 2002. Could widespread use of combination antiretroviral theapy eradicate HIV epidemics? *The Lancet Infectious Diseases* 2:487–493.

Weiser S, Wolfe W, Bangsberg D, Thior I, Gilbert P, Makhema J, Kebabetswe P, Dickenson D, Mompati K, Essex M, Marlink R. 2003. Barriers to antiretroviral adherence for patients living with HIV infection and AIDS in Botswana. *Journal of the Acquired Immune Deficiency Syndrome* 34(3):281–288.

WHO (World Health Organization). 2003a. *Emergency Scale-up of Antiretroviral Therapy in Resource-Limited Settings: Technical and Operational Recommendations to Achieve 3 by 5*. [Online]. Available: http://www.who.int/3by5/publications/documents/zambia/en/ [accessed June 30, 2004].

WHO. 2003b. *Scaling up Antiretroviral Therapy in Resource-Limited Settings: Treatment Guidelines for a Public Health Approach. 2003 Revision*. [Online]. Available: http:// www.who.int/3by5/publications/documents/arv_guidelines/en/ [accessed June 30, 2004].

WHO. 2003c. *Guidelines for Implementing Collaborative TB and HIV Programme Activities*. [Online]. Available: http://www.who.int/gtb/publications/tb_hiv/2003_319/tbhiv_ guidelines.pdf [accessed June 30, 2004].

WHO. 2003d. *Nutrient Requirements for People Living with HIV/AIDS: Report of a Technical Consultation*. Geneva: WHO.

WHO. 2003e. *Adherence to Long-term therapies: Evidence for Action*. Geneva: WHO.

WHO. 2003f. *Access to Antiretroviral Treatment and Care: The Experience of the HIV Equity Initiative in Cange, Haiti*. [Online]. Available: http://www.who.int/hiv/pub/prev_ care/en/Haiti_E.pdf [accessed June 30, 2004].

WHO. 2004a. *Draft Guidelines*. [Online]. Available: http://www.who.int/3by5/publications/ documents/en/pmtct_2004.pdf [accessed May 28, 2004].

WHO. 2004b. *A Community Health Approach to Palliative Care for HIV and Cancer Patients in Africa*. [Online]. Available: http://www.who.int/cancer/palliative/ projectproposal/en [accessed June 30, 2004].

WHO. 2004c. *Stop TB Working Group on TB/HIV*. Available: www.stoptb.org/Working_ Groups/TBHIV/ [accessed August 24, 2004].

WHO Collaborative Study Team on the Role of Breastfeeding on the Prevention of Infant Mortality. 2000. Effect of breastfeeding on infant and child mortality due to infectious diseases in less developed countries: a pooled analysis. *Lancet* 355:451–455.

Wilkinson D, Squire SB, Garner P. 1998. Effect of preventive treatment for tuberculosis in adults infected with HIV: Systematic review of randomized placebo controlled trials. *British Medical Journal* 317:625–629.

5

Managing Scale-up of Antiretroviral Therapy

A ntiretrovirals (ARVs) alone are not the answer to the HIV/AIDS pandemic. Linked inextricably to the ultimate success of these drug interventions are logistics systems that ensure the safe and timely procurement and delivery of the drugs and other commodities to their intended destinations, and to the people whose lives depend on them. Antiretroviral therapy (ART) scale-up will require tens of thousands of health care workers with the experience and training needed to treat so many people with a complex medical intervention. Well-functioning countrywide ART programs will also require significant investments to build the capacity of a broad range of other technical and managerial expertise, from data analysts to procurement strategists to supervisory personnel. Additionally, ART scale-up will require dedication of the necessary funds and other resources to the enormous task of securing and delivering effective drugs. Finally, both dedicated resources and processes will be needed to establish and maintain harmonized monitoring and evaluation systems that will not only measure the effectiveness of ART programs and outcomes, but also inform the ongoing improvement and optimization of the clinical and management operations of scale-up. An integrated management structure that includes these principal components will be necessary for the long-term success of ART programs.

BUILDING HUMAN RESOURCE CAPACITY

Although scientific data on health care personnel in resource-constrained settings, particularly sub-Saharan Africa, are extremely difficult to collect, WHO surveys and general reports indicate that human resource capacity is generally extremely weak in such settings and in many places is a critically limiting factor in providing access to ART. In fact, some evidence suggests that ART scale-up could fail on these grounds alone (Kober and Van Damme, 2004). Many of those countries with the highest numbers of people living with HIV/AIDS have very few health care providers trained in comprehensive care for the disease (Liese et al., 2003; USAID, 2003). Many health workers have died as a result of untreated AIDS, and others have moved to wealthier countries in search of better pay and job security (Padarath et al., 2003; Pang et al., 2002; Tawfik and Kinoti, 2001). (For an extended review of human resource capacity considerations, see Appendix C.)

In acknowledgment of this situation, WHO's 3-by-5 plan calls for the rapid training of tens of thousands of workers to aid in the delivery of ARVs. However, the medical complexity of HIV/AIDS therapy cannot be overestimated. Nor can the logistical complexity of reliably delivering ARVs to their intended destinations—a recurring process that can demand significant organizational skill and infrastructure—be ignored. Rapid scale-up will require sufficient expertise in all of the various nonmedical components of ART programming, as well as the more obvious health-sector roles. The problem is compounded not only by the shortage of trained workers with specific HIV/AIDS experience or expertise, but also by severe shortages in many resource-constrained settings of the well-trained professionals needed to handle other critical functions, such as commodity logistics, pharmaceutical regulation, laboratory support, information management, and operations research.

The seriousness of the situation is illustrated by an October 2003 report analyzing the cost and resource requirements associated with providing ART through the Zambian public health sector (Kombe and Smith, 2003). Despite key findings indicating that the provision of highly active antiretroviral therapy (HAART) to all clinically eligible patients will be prohibitively expensive, the report suggests that human resource capacity may become the most critical rate-limiting factor.

In the report, the estimated per-patient cost of the health care training necessary for public-sector ART scale-up in Zambia, with an initial goal of providing ARVs to 10,000 people, is US$3.70, which amounts to a total overall cost of $37,000 per year. That amount, which represents less than 1 percent of the estimated total per-patient cost (i.e., $488), would cover the marginal requirement for the estimated additional 13 full-time equivalent (FTE) doctors and nurses, 15 FTE pharmacists, and 32 FTE laboratory technicians needed to provide ART to 10,000 patients. Although the demand for laboratory technicians poses a challenge, meeting the overall workforce needs for achieving Zambia's initial scale-up goal is quite feasible, and the amount of funding necessary to bring the workforce to full capacity is relatively minimal. The low per-patient cost of training compared with the cost of the drugs and other components of scale-up suggests that serious, well-planned investments in health worker training would be an extremely cost-effective move.

On the other hand, 10,000 people still represent only about 10 percent of the total number of Zambians currently in need of ART, and many more infected but currently immunocompetent Zambians will join these ranks over the next decade. Providing full ARV coverage for the entire clinical population in need, as it stands now (i.e., about 100,000 people, rising to about 330,000 in 5 years, but also assuming a 20 percent mortality rate), would marginally require an additional 130 FTE nurses and physicians in the first year and 429 by the fifth year, and 316 laboratory technicians in the first year and more than a 1,000 by the fifth year. And these estimates do not even begin to address additional voluntary counseling and testing (VCT) staffing needs. Clearly, the human workforce needs for full coverage are immense.

Throughout sub-Saharan Africa in particular, the reality of the human resource situation is sobering, as these accounts and a wealth of qualitative reports attest (Kober and Van Damme, 2004). Recent data related to the overall health-sector human resource crisis in Africa and collected for the U.S. Agency for International Development (USAID) reveal that newly constructed health facility structures, including clinics and hospitals, remain unstaffed or understaffed throughout sub-Saharan Africa, as general efforts to expand the network of such facilities have greatly outpaced efforts to build human resource capacity. For example, despite vigorous efforts by the government of Mali to expand the number of its community health centers to 533, 43 percent of these centers were not functioning as of January 2001, with the remainder not operating because of a shortage of personnel to staff them (Lynch and Diallo, 2001; USAID, 2003). As it takes 3 to 4 years to train and deploy nurses and 5 or more years to train and deploy physicians, it is clear that without sufficient and aggressive training initiatives, this gap between physical infrastructure and human resource capacity will continue to widen.

Given the desperate and growing demand for health workers and the losses of trained workers to better jobs in more well-to-do countries, many African nations have reportedly been encouraged to adopt human resource policies that lead to the deliberate overproduction of health workers to fill the growing gaps in human resource capacity. Filling these gaps is not a simple task, however, as the African health sector's human resource crisis is multidimensional and involves a complex set of underlying upstream and more-proximal causal factors (Puku, 2002; Narasimhan et al., 2004; Schwab, 2001). The problem encompasses not just the scarcity of well-trained health workers, but also generally poor morale and staff motivation, insufficient management, an imbalance between urban and rural workforces, and strains on human resources caused by infrastructure changes and new, unfamiliar practices and technologies (see Table 5-1).

The burden of HIV/AIDS, which amounts to nearly one-fifth of the disease burden in sub-Saharan Africa, has not only dramatically increased the patient volume and associated workforce needs, but also led to the death of many health workers. According to one report, AIDS-related mortality accounts for 19 to 53 percent of all deaths among government staff, including public-sector health workers, in most African countries (USAID, 2003). Moreover, the number of hours or days of work lost due to AIDS-related illness can be substantial, further reducing actual workforce capacity.

Unfortunately, quantitative data and objective analyses of the situation are scarce. Most available data come from only three countries (Malawi, Zambia, and Zimbabwe), although these are by no means the only countries facing this critical problem. The lack of data is due in large part to a generally nonexistent personnel information system, which itself is indicative of how seriously neglected the issue is.

The human resource crisis in the health sectors of resource-constrained settings reflects the underlying crisis in tertiary education throughout the developing world, particularly in sub-Saharan Africa. The quality of such education tends to be low; access is limited; and as most health professional training is conducted under the auspices of national governments (through their ministries of health), there is not enough public money available to fund the numbers and types of formal preservice training programs that are needed (an issue discussed further below). In short, the production of new workers has not kept pace with the growing demand for greater workforce capacity. A recent report indicates that when countries do receive aid to build schools and training hostels, they often do not receive the funds needed to support the organizational programs those facilities house. Malawi, for example, has reportedly closed medical and nursing schools during midterm because of a lack of funds to support faculty and student services. Between 1996 and 1999, two of Zambia's public universities reportedly only received 45 percent of expected funds from the treasury (USAID, 2003).

Over the last decade, the underfunding of preservice training for nurses, physicians, and other medical and allied professionals has contributed to a generally limited teaching capacity, significant curriculum gaps, and greater difficulty in enforcing qualification and practice standards. Graduates often are not well prepared to work in the field or at the front lines of public health services. Box 5-1 describes one intiative aimed at addressing this

TABLE 5-1 African Countries by Health Care Worker/Population Ratios, late 1990s

Population per Doctor	Countries
1 per 30,000 or more	Burkina Faso, Central African Republic, Chad, Eritrea, Ethiopia, Gambia, Malawi, Mozambique, Niger, and Tanzania (10)
1 per 20,000	Angola, Benin, Comoros, D.R. Congo, Lesotho, Mali, Rwanda, Sierra Leone, Somalia, Togo, Uganda, and Zambia (12)
1 per 10,000	Burundi, Cameroon, Cote d'Ivoire, Djibouti, Ghana, Madagascar, Senegal, Sudan, and Swaziland (9)
1 per 5,000	Botswana, Cape Verde, D.R. Congo, Equitorial Guinea, Gabon, Guinea, Guinea-Bissau, Kenya, Mauritania, Mauritius, Namibia, Nigeria, Sao Tome and Principe, Seychelles, South Africa, Swaziland, and Zimbabwe (16)

Population per Nurse	Countries
1 per 10,000 or more	Central African Republic, Gambia, and Mali (3)
1 per 5,000	Benin, Burkina Faso, Chad, Eritrea, Madagascar, Niger, Senegal, Togo, and Uganda (9)
1 per 2,000	Cape Verde, Comoros, Cote d'Ivoire, D.R. Congo, Equitorial Guinea, Ghana, Guinea, Lesotho, Sierra Leone, and Sudan (10)
1 per 1,000	Angola, Botswana, Djibouti, D.R. Congo, Guinea-Bissau, Kenya, Mauritania, Mauritius, Namibia, Nigeria, Sao Tome and Principe, Seychelles, South Africa, Tanzania, Zambia, and Zimbabwe (16)

Population per Midwife	Countries
1 per 20,000	Angola, Burkina Faso, Central African Republic, Chad, Equitorial Guinea, Eritrea, Guinea, Mali, Niger, and Sierra Leone (10)
1 per 10,000	Benin, Gambia, Madagascar, Mauritania, Senegal, and Togo (6)
1 per 5,000	Comoros, Congo, Cote d'Ivoire, Guinea-Bissau, and Uganda (5)
1 per 2,000	Ghana, Lesotho, Namibia, Nigeria, Sao Tome and Principe, Seychelles, Tanzania, and Zimbabwe (8)

Overall, the population per doctor in the developing world is 1:1,400; in industrialized nations, it is 1 per 300. Population per nurse in the developing world is 1:1,700; in the industrialized world, it is 1 per 170.

SOURCE: USAID, 2003.

BOX 5-1
The International Training and Education Center on HIV

The U.S. Health Resources and Services Administration and the Centers for Disease Control and Prevention established the International Training and Education Center on HIV (I-TECH) in 2002 to address human capacity development for care and treatment in the countries hardest hit by the AIDS epidemic. One goal of I-TECH is to support health care worker training programs that are locally determined and self-sustaining. Together with its domestic and international partners, I-TECH conducts needs assessments in high-priority areas; develops standards for education, training, and evaluation; disseminates best practices in human capacity development; assists local partners with training; and hosts study and exchange visits. I-TECH uses experienced clinicians, trainers, and program planners for a host of activities, including the following:

- Needs and capacity assessment
  — Identifying local service and training resources and needs
- Clinical care and treatment
  — Developing local capacity
  — Developing protocols
  — Providing technical assistance
  — Providing clinical education
- Training and instructional design
  — Training trainers
  — Writing or adapting curricula for country-specific applications
  — Producing multimedia curriculum components to enhance training and provide programming for distance-learning systems
- Monitoring and evaluation
  — Evaluating training plans
  — Analyzing costs/benefits
  — Translating standards of care into indicators
- Organizational development
  — Assisting with recommendations
  — Assisting with short- and long-term strategic planning
  — Assisting with national tuberculosis (TB)/AIDS program development

I-TECH currently works with the CDC Global AIDS Program and its collaborators in the Caribbean region, as well as in additional countries including Botswana, Ethiopia, India, Malawi, Namibia, South Africa, Thailand, and Zimbabwe.

SOURCE: International Training and Education Center on HIV, 2004.

---

need, while Box 5-2 reviews how the factors discussed above affect the potential role of nurse-based care.

To aid in the effort to bolster human resource capacity in resource-constrained settings, multinational participation is encouraged. Although partnerships between institutions in the developed and developing worlds

---

BOX 5-2
Nurse-Based Care

It is estimated that some two-thirds of the burden of care for HIV/AIDS in Africa could potentially be addressed by community health nurses. The Médecins sans Frontières (MSF) program in Khayelitsha, South Africa, is a good example of a successful heavily nurse-based prevention and ART program. (For more detail on this program, see Chapter 2.) Each clinic team consists of one physician, two nurses, and two counselors. Although the physician plays a more prominent role initially, the nurses are becoming increasingly responsible for patient follow-up visits to the clinics (every 1 to 2 months), particularly as the number of people being treated increases. As of December 2003, there were 750 patients receiving ARVs through MSF; an additional 550 are expected to become part of the program this year.

Another South African MSF program in Lusikisiki, which was initiated in January 2003 and aims to have 400 people on ART by December 2004, is operated entirely by nurses, counselors, and volunteers. Prior to MSF's arrival, none of the country's 12 rural nurse-run clinics had been visited by a physician in 5 years. Now doctors are responsible for training the nurses in ART, as well as OI therapy, prevention of mother-to-child transmission (PMTCT), and VCT, and for supervising newly trained nurses for 1 to 3 weeks before they work by themselves. Thereafter, doctors rotate through the clinics fortnightly.

Yet despite this potential for nurse-based care to play a key role in ART scale-up, there are serious nursing shortages and problems with nurse training. Providers must be able to determine when to start, stop, or switch therapy; to explain the often complex dosing regimens and the side effects that may result; and to manage appropriate and adequate monitoring to slow the emergence of multidrug resistance. Knowledge and training for ARV providers are particularly important in settings not well equipped with sophisticated laboratory and monitoring equipment and resources. Although adherence and treatment success are possible based on clinical criteria alone, this is true only if health care providers are knowledgeable and capable with regard to monitoring and evaluating patient response to treatment in the absence of laboratory monitoring. There is an urgent need for an objective evaluation of the extent to which nurse-based care can fill the gaps in human resource capacity.

---

will undoubtedly play a significant role in training, mentoring, and transferring knowledge, the value and usefulness of south–south partnerships should also be recognized.

Recommendation 5-1. Efforts should be made to augment mechanisms that can be used to mobilize larger numbers of trained professionals from resource-rich countries with extensive and relevant expertise to provide technical assistance and training to countries in need. *Such an HIV/AIDS corps would serve to strengthen long-term ties among health professionals working to fight HIV/AIDS in all countries. A variety of* *innovative governmental and private-sector mechanisms should be designed and expanded to bring qualified volunteer medical professionals into both urban and rural areas to support prevention, care, and training programs relevant to ART scale-up. The required expertise and skills and the areas for placement in country should be determined by local programs.*

Recommendation 5-2. Donors and organizations with relevant expertise (e.g., academia, industry, public health agencies, nongovernmental organizations) should support active partnerships among all institutions possessing such expertise and those seeking to acquire the benefits of training; mentoring; and the transfer of antiretroviral therapy–related medical, technical, and managerial knowledge and skills. Partnerships among medical institutions within and across national borders should be encouraged by donors and governmental authorities. *These twinning relationships should support the transfer of appropriate technology; expertise in medicine, monitoring and evaluation, and applied and operations research; and lessons learned. Physical and electronic means should be used to provide ongoing support for these partnerships.*

Recommendation 5-3. Expertise within the AIDS Education and Training Center networks sponsored by the U.S. government and similar initiatives by other countries should be utilized to support the development of effective training programs in HIV care in order to prepare local physicians, nurses, community health workers, laboratory professionals, pharmacists, and logisticians in heavily HIV-afflicted countries facing severe human resource shortages.

DEVELOPING A SUSTAINABLE WORKFORCE

The Brain Drain

The brain drain (i.e., the departure of trained and educated individuals from one place to another) has had severe impacts on the health care sector of developing countries. Higher wages, better living conditions, and increased chances for career advancement are a few of the main reasons that health care workers are leaving their native countries (Dovlo, 2003; Padarath et al., 2003). The brain drain can occur domestically or internationally, with effects being felt at either the regional or national level. Not only are there not enough trained health care workers in most resource-constrained settings, but the numbers are rapidly declining. As noted above, well-trained workers are leaving in search of better-paying jobs, both locally and abroad and in both the private and nongovernmental organization (NGO) sectors, thus creating an even greater need for more trained personnel in the most resource-constrained settings (see Box 5-3). According to a recent USAID-sponsored report, data from Ghana, Zambia, and Zimbabwe show that annual losses from the public health sector range from 15 to 40 percent (USAID, 2003). These losses are due to emigration (in search of better-paying jobs), shifts from the public to the private sector, deaths from HIV/AIDS, and early retirement. The situation varies regionally and even within single countries, as the distribution of health workers is heavily skewed toward urban areas (see below). An even greater problem may be the loss of African-trained (and -financed) workers to industrial countries, where shortages of health-sector workers, particularly nurses, appear to be fueling the demand (Bundred and Levitt, 2000; Pang et al., 2002).

Although the loss of nurses and physicians may be the most obvious and commonly cited aspect of the human resource crisis in Africa and in the developing world generally, some experts argue that the loss of pharmacists is an even greater problem (Katerere and Matowe, 2003). Pharmacies are commonly considered the "poor man's clinic" because they offer free consultations and are usually more accessible than primary health care facilities. As indicated in the previous chapter, pharmacist-led counseling is one of the few adherence interventions that are actually evidence-based. Thus the loss of pharmacists not only forces the closure of pharmacies, thereby reducing the accessibility of ARVs, but also comes at a time when the management and counseling skills of pharmacists are desperately needed to ensure the rational use of ARVs.

For example, the South African Pharmacy Council recently reported that 600 registered pharmacists emigrated in 2001 alone (Katerere and Matowe, 2003). This is alarming, as only 1,000 students graduate from South African pharmacy schools each year. Also in 2001, more than 60 pharmacists left Zimbabwe—an even more alarming statistic as that country produces only 40 pharmacists a year. Not only are practicing pharmacists and pharmacy school graduates emigrating, but so, too, are pharmacy school academic staff. According to one anecdotal report, many nonpharmacy graduates are teaching courses in South African pharmacy schools, and almost all of the academic staff of the University of Zimbabwe department of pharmacy have emigrated.

As most African governments already allocate 50 to 70 percent of their overall public health expenditures to salaries and wages, there is little money left over to address the problematic salary differences between local civil service and private, NGO, or foreign employment opportunities for physicians and other highly trained workers (Over, 2004; USAID, 2003). The pandemic of HIV/AIDS in developing countries has placed enormous strain

BOX 5-3
The Brain Drain: Facts and Figures

According to a USAID-sponsored report on the human resource crisis in Africa's health sector (USAID, 2003), only 360 of the 1,200 doctors trained in Zimbabwe during the 1990s continue to practice within the country. A July 2003 article in *Lancet* (de Castella, 2003) reports that this country's brain drain is particularly prevalent among doctors and anesthetists, who flee the country for the United Kingdom, New Zealand, and South Africa. A recent survey found that two-thirds of University of Zimbabwe medical students intended to leave the country after graduating, and one of the country's major 1,000-bed hospitals lacks even a single qualified pharmacist. As the author of the *Lancet* article writes (p. 46), "If HIV/AIDS is the deadly cancer gnawing away at a population, then the brain drain is the medical profession's own wasting disease—with particular specialists like pharmacists in very short supply, and an average vacancy rate of 24 percent across the medical spectrum."

The grounds for this exodus can be found in the current working conditions for members of the health professions. The monthly salary for a senior house officer working a 70- to 80-hour week, for example, is the equivalent of US$187, leading most to supplement their public-sector employment with private work. Many doctors report shortages of even basic drugs and medical supplies, such as needles and suture materials. Patients must pay out of pocket for some services, often forcing providers to withhold treatment until at least some level of payment has been provided. In addition to the demoralizing effects of working for so little money and with so few resources, there is the perceived threat of becoming infected oneself with HIV, as is believed to have happened to two doctors through needle-stick accidents at the university's medical school.

In an attempt to address medical staff shortages, the Ministry of Health recently ordered a two-fold increase in the number of medical students in training at the University of Zimbabwe. However, no corresponding increase was made in the size of the teaching staff.

The situation in Zimbabwe is paralleled to varying degrees elsewhere on the continent. In other African nations, the USAID-sponsored report finds that:

- In Zambia, only 50 of the 600 doctors trained locally since independence have remained in the country.
- In Kenya, 100 advertised vacancies for physicians in 2001 brought applications from only 8 individuals.
- In Ghana, 328 nurses are recorded to have been lost in 1999, roughly equivalent to the country's annual output of nurses. Estimated losses for the year 2000 totaled 600. Even for earlier periods, another study found that 61 percent of the graduates of one of Ghana's medical schools left the country between 1986 and 1995 (Dovlo, 2003).

As a result of these losses, many African countries are now actively trying to recruit health professionals through advertisements in foreign publications. This is a crisis that, at the very least, deserves further objective assessment so that the scope and urgency of local needs can be identified and addressed.

on health care systems that are already severely underfunded; the brain drain is only worsening the problem.

Urban–Rural Imbalance

The well-known health care disparities between the "urban poor" and the "rural poorer" that exist throughout the developing world are pronounced in sub-Saharan Africa. These disparities are due in part to a within-country brain drain. Most doctors and nurses are trained to work in hospitals (as opposed to rural clinics) and often find urban areas much more desirable than rural. Urban settings provide physicians with greater camaraderie, increased chances for promotion, and better living conditions (e.g., schools, housing, technology) than are available in rural areas (USAID, 2003). Also, many physicians moonlight from their low-paying daytime jobs with more lucrative private-practice appointments with those patients who are able to pay. This type of work is often easier to find in more heavily populated urban areas (USAID, 2003). Finally, as discussed above, the AIDS pandemic further infiltrates societies, health care workers themselves are often infected, and prefer to remain close to urban hospitals for their own treatment.

According to data from Malawi, Zambia, and Zimbabwe, in the late 1990s there were 2 to 10 times more professional health workers in central and provincial hospitals than in rural health centers (USAID, 2003). According to the Ghana Ministry of Health, in 2000 there were nearly 11 times as many doctors and more than 12 times as many nurses working in Greater Accra than in the Upper Western Region, even though there are more than 5 times as many people living in the latter (Ghana Ministry of Health, 2000).

Addressing such dramatic imbalances will not be an easy task, as urban settings are generally much more profitable, both salarywise and professionally, for practitioners. According to a survey conducted among government-employed Portuguese-speaking African doctors, their median monthly salary is equivalent to what they would earn from just 7 hours of private practice (Ferrinho et al., 1998). Thus it is clear that ART scale-up programs targeting rural areas will need to allocate funds specifically to ensure the availability of the necessary health care personnel. The need for rural service programs and incentives for health care workers to relocate or remain in traditionally underserved rural areas needs to be further evaluated and appropriately addressed.

In the developed world, various incentive programs are employed to maintain physician presence in rural areas. Some state-funded U.S. medical schools offer significant financial relief in the form of tuition benefits in exchange for the student's future service in a rural part of the state. The

National Health Service Corps, run by the U.S. Department of Health and Human Services (DHHS), has a similar program designed to place future physicians in underserved areas in exchange for tuition scholarships. Large-scale efforts in this regard have not yet been tried in Africa (USAID, 2003). Inevitably, such staff retention programs and incentives will be necessary if trained personnel capacity is to be expanded and sustained in developing countries, particularly in rural areas.

Laboratory Technicians

In addition to physicians, pharmacists, nurses, and other health care workers directly involved in care and treatment for HIV/AIDS patients, laboratory technicians are essential to the actual administration and monitoring of ARVs. For example, as noted above, Zambia has estimated that its initial ART scale-up program (for 10,000 patients) will require 32 FTE laboratory technicians in addition to an estimated 13 FTE doctors and nurses and 15 FTE pharmacists.

The important role of laboratory technicians in ART scale-up suggests the need for more of these personnel and improvements in their training. Compliance with good laboratory practices is critical. Generally, problems with inaccurate laboratory analyses fall into one of three categories: preanalytical (e.g., improper labeling, specimen mix-ups), analytical, and postanalytical (i.e., when a test is done correctly, but the results are recorded incorrectly). It is essential to identify and evaluate deficiencies in training programs for laboratory technicians whose correction would minimize these errors. Other factors that may be contributing to poor laboratory compliance, such as not having clear laboratory procedures in place, should also be addressed.

Private Versus Public Sector

In resource-constrained settings, many people who suspect that they have a sexually transmitted disease seek care in the private sector, including private medical practitioners, pharmacists, traditional providers, and drug vendors. This fact raises several concerns about the regulation of the behavior of private providers and the proper use of ARVs. The report of a recent study in Zimbabwe, for example, describes prescribing practices as "therapeutic anarchy" (Nyazema et al., 2000). Reflecting a system without suitable controls, physicians and private pharmacies were found to be prescribing mono therapy to many patients, and most of the interviewed patients believed that the drugs actually cured HIV infection. In another survey of Ugandan private medical facilities, only 4 of 17 facilities prescribing ARVs had received CD4 and viral load results in the previous 2 months (i.e., for only 38 of 450 patients) (Brugha, 2003). Even when users recognize that public services may be superior, they often select private providers for the sake of privacy and as a way to avoid the stigma associated with seeking treatment for HIV infection.

To circumvent such improper use of ARVs, better controls need to be instituted. Strategies need to be developed for providing treatment guidelines for private-sector practitioners, establishing links between private practitioners and specialists, and increasing private-sector access to information and research evidence. National tuberculosis programs have faced similar problems, presenting a potential opportunity to learn from those experiences (Caminero, 2003). (On the other hand, it should be noted that at least one study has indicated that private-sector care and ARV prescribing practices are consistent with international standards [Macharia, 2002].)

General Health-Sector Training

Clearly, given the decreasing number of well-qualified and highly trained health workers in resource-constrained settings, there is a need for cost-effective training programs that better prepare graduates for working in the field and on the front line. Ironically, however, donor support has generally tended to be overly skewed toward training as opposed to staff retention and human resource system improvement, such that the already financially strapped national governments are often left with the burden of bearing recurrent costs, such as salaries. Moreover, donor-supported training programs generally are not very well coordinated, are focused too heavily on in-service training as opposed to much-needed preservice training, and do not address the underlying causes of poor staff morale. In Malawi, 10 percent of all donor expenditures in fiscal year 1997 were dedicated to training (amounting to US$4.5 million, including $2.2 million for out-of-country workshops, $1.5 million for out-of-country short- and long-term training, and $0.8 million for other training initiatives). Alternatively, if this amount had been devoted toward supplementing the meager salaries of the civil service health-sector workforce, it would have translated into a US$473 salary increase for 1 year for each of Malawi's 9,500 health-sector civil servants (a roughly 50 percent raise over the typical salary)—a comparison that did not go unnoticed among these civil servants (USAID, 2003).

Although there have been few quantitative assessments of the relative cost-effectiveness and value of preservice versus in-service training programs, the focus on in-service training (e.g., conferences, workshops, site visits) is questionable despite providing short-term solutions:

- In-service training diverts attention away from preservice training programs that create new practitioners and from the urgent needs of those programs.

- It tends to cover only a certain proportion of the workforce.
- It is usually not sustainable after donor funding ends.
- In-service workshops tend to be held in hotels rather than out in the field, and are not exam based.
- These workshops can be disruptive as they require workers to leave their posts in the field (although it can also be argued that the workshops could, if conducted appropriately, improve morale and provide a much-needed break for overworked staff).

Box 5-4 describes the efforts of one country—Botswana—to build health-sector human resource capacity to address the HIV/AIDS epidemic.

Donor-sponsored training programs tend to be focused on specific disease interventions while neglecting the support skills and services needed for the effective implementation of those interventions. These skills and services include pharmacy and pharmaceutical management, health facility management, health planning and administration, human resource planning and systems, accounting and finance, and procurement and logistics—in short, all of the components of ART scale-up not directly related to actually administering the drugs. Finally, the development of new technologies requires the acquisition of new skills and new training, creating yet another burden for already overtaxed training programs.

Management Challenges

The need for more trained workers with the skills necessary for administering and monitoring ART is not the only manpower demand related to scale-up. The managerial and supervisory capacity of the health care sector in many resource-constrained settings is also seriously lacking and in urgent need of improvement. Qualitative reports have pointed to various personnel-related and systematic causal factors:

- As is the case with medical and technical positions, the above-noted loss of workers due to either death from HIV/AIDS or migration to higher-paying jobs, coupled with the slow production of new workers to fill open and needed positions, has resulted in many medical, technical, and managerial positions remaining vacant.
- Already scarce medical personnel from other sectors, including physicians, are often misused for management tasks.
- Health care management tends to be highly centralized, with little or weak supervision, monitoring, or communication with local providers. Consequently, local needs often go unnoticed.

BOX 5-4
Botswana's HIV/AIDS Human Resource Capacity Building

Much of the HIV/AIDS-related human resource capacity building in Botswana is done through the African Comprehensive HIV/AIDS Partnerships (ACHAP). ACHAP runs several training programs throughout the country at many levels of the HIV/AIDS health care workforce.

Teacher Capacity-Building Program—developed by ACHAP, the United Nations Development Program (UNDP), the United Nations Population Fund (UNFPA), the Bostwana Ministry of Education, and Botswana Television. The program is designed to improve schoolteachers' ability to facilitate stigma reduction and HIV/AIDS discussion among their students.

National Behavior Change Interventions Training Program—developed by ACHAP and the National AIDS Coordinating Agency (NACA) to provide behavior modification intervention skills to government workers, civil servants, and district level employees. The program encompasses six training sessions per year over 3 years.

HIV/AIDS Training Clinical Preceptorship Program—developed by ACHAP to bring international experts to Botswana to provide hands-on training to local health care providers. Participants spend at least 3 months in the program.

KITSO AIDS Training Program, Harvard—developed by the Botswana Ministry of Health, the Harvard AIDS Institute, and the Botswana–Harvard AIDS Institute Partnership to train health care professionals in HIV/AIDS care and ART. The program uses both classroom and clinic-based instruction. Participants must complete the four core modules and one of three elective modules, at which point they are awarded a certificate from the Harvard School of Public Health's Center for Continuing Professional Education.

KITSO AIDS Training Program, Baylor—developed by ACHAP, Baylor College of Medicine, and the University of Botswana to further enhance the existing KITSO curriculum. This program is currently in the development stages and is expected to begin in July 2004.

SOURCES: See http://www.achap.org/Programmes.htm; http://www.hsph.harvard.edu/hai/kitso/; http://bayloraids.org/africa/kitso.shtml.

• Problems of favoritism and a lack of clear expectations and performance appraisal contribute to the problem. According to one report, many African countries foster a "supervisory culture of control, instruction-giving, and fault-finding . . . rather than one of facilitation and understanding what is happening so that the problems can be addressed" (USAID, 2003:20).

• Weak personnel information systems technology and capacity contribute to the problem by making it difficult to retrieve data on employed staff, including their location. Although lower-level facilities often have more complete information, the data are not typically sent to or available at central management locations.

The fact that personnel data are so incomplete not only creates management challenges, but also severely constrains efforts to change or develop human resource policy in ways that will maximally benefit the health care infrastructure. The lack of such data is also one of the reasons for the paucity of quantitative data on and objective assessment of the current human resource crisis in general.

Sometimes, deficiencies in management (and technical) expertise are addressed by hiring outside consultants or providing donor-sponsored advisors (e.g., World Bank implementation units). Although this type of quick fix may be necessary to address immediate crises, it is not sustainable over the long term and often complicates problems of motivation and morale by engendering jealousy (e.g., consultant and advisor salaries are often much higher than those of local workers). The number of such outside advisors is not trivial. In Zambia in the mid-1990s, there were apparently as many donor-funded positions as senior positions on the government payroll.

The current general move toward decentralization of health services, a strategy embraced by many African countries, may help alleviate some of these management problems. However, it also raises other, at least equally important, issues regarding local capacity and the need to develop new structures (e.g., budgeting and reporting mechanisms, new relationships among central ministries).

Given the critically important role of logistics, communications, and information management systems in ART scale-up, moreover, having people in place who can operate and manage such systems is critical. Additionally, the capacity to conduct credible monitoring and evaluation programs (described later in this chapter) requires human resources not involved with the operational aspects of scale-up. The people collecting and analyzing the data should not be those who are administering treatment and managing programs. Thus there is a need to mobilize data analysts and others to support monitoring and evaluation and to address associated operations research issues. The nature and extent of these skills will vary among different settings.

ART scale-up will rely on expertise from outside the clinical health sector as much as from within. Identifying specific deficiencies and needs is difficult, as there are scarce data from which to draw evidence-based conclusions. It is clear, however, that expertise will be needed in all areas of ART scale-up, including physicians; nurses; clinical officers; pharmacists; counselors; laboratory technicians; management personnel; information technologists; procurement and distribution professionals; drug regulatory experts; data analysts; and experts in monitoring, evaluation, and operations research.

Recommendation 5-4. Countries should establish information systems at the regional and national levels so they can regularly assess and coordinate their evolving human resource needs. *Both countries with relatively adequate human resources and those that are more resource-constrained must pursue appropriate policies and programs to stem the "brain drain" of local expertise that is critically needed for the scale-up of ART programs. The current shortage of trained, dedicated personnel for monitoring and evaluation programs should be rectified in conjunction with meeting other training and personnel needs.*

SECURING AND DELIVERING EFFECTIVE DRUGS

Purchasing drugs is about more than the price of the pills. Continuous drug availability and the safe, timely distribution of quality-assured drugs to the people who need them will be critical to the viability of any ART program, as interruptions in the drug supply can rapidly lead to treatment failure and the emergence of drug resistance even in the most motivated patients who are otherwise receiving good care. In many resource-limited areas, the requisite infrastructure for the regular procurement, distribution, regulation, and safe storage of ARVs may not be functional. The numerous problems currently facing many resource-limited countries include weak procurement strategies; a lack of sufficient and appropriate warehouse space for stocking drugs; too few people and vehicles to deliver the drugs to their intended, often remote, destinations in a timely manner; and poor communication along the drug delivery line. Addressing each of these components and ensuring the safe delivery of quality ARVs and related products to a number of sites across different sectors and for a growing number of people presents a much more complex set of challenges than those faced by pilot projects. Even in such projects, reports abound regarding the complications associated with the safe procurement, storage, and delivery of products. A well-planned and -executed logistics system can help alleviate many of these problems.

Procurement

For a number of reasons, ARV procurement is more challenging than is the case for other types of essential medicines. Cost issues aside, stock management is crucial for maintaining uninterrupted drug supplies; procurement systems must be flexible enough to adapt to the rapidly changing and wide range of treatment regimens; and a lack of quality reference standards makes it difficult to assess the quality of generic ARVs (Médecins sans Frontières et al., 2003).

The main findings of a report examining the 2-year purchasing experience of Médecins sans Frontières (MSF) in 10 countries reveal that procurement works best when there is a well-supported and well-funded national HIV/AIDS strategy that includes ART. Although MSF advocates no single or best strategy for procurement, their experience suggests that the easiest and most effective procurement strategies involve a strong public procurement agency (e.g., as in Cameroon), local drug production (e.g., as in Thailand), and/or dynamic private-sector distributors (e.g., as in Malawi) (Campaign for Access to Essential Medicines, 2004; see also Box 5-5).

BOX 5-5
World Health Organization's AIDS
Medicines and Diagnostic Service

The World Health Organization's (WHO) AIDS Medicines and Diagnostic Service (AMDS), operational since December 2003, is the access and supply arm of the UNAIDS/WHO 3-by-5 campaign. The AMDS was created to expand the access of developing countries to quality drugs and diagnostic services. To this end, it offers the following support:

• Provides manufacturers with information about the global market demand for drugs and diagnostics, and provides technical support to countries for procuring and supplying these goods.
• Provides technical support to local production operations in developing countries.
• Assists countries in obtaining information on the patent and regulatory status of quality ARVs and diagnostics and the best prices for products.
• Assists countries in relationship building with alternative sourcing options, such as existing procurement agencies.
• Provides countries with guidance on:
— Selection of core ARVs
— Registration and quality assurance
— Product specifications
— Prequalification of ARVs and diagnostics
— Market intelligence on sources, prices, and raw materials
— Import taxes and margins
— Supply management and monitoring
— Local production and quality assurance

As of mid-2004, 20 countries were using the AMDS for procurement and/or distribution of drugs and diagnostics. The AMDS is inviting participation by nongovernmental organizations, foundations, and governments.

SOURCE: WHO, 2003c.

BOX 5-6
Important Elements of the
William J. Clinton Foundation Procurement Strategy

• Volumes are combined across multiple participating countries. Combining the number of laboratory tests needed over a 5-year time period and in several different countries leads to a significantly large volume of product. The same is true for the amount of ARV medication needed over that period of time.

• The foundation makes every effort to establish multiyear tenders (i.e., 3 to 5 years, instead of the usual 6 months to 1 year). Shorter tenders make it difficult for suppliers to predict demand, and therefore to consider investments in production capacity and negotiate lower prices with suppliers of raw materials and active pharmaceutical ingredients (APIs). Tenders are issued for the number of patients who will require ARVs, not the number of ARVs required. Thus, for example, if a program intends to provide ARVs to 5,000 patients, a tender is issued for those 5,000 patients for 3 to 5 years. If the program is scaled up to 10,000 patients in the second year, a second tender for those additional patients will need to be submitted. The tendering process results in not just one but three suppliers winning bids so as to encourage competition, with the Clinton Foundation price serving as the ceiling price under which prequalified suppliers must bid.

• Participating countries back up their payment with a letter of credit or other secure instrument (since the potential for nonpayment is of concern to some suppliers).

• As an integral part of its procurement strategy, the foundation conducts extensive site evaluations and analyses of the capacity for generic suppliers to ensure long-term sustainability and of opportunities for additional cost reductions. The production process is mapped in detail, step by step; the cost, time, and labor associated with each component of the process are determined; and the overall production cost is calculated. Major cost drivers are then identified so that ways to reduce costs at that level can be predicted and the impacts of increased volume evaluated.

SOURCE: Margherio, 2004.

The development and implementation of procurement strategies should be informed by the market status of the desired drugs (i.e., generic, limited-source, or single-source, with the latter two indicating some degree of market exclusivity or patent protection); the characteristics of the medicines and associated suppliers (i.e., quality assurance, susceptibility to resistance, required cold-chain and expiration issues, need to monitor side effects); and the supplier's timetable for drug delivery to ensure a match with treatment initiation and maintenance schedules. Key factors to which the Clinton Foundation attributes its recent success in procurement are described in Box 5-6 (see also the discussion of the the foundation's program in Chapter 2).

Commodity Security

Commodity security, which ensures the long-term, continuous, and reliable availability of essential commodities (drugs, diagnostics, laboratory supplies, etc.) to those who need them, will be critical to the long-term sustainability of ART scale-up. At the program level, the consistent and secure delivery of high-quality drugs depends on five key components, a breakdown in any one of which could cause the entire system to collapse (Chandani, 2004; World Bank, 2004):

- The capacity to *forecast* programmatic needs
- The capacity to *finance* product requirements and to effectively coordinate funding for the purchase of required commodities
- The capacity to *procure* the products in a timely and efficient manner
- The capacity to *deliver* the products to those who need them on a reliable basis
- The availability of good *logistics data* and an information system (e.g., to enable accurate forecasting)

The ability to forecast is particularly problematic, as there is a paucity of data on which to base accurate forecasting, and most programs have very little experience to guide their initial forecasts. Many assumptions must be made regarding not just the estimated need for first-line-regimen drugs, but also drug substitutions that will be required because of toxicity, treatment failure, and other problems.

As programs expand, it will be vital for logistics data to be collected, appropriately analyzed, and routinely available for the updating of forecasts so as to minimize the use of assumptions and maximize the utility of ARV purchases. The physical security of the supply chain in terms of protecting commodities from pilferage is another area of vital concern. Again, there are several ways in which a well-functioning logistics system can minimize this problem. For example, guidelines can be developed for transparency in such areas as procurement, inventory management procedures, routine tracking of stock levels and use, the use of secure vehicles, and requirements for storage conditions. Although an in-depth discussion of corruption is beyond the scope of this report, there is some concern that the problem, already entrenched in so many institutions worldwide, may become exacerbated as the global AIDS response infuses such large amounts of money and resources into communities with large, unemployed, desperate populations. A well-functioning logistics system (see below) can detect discrepancies and identify when and where leakage occurs.

Logistics Systems

DELIVER defines logistics as "the set of activities that move products through the supply chain to the ultimate customer" (DELIVER, 2000, 2004). These activities include the following:

- Ensuring that ARVs reach the people being targeted
- Providing a buffer against uncertainties in funding and procurement
- Ensuring an uninterrupted supply of products so as to guard against the emergence of resistance, enhance treatment outcomes, and maximize investments
- Securing the supply chain to minimize wastage or leakage of drugs
- Providing data on ARV use for donors and program and logistics managers
- Managing and delivering the approximately 120 other commodities necessary for ARV treatment (e.g., laboratory reagents and supplies, HIV diagnostic test kits)

Box 5-7 describes lessons learned about logistics systems during efforts to improve the delivery of drugs for sexually transmitted infections (STIs) in Kenya.

The importance of logistics systems to a smoothly operating drug supply chain raises questions about what can be done to improve already existing systems in some countries. In developing or assessing logistics systems, short- and long-term demands must be appropriately balanced. Although developing multiple parallel or separate systems may not be a desirable long-term solution, an emergency response may require initially bypassing existing structures or systems (e.g., those without the capacity to assume more responsibility). At the same time, ways to integrate the new parallel system, or components of that system, should be considered so that within 5 to 10 years, multiple systems will no longer exist. Several steps can be taken to improve existing logistics systems (Attawell and Mundy, 2003; Chandani, 2004):

- Streamline supply chains, particularly public-sector systems, which tend to have many levels of authority, so that the system is more responsive, opportunities for leakage are minimized, and costs are reduced.
- Limit the number of logistics systems by establishing partnerships (i.e., public–private partnerships among different donors and national governments). The more systems are in place, the greater will be the overall cost and the extent of regulation required, and the less efficient will be the operation of the country's overall drug supply.

BOX 5-7
Lessons Learned: Improving Drug Delivery for
Sexually Transmitted Infections in Kenya

Although not a "how-to" guide for logistics practitioners, DELIVER's *Programs That Deliver: Logistics' Contribution to Better Health in Developing Countries* is intended to serve as an overview for policy makers on all of the various components of a logistics system. While its focus is on family planning programs, the concepts, approaches, and lessons outlined provide a strategic framework that could readily be adapted to ART scale-up.

The following example illustrates how improving just one aspect of a country's logistics system can improve program outcomes. In 1995, Kenya received a US$600,000 donation of more than 2,500 sexually transmitted infection (STI) kits from the British Department for International Development. At that time, it was estimated that the kits could supply 163 sites for 1 year (i.e., all of Kenya's hospitals and one-third of its health clinics). Meanwhile, also in 1995, the Family Planning Logistics Management Project, the predecessor to DELIVER, started providing technical assistance and software to Kenya for the tracking of customer symptoms and the number of STI drugs consumed by each customer. The resulting information was used to estimate when each site would need its next supply of drugs. Within 5 months of implementation, this new tracking system had produced enough information to permit redesign of the kits such that they, and the drugs they contained, could be redistributed. Instead of serving 163 sites for 12 months, the kits ended up serving 500 sites for 29 months for the same amount of money. Thus the same budget was used to serve three times as many people for twice the amount of time—all because of the implementation of a logistics management information system. (The cost of the logistics and additional clinical support was estimated to be 22 percent of the cost of the drugs themselves.)

SOURCE: DELIVER, 2003.

- Invest in building logistics information systems that provide the necessary data for forecasting and long-term planning.
- Develop flexible procurement mechanisms, such as framework contracts, so that countries are not stuck with unneeded products when uptake is low, while countries in need can readily obtain more products.
- Consider logistics issues when selecting products. For example, the use of fixed-dose combinations (FDCs), blister packs, and cold-chain independent drugs will greatly enhance program implementation.
- Consider the regionalization of logistics system and whether and how that strategy could strengthen country systems.

Information Systems

ART scale-up is a complex systems problem involving a multitude of interacting components, people, and sectors. Consequently, the vital but often overlooked role of data and information must not be underestimated. Data and information necessary for managing all aspects of ART scale-up will need to be standardized, compiled, and made easily accessible. Information systems will be essential to meet these needs.

Information systems comprise two main components. The first is information management, which encompasses data collection and analysis. The second is information technology, which includes the telecommunications network in the country in which the system is being implemented (e.g., telephones, fax service), Internet access technologies (varying, for example, between capital cities and remote locations), bandwidth, and service reliability. Also, at a more basic level, power supply availability and stability are critical; anecdotal reports about having all of the pieces in place but no power to run the system abound. Finally, the cost of information technology and cultural considerations (e.g., attitudes toward the use of technology) need to be addressed.

Brazil provides an excellent example of how a well-functioning information system can dramatically ease ART scale-up (see Box 5-8). A key component of scale-up in that country was a targeted effort to address and strengthen the country's information management and information technology needs. There was an awareness that, in a country the size of Brazil, the logistical demands of ART scale-up would require the ready availability and usability of valuable, accurate information pertaining to all aspects of drug delivery—from procurement to patient adherence. Thus the demand was recognized for the creation and implementation of two computerized systems: SICLOM (Sistema de Controle Logistico de Medicamentos, or System of Logistical Control of ARV) (Viols et al., 2000), to register and track the distribution of ARVs; and SISCEL (Sistema de Controle de Exames Laboratoriais, or Systems for Control of Laboratory Exams) (Lima and Veloso, 2000), to track CD4 and viral load laboratory test results.

The design and implementation of appropriate information systems requires a thorough information technology site assessment beforehand. This effort must include obtaining any special licenses needed for uplinking and permission for using the Internet, forming strategic partnerships when possible, conducting on-site evaluations in person, verifying customer service satisfaction, and evaluating met and unmet financial needs.

Recommendation 5-5. To provide continuous, secure delivery of quality drugs, diagnostics, and other products, national and international program managers of antiretroviral scale-up efforts should ensure that

---

BOX 5-8
Brazil's Use of Information Technology

SICLOM: Sistema de Controle Logistico de Medicamentos

In 1998, the National AIDS Programme in Brazil developed a computerized system to control drug logistics. This system allows for the registration of drug distribution, which helps authorities maintain stock information and track prescriptions. The drug dispensing unit has at least one computer and one attendant staff person to run SICLOM.

By registering the distribution of ARVs, SICLOM helps maintain needed stocks at 486 AIDS drugs dispensing units (ADDUs) located throughout the country and assists in tracking prescriptions (Lima and Veloso, 2000; Veloso et al., 2000). The largest unit, in San Paulo, serves 7,000 enrolled people living with HIV/AIDS. Some 285 ARV-dispensing units use SICLOM to track about 118,000 enrolled patients.

The system tracks prescriptions issued to establish whether they fall within treatment guidelines established by the National AIDS Programme. At the end of each day, the prescription information from each drug dispensing unit is sent via modem, online connection, email, or CD-ROM to the office of the National AIDS Programme in Brasilia. At this main center, the data are synchronized, allowing analysis of problems or errors in drug prescriptions; a report indicating any problems or errors detected is generated.

For example, from November 1999 to January 2000, SICLOM detected and rejected 9 percent of prescriptions as being outside the Brazilian guidelines for ART. If 5 percent of these rejected prescriptions had been filled as written, patients could have developed serious side effects. Not only do the data indicate correctable errors and thereby aid in reducing side effects or other complications that might have resulted from the incorrect or nonrecommended use of ARVs, but they are also used to indicate areas in which further training of health care providers is needed.

SISCEL: Sistema de Controle de Exames Laboratoriais

One year after instituting widespread and free access to ART, the Brazilian Ministry of Health established a network of public laboratories to monitor patients clinically. Patients could use these laboratories to receive CD4 and viral load testing free of charge. As of 2004, 94 of these public laboratories were in operation and had issued more than 500,000 test results. The data gathered from these laboratories are sent via online Internet connection or dial-up modem to the National AIDS Programme in Brasilia. Clinicians can access the database to review SISCEL-generated graphs of changes in CD4 and viral loads. SISCEL maintains Brazil's guidelines for laboratory testing and also is integrated with SICLOM.

SOURCES: Galvão, 2002; Lima, 2004.

well-coordinated commodity and logistics systems are in place from the outset of program initiation. *Technical leadership, governmental commitment, and institutional support are needed to ensure the secure delivery of quality drugs and supplies. Methods to avert the interruption of drug supplies include information systems to facilitate the projection of needs and track the distribution of available stocks. Such planning and investment should also account for the consequences of civil disruption or natural disasters, which would require adequate contingencies to avoid disruption to the supply and treatment systems.*

Quality Assurance of Antiretroviral Drugs

The benefits of high levels of adherence to ARV regimens would be illusory if those drugs were not themselves efficacious, safe, and of consistent quality. The extension of these treatments to millions of persons in need over the next several years will involve a growing number of established and new manufacturers. Ongoing, rigorous quality assurance throughout the manufacturing and distribution chain is essential, especially as less experienced manufacturers enter the global market to produce ARVs. As more and more drug producers enter the market to produce ARVs at the lowest possible cost, the oversight system will need to be especially vigilant to ensure that cost savings are not routinely or intermittently sought at the expense of quality.

As noted in the World Bank's 2004 technical guide on ARV procurement, an additional risk faced in dealing with commodities of significant market value such as ARVs is that of counterfeit products (World Bank, 2004). Counterfeit products may contain the wrong components or insufficient active ingredients, or may be contained in fake packaging. Temptations to divert very low-cost generic ARVs meant for use in resource-poor settings to more lucrative markets should be anticipated as a factor that could promote the downstream substitution of counterfeits and other forms of corruption. The World Bank guidelines emphasize that competent national authorities must have the capacity to enforce the laws and regulations designed to prevent fake or substandard medicines from reaching patients.

As noted by the World Bank, a systematic approach to procurement includes four elements: (1) prequalifying suppliers and products through evaluation of product dossiers and assessment of the use of good manufacturing practices; (2) well-crafted procurement contracts that detail supplier conditions, including technical specifications; (3) quality monitoring including laboratory testing; and (4) the installation of systems for continuous evaluation of supplier performance (World Bank, 2004).

The World Health Organization's (WHO) Essential Drugs and Medicines Policy Department embarked in 2001 on an important prequalification project to provide governments and pharmaceutical manufacturers with the first step toward establishing and maintaining mechanisms to ensure the quality, safety, efficacy, and rational use of pharmaceutical products (WHO, 2004a). The prequalification efforts have encompassed not only the assessment of pharmaceutical and diagnostics manufacturers, but also work on standards for procurement systems and quality assurance laboratories. Recognizing the extreme limitations of many resource-poor countries with respect to ensuring that their citizens obtain quality-assured pharmaceuticals and enjoy the advantages of consolidated and harmonized quality assessment procedures, WHO has laudably undertaken this prequalification endeavor. WHO does note, however, that its efforts are not a substitute for regulation by competent national authorities that need to address the remaining elements of procurement.

WHO does not regard inclusion on the prequalification list to be a warranty of the fitness of a product for treatment of HIV/AIDS with regard safety and/or efficacy. WHO also points out that its processes do not guarantee that "the products and manufacturing sites which have been found to meet the standards recommended by WHO, will continue to do so" (WHO, 2004a). In addition, WHO cautions that downstream issues such as the improper storage, handling, and transportation of drugs may affect their quality, efficacy, and safety (WHO, 2004a). For these reasons, national capacity building must be supported in parallel with the valuable first step taken by WHO.

As noted by WHO (2004a):

> . . . the [prequalification] process began with a public invitation, to suppliers of pharmaceutical products, for their Expression of Interest (EOI). Evaluation of the product quality [has been] based on product data and information provided by the suppliers, followed by inspections of manufacturing sites. Guidelines on the contents of product data dossiers for quality assurance and on inspection of manufacturing sites are available from special section of EDM web site and WHO publications, which are in the public domain. Quality control analysis of selected samples of drugs was carried out.

Products meeting all quality criteria can be prequalified within 120 days of application. When suppliers and products fail to meet standards, WHO offers the opportunity to improve dossiers or compliance with Good Manufacturing Practices.

Reflecting on the first few years of the prequalification program, WHO (2004a) found that "it took a long time for many of the suppliers to submit product data to the specifications requested. Data on product quality and on bioequivalence were often inadequate and some manufacturing sites requested postponement of scheduled site inspections." As the project has progressed, however, "an improvement in the quality of product dossiers submitted by suppliers and a voluntary willingness to upgrade manufacturing sites have been observed. This may result in an improvement in the quality of HIV/AIDS drugs that are being traded in international commerce" (WHO, 2004a).

A challenge for ARV assessment is the fact that publicly available quality control and analytic methods or reference standards generally are not available for these often relatively new medicines. As a result, original methods developed and validated by the manufacturer are frequently used. A common basis for concluding that these in-house assay methods are valid is necessary across these manufacturers. Periodically, product dossiers and manufacturers must be reassessed, while changes in manufacturing methods or facilities require immediate review. Samples tested for qualification and regulatory purposes should be from actual production lots rather than pilot test lots. Periodic random representative sampling and quality control analysis of production lots, preferably downstream near the end user, are an essential supplement to impressions drawn from the prequalification of suppliers.

Beyond proper manufacture critical to appropriate care will be the construction of reliable distribution systems to ensure that drugs flow steadily and in sufficient quantity and that consistent quality is maintained until the point of use. Also essential to quality assurance are a country's development of quality assurance laboratory resources and other regulatory mechanisms to guarantee quality across time and geographically dispersed distribution points, as well as the introduction of postmarketing surveillance programs. Some countries do not now possess the capacity to monitor ARV quality and need relevant training and other support. Box 5-9 describes one example of a strategy that can be employed by countries without established, reliable regulatory systems in place: the use of foreign procurement agencies.

FDCs raise some challenging quality assurance issues. While holding promise as means to simplify treatment regimens and improve patient adherence, FDCs add complexity to the quality assurance challenge because generic FDCs rarely can draw on experience with a fully evaluated, innovator-originated equivalent FDC product. At times, simultaneous use of the individual components has been characterized as safe and effective, but in other instances, the FDC represents combinations never before used together or used according to a novel dosing scheme. Moreover, an FDC might incorporate an entirely new molecule.

In recognition of the need for uniform principles to guide the formulation and evaluation of FDCs, WHO and DHHS have been developing guidelines or international standards to support FDC development. Reflecting the multidimensional complexity of the matter, WHO reports that

---

BOX 5-9
The Use of Foreign Procurement Agencies:
The Example of the Clinton Foundation

An option for countries lacking the regulatory systems necessary to provide quality assurance for ARVs is to rely, at least initially, on foreign procurement agencies. For example, an increasing number of countries are expressing interest in becoming involved with the Clinton Foundation's strategic procurement partnership program (described in Chapter 2). An important component of the foundation's procurement process is assuring good drug quality by prequalifying suppliers. To that end, the foundation focuses on manufacturers that meet drug quality criteria as defined by WHO and by the South African Medicines Control Council. The foundation also provides technical assistance through its country teams to ensure that drug distribution systems are secure and that inventory is properly maintained. It also reportedly is going to begin sample testing of shipped materials and is exploring the branding of the Clinton Foundation project so that drug leakage can be readily detected and addressed (Margherio, 2004).

Despite the success of the Clinton Foundation's procurement work thus far, as well as the initial value of WHO's prequalification guidelines and other similar resources and options, the capacity of national regulatory agencies to conduct ongoing quality monitoring both at the point of entry and throughout the supply chain must be enhanced as ART programs expand—particularly if national governments are expected to eventually procure ARVs on their own. It is not well understood whether sufficient procedures are in place to ensure ongoing drug quality after initial qualification (through such methods as random specimen inspection) or to identify the emergence of drug-related adverse events or ineffectiveness that could result from drug combinations or interactions (postmarket surveillance).

SOURCE: Margherio, 2004.

"work is proceeding to resolve a few remaining clinical, public health, adherence, patent, production, regulation, and other issues" (WHO, 2004a).

The WHO- and DHHS-coordinated guidelines should encompass the need in specific circumstances for microbiologic and toxicologic studies of the proposed combinations. Rigorous assessment of bioequivalence of the FDC to the individual components is central to the acceptability of FDCs. As noted by the World Bank, therapeutic equivalence, as determined through in vivo bioequivalence studies, is especially important for FDCs given the seriousness of the condition being treated and the complex pharmacokinetic and physicochemical properties of these drug combinations. Of course, the drugs used in these studies must be essentially the same as those used in actual mass production for sale. Moreover, when simultaneous use of the individual components of FDCs is not standard, one must consider not only the safety and efficacy of each component, but also the safety and efficacy of their simultaneous use and possible interactions—both favorable and unfavorable. The value of each component individually and in combined form must be clear. Inactive ingredients not present in single drugs may be a factor in the use of combinations as well.

> **Recommendation 5-6. The committee endorses as critical the use of the cheapest, safest, most effective high-quality antiretroviral drugs that can be procured. Fixed-dose combinations are recommended as most desirable if they are also of high quality, safe, effective, and inexpensive. The committee also strongly endorses a rigorous, standardized international mechanism to support national quality assurance programs for antiretroviral drugs. This mechanism should be timely, transparent, and independent of conflicts of interest; employ evidence-based standards; and provide ongoing assurance of consistent high-quality manufacture and handling. In particular, the pharmacological issues associated with fixed-dose combinations must be rigorously and rapidly addressed.**

This Institute of Medicine (IOM) committee was asked to discuss the essential components and related general principles of a systematic framework to achieve a balance between the development of resistance and the need to scale up ART rapidly in resource-constrained settings. Yet it was not constituted with the particular technical expertise nor did it have the time to provide the sort of in-depth, independent, evidence-based examination necessary to critique or endorse specific drug quality assurance programs. Nevertheless, the committee commends the efforts of WHO, the U.S. government, and other international partners to facilitate and expedite the manufacture, procurement, distribution, and administration of consistently safe quality pharmaceuticals. Now that attempts to assure the quality of FDCs for AIDS treatment have highlighted the need for specific guidelines for particular component scenarios, publication of final expert consensus guidance is urgently needed. Organizations and governments working toward this goal should collaborate energetically and with the highest possible level of transparency to support each other's efforts. The bottom line is that the approval process for ARVs must be swift while not compromising the quality and efficacy of the drugs.

MONITORING AND EVALUATION

Given the unprecedented magnitude of global ART scale-up and the paucity of data on how to provide ART safely and effectively in resource-constrained settings, scale-up programs must be based on a learn-by-doing approach as capacity is built and programs are continually reworked. The urgent need to deliver life-saving drugs to millions demands reliance on continuous monitoring and evaluation (M&E), rather than exhaustive up-front studies, to identify optimal outcomes and processes. One important function of M&E is to help ensure that programmatic goals are being met and, most important, that the greatest numbers of patients are being treated effectively to ensure that mortality and morbidity from HIV/AIDS are re-duced. M&E also helps identify efficient, effective programmatic activities that warrant expansion and underperforming programs that should be either discontinued or improved.

Another important role for M&E is to ensure that funded ART pro-grams are sensitive to ongoing country activities and are not negatively impacting HIV/AIDS prevention or other public health initiatives or pro-grams. Not only does well-planned and well-executed M&E benefit pro-grams in place, but a rigorous evaluation of the impact of initial ART efforts will be critical to the long-term sustainability of ART scale-up—particularly from a donor perspective, as there will be reluctance to con-tinue funding programs that are not cost-effective or otherwise successful. This point is especially important in light of the long-term commitment required for ART scale-up.

What exactly is M&E? As defined in the National AIDS Council's manual for use by practitioners in the design and implementation of M&E programs (National AIDS Council, 2002:3):

> Monitoring is the routine, daily assessment of ongoing activities and progress. In contrast, evaluation is the episodic assessment of overall achievements. Monitoring looks at what is being done, whereas evalua-tion examines what has been achieved or what impact has been made.

With regard to examining health outcomes and impacts for both pa-tients and services, M&E can be used to address any of a number of questions, depending on the specific goals of a program or intervention, as well as the needs and interests of the organization or authority requesting the information. For example:

- What is the impact of ART on the health of patients treated? This question is addressed using such indicators as weight gain, functional sta-tus, incidence of opportunistic infections, mortality, and CD4 and viral load measurements (when available).
- What is the impact of ART in reducing the age-specific HIV-related mortality rate, the mother-to-child transmission rate, and the age-specific prevalence of HIV infection?
- What is the impact of ART on the ability to return to work?
- What is the impact on both individual and societal productivity?

- What is the impact on health care utilization (e.g., hospitalizations, clinic visits)?
- What is the impact on prophylaxis for opportunistic infections?

Given that ART scale-up is only just beginning, it is difficult to find examples of how M&E could be used by treatment programs in resource-constrained settings to identify practices that are working versus those that need to be improved. Countries' efforts to evaluate their national AIDS programs have varied. Some experts have expressed concern that M&E for existing programs has generally been highly inadequate, and that programs in the process of being rolled out have no formal M&E mechanisms in place and insufficient staffing for evaluating programmatic impact. This situation may be due in part to the fact that until recently, the conceptual framework for M&E was not very solid, and there have been few M&E tools available for countries to use.

> **Recommendation 5-7. Monitoring and evaluation processes should be put in place by program managers at all levels at the start of scale-up initiatives.** *A fixed percentage (approximately 5–10 percent) of ART program funding should be budgeted strictly for monitoring and evaluation (exclusive of support for hypothesis-driven operations research).*

> **Recommendation 5-8. Program managers should measure the effectiveness of HIV prevention and treatment efforts by means of scientifically valid and systematically conducted surveys of HIV prevalence and incidence, HIV morbidity and mortality, and risk behaviors.** *ART programs should be designed to improve the quality of life and add many years of productivity for as many people as possible. The success of ART scale-up should be evaluated on the basis of the extent to which these specific goals are achieved.*

Monitoring and Evaluation Challenges

As described earlier in this chapter, the lack of trained health care and ancillary personnel is one of the greatest challenges to successful ART scale-up. In this regard, the dearth of M&E expertise is not an exception. Such expertise is not widely or uniformly available, and training at the outset of scale-up programs will be necessary to ensure that efforts and investments in M&E foster the expected returns.

Clearly, the reduction of AIDS-related morbidity and mortality is the most important outcome of ART programs, and the measure of this outcome is the most obvious indicator of program success. However, there are other important components of ART scale-up that require similar levels of M&E and financing, such as measurement of the cost-effective impact of certain projects, efforts, or decisions); issues related to commodities (e.g., how decisions impact the availability of certain commodities); the provision of services and coverage; the quality of service delivery; operations research (e.g., how scale-up impacts operations research, whether enough funds have been directed toward such research, how results of the research are being fed back into systems); behavioral components (e.g., adherence); biological and epidemiological components (e.g., prevalence, incidence); and policy. Much of the data needed to monitor these components of scale-up are generally not available or of poor quality in most settings. Where they are generated, few such data are actually used by program managers.

Related to these concerns is the current lack of effective mechanisms to rapidly apply the lessons learned from M&E to improve the quality of care and the effectiveness of clinical and procedural management and training programs within scale-up efforts. Information platforms that can be used to identify initial data and information needs, along with methods for effectively assessing and implementing improvements, have not been widely incorporated into developing-country settings. One such method that might be considered is the Breakthrough Series system for learning and improvement developed by the Institute for Healthcare Improvement (IHI) (2003)— a collaborative learning model that incorporates multiple sites (e.g., regional hospitals, primary health care centers, rural clinics) in the study, testing, and implementation of best-practice knowledge to produce rapid improvement in health care delivery or management systems. As noted earlier, effective ART scale-up in resource-constrained settings will have to rely heavily on a learning-by-doing approach. These programs must also ensure that they "do what they learn" (Massoud, 2004). (See Box 5-10 for further information on the IHI model.)

To address multiple challenges, M&E information systems should (Delay, 2004):

- Complement existing information systems.
- Utilize simplified, harmonized, and prioritized data and data collection techniques.
- Contribute to the improvement of patient management (in addition to providing useful information to the donor).
- Build local capacity and incentives to collect, interpret, and disseminate the data in an appropriate form.
- Support a culture of strategic information sharing (e.g., with respect to translating knowledge).
- Protect the confidentiality of all health information.
- Maintain individual patient records using unique patient identifiers.
- Involve people living with HIV/AIDS.

BOX 5-10
The Institute for Healthcare Improvement
Model for Improvement

IHI's Model for Improvement requires collaborative teams to ask three fundamental questions: (1) What are we trying to accomplish? (*Aim*), (2) How will we
know that a change is an improvement? (*Measures*), (3) What changes can we
make that will result in improvement? (*Changes*) (Langley et al., 1996; WHO,
2004b). By addressing these questions, teams establish which specific outcomes
they are trying to effect, identify appropriate measures to track their success, and
determine key changes they will implement for testing (*Plan*). Key changes are
then tested in a cyclical fashion that recognizes cultural and organizational characteristics. Change is implemented, and progress, problems, and unanticipated outcomes are documented (*Do*). The collaborative site teams complete data analysis
and comparison of outcomes and initial objectives (*Study*). (See the figure below.)

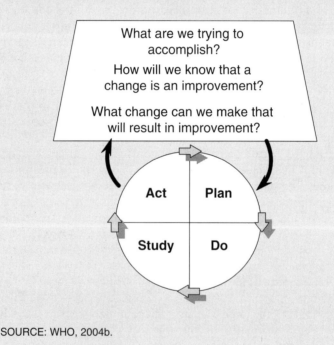

SOURCE: WHO, 2004b.

• Collect information from all providers of ART, including public,
private, NGO, workplace, and other sites.
• Ensure that the data gathering and analysis methodologies used are
flexible, adaptable, and acceptable.

It is essential to select good indicators for use in M&E—data that are

Decisions are then made regarding how to implement and refine successful changes and abandon unsuccessful efforts (*Act*). Critical to this collaborative improvement approach is that participating health care teams contribute to adapting the new approaches for care. Real-time interactive operations research is designed to capture local knowledge and experience by making health care teams active partners in the refinement and improvement of care process. (See the figure below.)

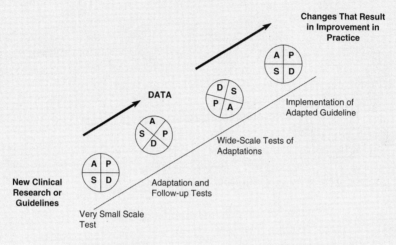

SOURCE: WHO, 2004b.

relevant, easy to collect, and easy to interpret and that reflect changes that are easy to track over time and can be quantified. Measures should reflect both quantitative and qualitative aspects of programmatic management and patient-level quality of care. A number of core ART evaluation indicators have been identified that, if measured every year or two, would probably be sufficient for donor-related evaluation purposes (see Box 5-11).

That having been said, depending on the specific scale-up objectives, even these core indicators may not be sufficient for all donors. The fact that different donors may have differing objectives, and thus differing M&E requirements, raises important concerns about the impact of the resulting lack of standardized metrics and harmonization of M&E procedures. The more donors have a presence in a country, the higher will be the potential transaction costs involved with M&E and the higher the burden on re-source-strapped host country programs.

WHO's Health Metrics Network, supported by the Gates Foundation, was developed in recognition of the fact that most developing countries are overwhelmed by reporting requirements. For example, the Tanzanian Ministry of Health once filed 5,000 pages of reports, including different sets of measurements for different donors in the same areas. WHO was asked by donors to serve as a secretariat and develop a single set of measurements such that satisfying the criteria of the Health Metrics Network would meet the requirements of multiple organizations (Kim, 2004) (see Box 5-12 for some recommended M&E outcome indicators).

The standardization and harmonization of foreign-donor M&E efforts is only one of several political challenges to collecting, analyzing, and interpreting accurate data and unbiased results:

• Because of widespread denial of the severity of the HIV/AIDS pandemic, data may be suppressed.
• The needs of funding agencies often conflict with those of program managers (e.g., the former may be interested in outcomes to which the latter does not give priority or vice versa).
• Collecting data on marginalized or illegal populations is difficult.
• There may be resistance to tracking resources, as doing so may expose corruption and inequitable distribution.
• Service delivery statistics are often perceived by staff as punitive.
• The selective use of evaluation data may skew M&E efforts and bias analyses.
• Performance-based disbursement policies can have a dramatic effect on data collection, analysis, and accuracy.

Another important challenge to M&E of ART scale-up will be monitoring long-term sustainability and impact. Tracking resources, including the cost per unit service and cost per commodity, will become more difficult as the number of people being treated increases. The same is true for tracking and monitoring staffing patterns (whether human resource capacity is really increasing, or ART scale-up is diverting staff from malaria control, childhood immunization, and other programs). Measures of logistics capacity, overall public health capacity, ARV resistance patterns, sur-

---

BOX 5-11
Program Process Indicators for Monitoring and Evaluation

Community Level
 • Number of primary health care clinics that have assessed community capacity
  • Number of districts with community training plans
  • Number of community persons trained to provide ART

ART Site Level
  • Number of sites with providers trained to provide ART
  • Number of HIV tests conducted
  • Number of positive HIV results
  • Number of test results received by clients
  • Number of HIV patients assessed for care
  • Number of HIV patients beginning care
  • Number of patients on ART at the beginning of a specified time period
  • Number of patients discontinuing ART during a specified time period
  • Number of patients referred to a higher care level for management of ART or second-line treatment

District/Region Level
  • Number of districts with evidence of HIV prevalence
  • Number of districts with data for 2-year mortality
  • Number of districts with a designated person(s) for data analysis and interpretation
  • Proportion of providers reporting data to district
  • Number of reports given by district to providers, stakeholders, communities, etc.

Central/National Level
  • Presence of a strategic information system
  • Presence of standardized data collection forms
  • Number of data collection forms disseminated to providers
  • Percent of patients assessed and prescribed ART who receive medications within 1 month
  • Percent of central, district, and dispensing site drug storage locations whose stock cards for ARVs are up to date and accurate
  • Percent of central, district, and dispensing site drug storage locations that experience ARV stock-out

SOURCE: Delay, 2004.

---

vival patterns, infection incidence, and economic productivity (i.e., whether the economic impact of HIV/AIDS is really changing over time) will also pose increasing challenges. Assuming that incidence is cut by half to 2.5 million cases per year and assuming that the goal will continue to be to treat only half of all clinically eligible HIV-infected individuals, the target will be

---

**BOX 5-12
Recommendations for Monitoring and
Evaluation Outcome Indicators**

- Number of persons screened under voluntary counseling and testing programs
- Gender and age of persons screened and testing positive
- Number of persons testing positive for HIV
  — Number of persons qualified for therapy
  — Number of persons initiating therapy
  — Date of therapy initiation
  — Regimen used
  — Number of persons receiving prevention counseling

- Number of persons hospitalized while on ART
- Indication of change in high-risk behaviors after therapy initiation
- Number of persons discontinuing therapy
- Reasons for discontinuation of therapy
  — Patient preference
  — Drugs not available
  — Lost to follow-up
  — Failed therapy
  — Drug toxicity
  — Death

- Reasons for persons remaining on therapy
- Number of persons continuing therapy despite clinical, immunologic, virologic failure
- Number of persons switched to a subsequent regimen
- Opportunistic infections (e.g., tuberculosis, cryptococcal meningitis)

---

to treat 6 to 9 million people by 2010. A global program of that magnitude will require extraordinary M&E efforts.

Finally, programs should be monitored at optimum frequency, which may differ for different types of interventions. And a mechanism for regular international communication of M&E results, inspired by the regular international rounds conducted during the SARS crisis, needs to be established. Box 5-13 summarizes some important features of M&E for ART scale-up.

Measuring Success

What defines programmatic success for ART? The number of drugs distributed is not the best measure, as the numerous problems elucidated earlier attest. There are too many things that can go wrong during the drug

---

BOX 5-13
Important Features of Monitoring and Evaluation
for ART Scale-up

- Complement existing information systems.
- Prioritize, simplify, and standardize data collection.
- Develop incentives to collect data.
- Build local capacity to collect, interpret, and disseminate data.
- Support a culture of information sharing.
- Protect the confidentiality of health information.
- Maintain individual patient records with unique patient identifiers.
- Involve people living with HIV/AIDS in M&E activities.
- Collect data from all sites providing ART (e.g., public, private, workplace, NGOs).

SOURCE: Delay, 2004.

---

delivery process and far too few management information systems in place to track drug delivery in a way that would provide meaningful information on the number of drugs distributed. Nor is measuring the number of people treated necessarily the best way to monitor progress, as both the individual clinical benefit (reduced toxicity and mortality) and population-level benefit (decreased morbidity and mortality) of therapy depend on adherence and the success of chosen adherence interventions.

A definition of treatment success needs to be formulated, with an awareness that it will likely change over time. It must also be realized that success can be defined from several different vantage points, including the patient, physician, community health system, nation, and donor agency.

What many U.S. clinicians considered successful a decade ago would not be considered successful today. Just 6 years ago, success was declared if 50 percent of ARV-treated patients showed complete viral suppression at the end of the first year or 18 months of treatment. Now, clinicians strive for 85 or 90 or even 95 percent as a sign of success. It is critical for ART scale-up programs in resource-constrained settings to strive for a very high— for example, 90 percent—success rate for initial regimens and that treatment regimens and care delivery systems be planned accordingly. Some experts argue that it is not fair to set the bar higher than it has been set in the United States or other resource-rich countries. If this is not done, however, the long-term sustainability of donor support in combination with the durability of inexpensive drug regimens will be at serious risk. Most resource-constrained countries simply cannot afford the flexibility in treatment regimen—in terms of both drug cost and the necessary expertise and human resource capacity—required to individualize treatment when complications arise, as can the United States and other resource-rich countries (Redfield, 2004).

Within 10 years, ART scale-up will have evolved into a US$30–100 billion annual effort, demanding an enormous amount of program success to meet donor goals. In the rush to achieve a quick fix, initial expectations should not be set too low such that they compromise the long-term sustainability of ART scale-up. At the same time, there can be no delay in responding to the ethical imperative to *act now*.

> **Recommendation 5-9. Monitoring and evaluation measures and requirements, as directed by various donors and other stakeholders, should be harmonized across programs to minimize time-consuming inefficiencies in data collection and program management.** *Additional efficiencies would be achieved if these efforts were coordinated by a single national ministry or agency. Donors should avoid attempting to ascribe results solely to individual funding sources in order to minimize the in-country confusion and inefficiency created by mandates to conduct multiple, uncoordinated monitoring and evaluation efforts in the midst of rapid scale-up.*

REFERENCES

Attawell K, Mundy J. 2003. *Provision of Antiretroviral Therapy in Resource-Limited Settings: A Review of Experience up to August 2003.* London: DFID Health Systems Resource Centre.

Brugha R. 2003. Antiretroviral treatment in developing countries: The peril of neglecting private providers. *British Medical Journal* 326:1382–1384.

Bundred P, Levitt C. 2000. Medical migration: Who are the real losers? *Lancet* 356:245–246.

Caminero JA. 2003. Is the DOTS strategy sufficient to achieve tuberculosis control in low- and middle-income countries? 2. Need for interventions among private physicians, medical specialists and scientific societies. *International Journal of Tuberculosis and Lung Disease* 7(7):623–630.

Campaign for Access to Essential Medicines. 2004. *Surmounting Challenges: Procurement of Antiretroviral Medicines in Low- and Middle-Income Countries.* [Online]. Available: http://www.accessmed-msf.org/prod/publications.asp?scntid=201120031530452& contenttype=PARA& [accessed January 5, 2004].

Chandani Y. 2004 (January 28). *Distribution of ARVs: Issues of Security, Logistics, and Quality.* Paper presented at the Institute of Medicine Workshop on Antiretroviral Scale-up in Resource Constrained Settings, Washington, DC. Institute of Medicine Committee on Antiretroviral Drug Use in Resource-Constrained Settings.

de Castella T. 2003. Health workers struggle to provide care in Zimbabwe. *Lancet* 362(9377): 46–47.

Delay P. 2004 (January 28). *Monitoring and Evaluation for ARV Programs in Resource Poor Settings.* Paper presented at the Institute of Medicine Workshop on Antiretroviral Scale-up in Resource Constrained Settings, Washington, DC. Institute of Medicine Committee on Antiretroviral Drug Use in Resource-Constrained Settings.

DELIVER. 2000. *Programs that Deliver: Logistics' Contribution to Better Health in Develop-ing Countries.* [Online]. Available: http://www/fplm.jsi.com/2002/Pubs/Pubs_Policy/ Programs_ That_Deliver/TOC/index.cfm [accessed August 30, 2004].

DELIVER. 2003. *In Kenya, Logistics Project Helps to Extend the Coverage of STI Drugs.* [Online]. Available: http://www.deliver.jsi.com/2002/PUBS/pubs_success/ontrack_ archives/index.cfm [accessed February 22, 2004].

DELIVER. 2004. *DELIVER Homepage.* [Online]. Available: http://www.deliver.jsi.com [accessed February 22, 2004].

Dovlo D. 2003 (September 23–25). *The Brain Drain and Retention of Health Professionals in Africa.* Case study prepared for a regional training conference on Improving Tertiary Education in Sub-Saharan Africa: Things That Work, Accra.

Ferrinho P, Van Lerberghe W, Julien MR, Fresta E, Gomes A, Dias F, Goncalves A, Backstrom B. 1998. How and why public sector doctors engage in private practice in Portuguese-speaking African countries. *Health Policy and Planning* 13:322–338.

Galvão J. 2002. Access to antiretroviral drugs in Brazil. *Lancet* 360(9348):1862–1865

Ghana Ministry of Health. 2000. *Consolidating the Gains, Managing the Challenges: 1999 Health Sector Review.* Ghana: Ghana Ministry of Health.

Institute for Healthcare Improvement. 2003. *The Breakthrough Series: IHI's Collaborative Model for Achieving Breakthrough Improvement (Innovation Paper).* Boston, MA: Institute for Healthcare Improvement.

International Training and Education Center on HIV. 2003. [Online]. Available: http:// ww.gotditech.org [accessed August 30, 2004].

Katerere DR, Matowe L. 2003. Effect of pharmacist emigration on pharmaceutical services in southern Africa. *American Journal of Health-System Pharmacy* 60:1169–1170.

Kim J. 2004. *The Challenge of HIV in 2004 and the UNAIDS/WHO "3 by 5" Program.* Paper presented at the Institute of Medicine Workshop on Antiretroviral Scale-up in Resource Constrained Settings, Washington, DC. Institute of Medicine Committee on Antiretroviral Drug Use in Resource-Constrained Settings.

Kober K, Van Damme W. 2004. Scaling up access to antiretroviral treatment in southern Africa: Who will do the job? *Lancet* 364:103–107.

Kombe G, Smith O. 2003. *The Costs of Anti-Retroviral Treatment in Zambia, Technical Report No. 029.* The Partners for Health Reformplus Project, Abt Associates Inc.

Langley G, Nolan K, Nolan T, Norman C, Provost L. 1996. *The Improvement Guide: A Practical Approach to Enhancing Organizational Performance.* San Francisco, CA: Jossey-Bass Publishers.

Liese B, Blanchet N, Dussault G. 2003. The Human Resource Crisis in Health Services in Sub-Saharan Africa. Washington, DC: World Bank.

Lima R. Information Management and Technology Considerations for ARV Programs in Resource-Constrained Settings. Paper presented at the Institute of Medicine Workshop on Antiretroviral Scale-Up in Resource Constrained Settings. Washington, DC. Institute of Medicine Committee on Antiretroviral Drug Use in Resource-Constrained Settings.

Lima RM, Veloso V. 2000. SICLOM: Fistruicao informatizada de medicamentos para HIV/ AIDS. *Acao Anti-AIDS* 43:6–7.

Lynch E, Diallo I. 2001. *Donor Mapping.* USAID. [Online]. Available: http://mali.viky.net/ usaid/mes_photos/donor_mapping_part3.doc [accessed August 30, 2004].

Macharia D. 2002. *Antiretroviral Chemotherapy in Resource Limited Settings: A Review of ARV Therapy in the Private Sector in Nairobi, Kenya.* Paper presented at the 9th Conference on Retroviruses and Opportunistic Infections in Seattle, WA. [Online]. Available: http://www.retroconference.org/2002/Abstract/13602.htm [accessed August 30, 2004].

Margherio L. 2004. *Perspectives on Purchasing First and Second Line ARVs.* Paper presented at the Institute of Medicine Workshop on Antiretroviral Scale-up in Resource Constrained Settings, Washington, DC. Institute of Medicine Committee on Antiretroviral Drug Use in Resource-Constrained Settings.

Massoud R. 2004. *Principles of Design and Scale-up for National Clinical Care Programs and Applications to the WHO 3×5 Targets.* Paper presented at the Institute of Medicine Workshop on Antiretroviral Scale-up in Resource Constrained Settings, Washington, DC. Institute of Medicine Committee on Antiretroviral Drug Use in Resource-Constrained Settings.

Médecins sans Frontières, World Health Organization, and UNAIDS. 2003. *Surmounting Challenges: Procurement of Antiretroviral Medicines in Low- and Middle-Income Countries. The Experience of Médecins sans Frontières.* Geneva: Médecins sans Frontières.

Narasimhan V, Brown H, Pablos-Mendez A, Adams O, Dussault G, Elzinga G, Nordstrom A, Habte D, Jacobs M, Solimano G, Sewankambo N, Wilbulpolprasert S, Evans T, Chen L. 2004. Responding to the global human resources crisis. *Lancet* 363(9419):1469–1472.

National AIDS Councils. 2002. *Monitoring and Evaluation Operations Manual.* Geneva: UNAIDS.

Nyazema NZ, Khoza S, Landman I, Sibanda E, Gael K. 2000. Antiretroviral (ARV) drug utilisation in Harare. *Central African Journal of Medicine* 46:89–93.

Over M. 2004 (January 28). *An Overview of Health Care Manpower, Health Care Infrastructure and Economics in Select Resource-Poor Countries.* Paper presented at the Institute of Medicine Workshop on Antiretroviral Scale-up in Resource Constrained Settings, Washington, DC. Institute of Medicine Committee on Antiretroviral Drug Use in Resource-Constrained Settings.

Padarath A, Chamberlain C, McCoy D, Ntuli A, Rowson M, Loewenson R. 2003. *Health Personnel in Southern Africa: Confronting Maldistribution and Brain Drain.* Equinet Discussion Paper #3. Regional Network for Equity in Health in Southern Africa.

Pang T, Lansang MA, Haines, A. 2002. Brain drain and health professionals. *British Medical Journal* 324(7336):499–500.

Puku N. 2002. Poverty, debt, and Africa's HIV/AIDS crisis. *International Affairs* 78(3):531–546.

Redfield R. 2004 (January 27). *Durability of ARV Therapy: US Experience and its Implications for Resource-Constrained Settings.* Paper presented at the Institute of Medicine Workshop on Antiretroviral Scale-up in Resource Constrained Settings, Washington, DC. Institute of Medicine Committee on Antiretroviral Drug Use in Resource-Constrained Settings.

Schwab P. 2001. *Africa: A Continent Self-Destructs.* New York: Palgrave, Macmillan.

Tawfik L, Kinoti S. 2001. *The Impact of HIV/AIDS on the Health Sector in Sub-Saharan Africa: The Issue of Human Resources.* Washington, DC: USAID.

USAID (U.S. Agency for International Development). 2003. *The Health Sector Human Resource Crisis in Africa: An Issues Paper.* Washington, DC: USAID.

Veloso V, Sudo E, Lima RM et al. 2000. *Promoting the Rational Use of Antiretrovirals through a Computer Aided System for the Logistical Control of AIDS Medications in Brazil.* Paper presented at the 13th International AIDS Conference in Durban, South Africa.

Viols V et al. 2000. *Promoting the rational use of antiretrovirals through a computer aided system for the logistical control of AIDS medications in Brazil.* Presentation at the 13th International AIDS Conference in Durban, South Africa.

WHO (World Health Organization). 2004a. *World Health Organization Prequalification Project.* [Online]. Available: http://mednet3.who.int/prequal/ [accessed August 2, 2004].

WHO. 2004b. *An Approach to Scaling Up: Using HIV/AIDS Care as an Example.* Draft Document.

WHO. 2004c. *3 by 5 Technical Brief: AIDS Medicines and Diagnostic Service (AMDS).* [Online]. Available: http://www.who.int/3by5/publications/briefs/amds/en/ [accessed August 24, 2004].

World Bank. 2004. *HIV/AIDS Medicines and Related Supplies: Contemporary Context and Procurement. Technical Guide.* Washington, DC: World Bank.

6

The Path Forward

There is no proven "right" way to scale up antiretrovial therapy (ART) and HIV prevention programming in resource-constrained settings worldwide, especially since the diversity of those settings will necessitate differing approaches. As noted in the preceding chapter, however, any delay in moving forward on a large scale while the answers are being determined would clearly be wrong, as ART scale-up has become an ethical imperative. Given the lack of experience on such a large scale and the paucity of relevant data, capturing lessons learned along the way will be critical to ensuring the long-term sustainability of newly implemented programs. To this end, this chapter sets forth critical operations, applied clinical, and behavioral research that will be crucial in a number of key areas. It concludes by emphasizing that even with iterative improvements obtained through solid research, the path forward will require sustained, long-term commitment. This commitment must be not only to acting, but also to using the information generated through sound research to act well.

OPERATIONS RESEARCH: CLOSING THE GAP BETWEEN RESEARCH AND CARE

Successful pilot programs are proof of effectiveness only in particular circumstances; their replicability in many other settings remains unproven. For example, although Haiti's GHESKIO program (see Chapter 3) demonstrates that ART programs can be successful in resource-constrained settings, it does not necessarily provide a replicable model that can be generalized to enable 3 million people to be on treatment by 2005. Indeed, one critique of a published evaluation of Haiti's success (Gilks et al., 2001) contends that the human resources and capacities employed (i.e., the logistics with regard to clinical input and staff time) were not clearly listed in the evaluation and that the criteria for selecting individuals for treatment were not stringent. These observations highlight the need for scientific evaluation criteria, without which important lessons that might be applied in other settings cannot be derived.

Pilot initiatives are by design relatively limited in size, often directed toward a small fraction of those in need and supported by unusually committed and resourced staff. Scale-up activities will introduce factors that may not be especially relevant in a pilot implementation. If a particular health resource is scarce in a country—for example, trained people who may already be staffing other essential health services—a large program scale-up effort may have collateral negative effects on already marginal health care systems by diverting a critical fraction of the limited human resource pool. These threats would not necessarily be evident in a pilot program whose relatively modest requirements were, in the grander scheme, absorbable or even resourced external to the underlying health care infrastructure. Various avenues might be pursued to mitigate this risk of collateral negative effects, although scientific evidence would likely be needed to assess the advisability of different options.

Vertical Versus Integrated Care as an Operations Research Issue

A common discussion in international health revolves around the relative advantages of "stovepiped" or "vertical" condition-specific implementation programs, versus the integration of condition-specific programs into a health sector–wide approach whereby the resources of various programs are effectively integrated into one system, usually under government leadership (see Box 6-1). The care of HIV/AIDS patients is not as easily "stovepiped" as that provided in, for example, an immunization program or even a tuberculosis (TB) program. Rather, HIV/AIDS patients require care that has longitudinal continuity, care that is often complex considering the myriad of opportunistic infections that can occur. The care they receive must also encompass reliable access to quality pharmaceuticals, attention to nutritional and psychosocial needs, counseling to prevent the spread of infection, and the requirements of palliative care. Thus the establishment of programs for HIV/AIDS care requires access to a wide range of services that need to exist for many other purposes as well.

On the other hand, while it would appear that the ideal HIV/AIDS care program would be integrated so as to strengthen the entire health care system, to accomplish such integration in a nondisruptive way takes time.

BOX 6-1
Some Theoretical Advantages of
Integrated and Vertical Programs

Integrated Programs
  • Minimize duplication in administration staffing, infrastructure, logistical, and procurement systems.
  • Often are more cost-effective.
  • Can be more efficient for patients through consolidation of care in a few places.
  • Involve less chance of gaps in care because of fewer referrals out of the program.
  • Are more responsive to local, decentralized management.
  • Foster the building of government capacity as opposed to management by donors.
  • Lower transaction costs between governments and donors as a result of harmonized administrative methods.
  • Unify government and donor priorities and funding targets.
  • Foster programmatic fiscal security through pooled funding.
  • May help avert resource imbalances and negative collateral effects that can occur with well-funded vertical programs.

Vertical Programs
  • May be easier to maintain quality and effectiveness with a narrower focus.
  • Require less complex operational planning and thus potentially less time-consuming.
  • Make use of more readily mobilized funding, which can be used more easily, reliably, and quickly.
  • Make it easier to protect key interventions (e.g., a TB program) where political commitment is weak.
  • May provide more comprehensive and linked monitoring and management response to problems.
  • Make it easier to target interventions specifically to places or populations with greatest needs.
  • Make it easier to maintain the technical quality of services.

SOURCE: Adapted with modifications from Brown, 2001.

And time is in particularly short supply under the stated President's Emergency Plan for AIDS Relief (PEPFAR) and World Health Organization (WHO) imperatives of placing millions of people under treatment over the next several years. Thus a focus of operations research must clearly be on how models of HIV/AIDS care in settings characterized by different underlying infrastructures can be rapidly established without seriously disrupting what previously worked well, and ideally with the potential for positive collateral effects on the broader system through leveraging of new resources.

Some have argued that tight integration with existing programs, such as those to diagnose and treat TB, may stretch limited resources in an efficient way. However, it has also been suggested that such integration with a long-established TB program may result in its being swallowed up by the bigger ART program, with negative consequences for TB control. Certainly the contribution of various factors to this issue will vary from country to country and even more locally. Rural health infrastructures may be more susceptible to negative collateral effects from new resource demands than urban systems, in which the concentration of trained providers is greater.

Operations research and the development of models to better understand the health system dynamics relevant to this issue should be priorities. The hoped-for outcome is that the infusion of resources to provide ART would, in a collateral fashion, strengthen the overall health care infrastructure. Indeed, this has been observed in some pilot projects, such as the GHESKIO program in Haiti. In that program, building on what already existed made it easier to scale up more rapidly while at the same time improving not only HIV/AIDS services, but also primary care (personal communication, Dan Fitzgerald, June 2004). There will clearly be a tension as PEPFAR, the WHO 3-by-5 campaign, and other donor-driven initiatives may tend to favor a vertical approach, as opposed to an approach emphasizing integrated sustainability based on health sector–wide government programs. While integration is the ultimate and indeed a necessary goal, the advantages of vertical programs should not be lost, as they also contribute to quality and effectiveness, two characteristics that must be part of the foundation of ART scale-up programs. In some settings, premature dependence on an integrated approach before capacity has been established could be disastrous.

Not infrequently, newly integrated health-sector programs have shown signs of failure due to such factors as lack of capacity among managers to deal with new tasks, inadequate technical supervision as hierarchies are removed, weak logistic support for carrying out necessary procurement, weak monitoring systems, misplaced foci in capacity building, change that was too swift with resultant gaps, and immature planning systems. Sometimes resources to support a particular activity end up reduced as vertical programs are integrated and resources shifted. Critical programs can also suffer from "invisibility" and slippage in their priority as they disappear into the larger health system (Brown, 2001). Understandably, it can be difficult for donors to cede control of programmatic responsibilities, such as drug procurement, to inexperienced or overburdened host government agents. This is the case in part because local government shortcomings in the management of donor funds may open donors up to criticism from their constitutiencies, and in part because gaps in performance can have serious consequences, as is certainly the case with ART. Nongovernmental organizations (NGOs) frequently represent a large proportion of the existing capacity for providing ART, and this adds complexity as their valuable initiatives are coordinated with sector-wide governmental efforts. Striking a proper balance between vertical and integrated approaches and between governmental and nongovernmental mechanisms will depend on particular local and national circumstances, offering fertile ground for documenting and disseminating lessons learned.

Learning by Doing Through Operations Research

Regardless of whether specific pilot initiatives prove to be replicable or integrated programs become the favored option, the complexities and challenges of implementing ART programs countrywide and on a much larger scale than that of any pilot initiative conducted thus far highlight the reality, emphasized earlier, that ART scale-up will largely be a learn-by-doing process. By feeding lessons learned back into the treatment and care systems, ART scale-up can be accelerated; become more effective in terms of improving both patient and population health, as well as increasing cost-effectiveness; and achieve the success needed to ensure continued donor support.

The only way lessons will be learned, however, other than through a generally intuitive sense of what might work, is for ART scale-up programs to have the funds and capacity needed to conduct rigorous, data-based operations research. Operations research is not the same as monitoring and evaluation (discussed in Chapter 5), and funds budgeted for one are not necessarily available for the other. Also, although many organizations and institutions, particularly academic institutions where research expertise is concentrated, can conduct operations research, the funding for such research must be clearly set aside in ART scale-up budgets. It must be recognized that many donors, who are focused on supporting care, group operations research with other more basic and clinical research activities that they view as outside of their mandate. Similarly, funders of traditional basic, epidemiologic, or clinical research often see operations research as beyond their focus. Hence operations research can fall into a funding gap.

Operations research (also known as management science) involves the use of advanced analytical techniques to achieve better outcomes, define optimal processes of service delivery, and develop more cost-effective systems. It encompasses a wide range of studies, including observational and outcome studies, epidemic modeling, and cost-effectiveness studies. Observational studies, for example, have been used a great deal in the United

States for determining the best way to deliver HIV/AIDS care. Such research must be seen as a routine, essential dimension of effective program management. The capacity—both financial and operational—to conduct integrated operations research should be put into place explicitly at the start of scale-up even if the actual research is not yet under way. At the very least, the capacity to collect the data necessary for operations research should be in place. Box 6-2 provides additional detail on operations research and its role in ART scale-up.

Given the magnitude of the HIV/AIDS problem, there have been few operations research studies, clinical or otherwise, conducted in sub-Saharan Africa or other resource-constrained settings. But as scale-up proceeds and as ART programs expand, so will the need and opportunity to conduct such research in parallel with program implementation. As noted, one of the most critical concerns with regard to operations research pertains to funding and the reality that most medical research worldwide is not linked to the provision of health care. Clearly, from both public health and ethical perspectives, research and care should be linked in the optimization of ART programs. Yet in most budgets, research and care are funded separately, and dedicated funds for one cannot be used for the other. Thus the need for dedicated operations research funding is again highlighted.

Recommendation 6-1. Operations research should begin at the initiation of scale-up and continue to inform the future direction and sustainable success of antiretroviral treatment and HIV prevention programs in resource-constrained settings. *Priorities for operations research should be identified by national programs and funded by donors through an explicit allocation that will address the need for rapid development of evidence for policy. Input from national authorities working with donors should be supplemented by consultation with WHO and other multilateral agencies to obtain technical advice and to help maximize regional synergies, share information, and avoid unnecessarily duplicative studies within a given region.*

Recommendation 6-2. Research priorities should be informed by the perspectives of local researchers, health workers, and community representatives and reflect respect for the cultures of affected communities. *Just as every pilot initiative functions uniquely, every scale-up initiative and national program will have its own way of functioning and should be shaped by the perspectives of those with a stake in its success. Ideally, if a well-developed operations research agenda is established early on, these different ways of functioning can be objectively evaluated in a timely fashion and the results used to inform managers of other scale-up programs about newly identified best practices. Collabo-*

BOX 6-2
The Role of Operations Research During ART Scale-Up

Given the incomplete evidence base on how to scale up ART in resource-constrained settings, a learn-by-doing approach will be necessary. As ART programs are rolled out and scaled up, continual process and program evaluation will need to be done to assess success and identify obstacles and failures. Guiding questions will be what works, what does not work, and why.

Operations research is a means of carrying out these evaluations and has been used in many health and development fields. Its overall aim is to improve the delivery of services (i.e., the operations of programs) by identifying problems and focusing attention and resources on searching for solutions. There are five basic steps in the process:

1. Problem identification and diagnosis
2. Strategy selection
3. Strategy testing and evaluation
4. Information dissemination
5. Information utilization

Policy makers, program managers, and donors will face many operations research questions as ART is scaled up. Examples of such questions include the following:

• What is the best way to ensure that a logistics system provides an uninterrupted supply of drugs?
• How can high levels of adherence to ARVs be maintained among patients?
• What is the role of community-based organizations in ART programs?
• When should ARVs be administered?
• Can nonphysicians administer ARVs safely and with high standards of care?

rative partnerships and endeavors between the research and health care communities should be encouraged.

Although the most obvious unanswered question to be addressed by research may be "What is the best ARV regimen?" with respect to ART in resource-constrained settings, it is by no means the only or even the most important one. Moreover, even that single question involves many nuances and complexities, as the best regimen in one set of circumstances (e.g., biological, medical, behavioral, social, economic, ethical) may not be the best in other contexts. For example, a multitude of operations research questions are raised by the critically important role of human resource capacity in ART scale-up and the urgent need to find innovative ways of

Engaging program managers, health care workers, community members, and people living with HIV/AIDS in operations research projects should help those in the field recognize such research as a valuable tool for decision making. Additionally, involving stakeholders throughout the process may heighten their interest in reviewing and using the results of the completed research. By engaging in operations research before and during program implementation, it is hoped that efficiency, effectiveness, and quality will be achieved.

The World Health Organization's 3-by-5 campaign has focused on six areas of activity for operations research during the scale-up of ART programs (WHO, 2004):

• To coordinate and help develop an appropriate operations research agenda relevant to the needs of ART programs.

• To seek data on the impact of scaling up ART on prevention and risk behavior, on mitigation, and on stigma and discrimination.

• To identify ways of defining the externalities of ART scale-up with regard to health system performance.

• To identify ways of costing ART programs and to link costs to impact and effectiveness.

• To improve program design and find better tools for reducing risky behavior and the evolution of drug resistance based on the analysis of data.

• To rapidly incorporate new knowledge back into ART program policy and practice.

SOURCES: Fisher and Foreit, 2002; WHO, 2004.

addressing human resource deficiencies and improving training programs (see also Chapter 5):

• What is the best way to strengthen workforce capacity?

• What are the most effective ways to train health care and other workers involved with ART scale-up?

• How can the utility of community-based and nurse-based care be maximized given the medical complexities associated with ART?

• How can laboratory training be improved to minimize worker-related errors?

• What are the best programmatic mechanisms to minimize negative collateral effects of scale-up on other essential programs?

- What are the most effective mechanisms to retain critical health care workers who might either be subject to "burnout" or enticed by lucrative overseas offers of employment?

Although some competition is healthy to encourage rigorous research and rapid results, having too many ongoing studies within a country, particularly within a concentrated area, can become confusing and even counterproductive. Thus the question arises of how operations research can be coordinated in a way that best suits the needs of the country in which it is being conducted. Another issue is how the conclusions drawn from operations research results should be shared and disseminated. Operations research must be designed such that comparisons among different approaches and outcomes can be readily distinguished from the inevitable differences that exist among the various populations in which the approaches are being tested. For example, if one intervention has an 85 percent success rate in one population and another only a 65 percent success rate elsewhere, how can it be determined to what extent the difference is due to the intervention or the population?

As the number of research studies increases worldwide, there is a growing need to establish common research protocols so results will be more comparable and the exchange of information more efficient. HIV-NAT (The Netherlands, Australia, Thailand Research Collaboration) has been cited as one example of a program specifically developed to facilitate and coordinate the exchange of clinical research information, in this case between scientists in The Netherlands and Australia and Thai investigators in an effort to address treatment questions of particular relevance to Thailand (The HIV Netherlands Australia Thailand Research Collaboration, 2004).

As new evidence regarding the safest and best use of ARVs in resource-limited settings accumulates, the need to integrate new policies or recommendations into already existing and implemented guidelines and protocols will grow. Thus questions arise regarding how existing guidelines, including those of WHO and others, allow for the ready adoption of important new evidence and how revised guidelines will be disseminated and integrated into community health programs worldwide. Moreover, greater clarity is needed regarding the ethical imperative to ensure that clinical guidelines for ARV usage in resource-constrained settings adhere to the same type of evidence-based criteria required for guidelines of the United States and other resource-rich countries.

Given the likely but still largely unknown (i.e., unsupported by a detailed evidence base) impacts of nutrition, coinfection with other endemic diseases, concurrent treatment for TB, and other factors on adherence to medications and the efficacy of ART, issues surrounding the need to test newly developed ARVs in resource-constrained settings need to be clarified and appropriately addressed. More broadly, in light of the larger social, cultural, environmental, and economic context of the HIV/AIDS pandemic, how can the research agenda be expanded such that the upstream determinants of infectious disease emergence, including poverty, are addressed in a meaningful and adequate way? Can poverty-reduction programs and ART programs be coordinated so as to be complementary and synergistic? Other cultural dimensions must also be considered. For example, in South Africa the majority of HIV-infected people use traditional medicines. Thus the consequences and effectiveness of using these treatments (as well as other non-ARV immune regulators) need to be objectively examined to better inform those prescribing ARVs about how to treat these patients.

It must be recognized that HIV/AIDS is not just a medical problem. Rather, to address the problem it is necessary to examine the total system—with its many complex negative and positive feedbacks—from a systems perspective. The question arises, however, of how this framework can and should be applied to research in the field. What are the practical implications of this type of thinking for budgeting for operations research to support ART scale-up?

Finally, the importance of modeling cost-effectiveness considerations and incorporating them into operations research questions should be neither underestimated nor overestimated. Models that can be used to predict demand for drugs and other resource requirements need to be developed and validated so that planners can ensure continuity of drugs and care in the face of changing needs. Regardless of how important the immediate health outcomes of any intervention or practice may be, the more cost-effective a process is, the more people will benefit. For example, although the expensive state-of-the-art laboratory monitoring standards applied in the United States may minimize treatment failure, reliance on such standards in resource-limited settings would also minimize the number of people who could receive treatment. Thus it is important to consider cost-effectiveness in addition to clinical outcomes when testing various treatment or other ARV-related interventions.

APPLIED CLINICAL RESEARCH

The WHO guidelines provide an excellent, evidence-based set of criteria for determining when to initiate therapy, how to monitor therapy, when to change drugs or regimens, how to incorporate care and treatment for opportunistic infections into ART, and so on. Nonetheless, the recommendations are intended to serve only as a starting point for the development of national guidelines. Some of the WHO guidelines are necessarily vague because of incomplete clinical knowledge. An example is the recommended treatment for women of childbearing potential or those who are pregnant.

Because of mutations associated with resistance to nonnucleoside reverse transcriptase inhibitors (NNRTIs), the use of nevirapine for the prevention of mother-to-child transmission of HIV could potentially limit subsequent treatment of the mother and her infected infant. Similar concerns exist for 3TC-containing regimens. As stated in the guidelines:

> The clinical consequences of selection of these resistance mutations in terms of response to future antiretroviral therapy of the woman or the infected infant are unknown. . . . This is one of the most pressing operational research questions facing the field and must be answered with appropriately conducted studies. . . . Until definitive data are available to answer these questions, treatment of women who have previously received single dose [nevirapine] prophylaxis or 3TC prophylaxis for prevention of MTCT [mother-to-child transmission] should be considered eligible for NNRTI-based regimens and not be denied access to life-sustaining therapy (WHO, 2003a:23).

This example illustrates the need for immediate applied research to inform national and international guidelines with regard to certain clinical components of ART scale-up in resource-constrained settings. Attendees at a 2001 conference held in San Francisco, California, to develop a research agenda on HIV/AIDS therapy for resource-limited countries identified three categories of topics: when therapy should be initiated, what therapies should be used, and what methods are most appropriate for patient monitoring when CD4+ cell count and viral load tests are not available. (A summary of the recommendations from that conference is provided by Vermund and Powderly [2003].) Moreover, the need for patient monitoring raises the question, especially in resource-constrained settings, of how frequently that monitoring should be done. Operations research can also help develop optimal programs for ARV resistance screening in individuals and surveillance in larger community populations.

Several different methodological approaches could be used in applied clinical research. For example, to address the question of when to start therapy, investigators could conduct prospective randomized trials (e.g., to compare the effectiveness of different times of treatment initiation), conduct observational database studies, or pursue pathogenesis studies (e.g., to identify lower-cost, clinically significant immunological parameters to track). Because prospective randomized trials are costly and lengthy and involve large sample sizes, they would need to be conducted in countries with the necessary infrastructure. Observational studies would be ideal for countries with widely available ART, such as Brazil, where a variety of patient groups and treatment regimens are available for comparison.

Priority Clinical Research Questions

In addition to questions about whether single-dose nevirapine impacts future therapeutic options for either mothers or their babies, critical areas of concern in which further evidence-based knowledge is needed include pediatric formulations; the treatment of HIV–TB coinfected patients; and the efficacy of various regimens for both adults and children, TB coinfected or otherwise, in resource-constrained settings.

As discussed in Chapter 5, there has recently been a focus on fixed-dose combinations (FDCs) as a means of facilitating the treatment of as many people as possible worldwide with ARVs. As FDCs are introduced, there may be an opportunity to conduct large, simple, randomized trials quantifying their effects on health outcomes and adherence. Moreover, as there are currently no direct comparisons of FDCs and blister packaging of the same medications, such a comparison could be incorporated into the same trials when possible. Quantifying the relative benefits of FDCs, blister packages, and loose drugs in this manner could better inform choices about delivery.

Other important clinical questions in need of answers include the following:

- How effectively can treatment failure be assessed in the absence of CD4 and viral load testing?
- What clinical or laboratory parameters should be monitored to determine treatment efficacy and failure?
- What is the clinical utility of viral load testing for therapy initiation and monitoring?
- What minimum laboratory testing should be done to monitor for adverse drug effects?
- What are the optimal methods for detecting and treating other HIV subtypes (i.e., HIV-2, Type O)?
- Can alternative regimens for initiation and salvage be developed?
- What are the mental health sequelae associated with treatment, and how can they be addressed?

Recommendation 6 3. Development and field evaluation of simple, rapid, inexpensive laboratory tests for diagnosing HIV infections and for monitoring therapeutic responses should be a high priority. *The shortage of laboratories and laboratory technicians in resource-poor countries, together with the millions in need of HIV testing and treatment monitoring, underlines the priority of developing tests with these characteristics. In relatively well-resourced countries, critical monitoring for toxicity and viral response utilizes generally expensive assays,* *whose annual costs could themselves be comparable to those of the ARVs to be used. For resource-constrained countries, less-costly measurement tools, such as viral load and CD4 counts, are needed to stretch limited budgets and enable technicians trained at a more basic level to perform the tests.*

Another priority for applied clinical research arises from the vital role of prophylaxis for opportunistic infections, including TB, in reducing AIDS-related mortality, at least in the short and medium terms. This point is illustrated by the experience of both Brazil and South Africa. Thus there is an urgent need for more research on related topics, including the wider applicability of cotrimoxazole and its use in children and infants, care for Kaposi's sarcoma in resource-constrained settings, the use of isoniazid in treating TB, and the use of antifungals.

Finally, as many of the clinical trials and prospective studies of ARVs and their effects have been conducted in the developed world, the extent to which the relationships among disease, drugs, and nutrition are a factor of the developed world's diet and nutritional status is unclear. At this time, therefore, the effect malnutrition will have on the success of ART scale-up on a broad scale is unknown. It is clear that many people living with HIV/AIDS in the developing world lack access to sufficient quantity and quality of nutritious foods (see Chapter 4). WHO (2003b) has recognized the limited research done on this issue—specifically in resource-constrained settings—and identified research questions it believes to be crucial for gaining a better understanding in this area (see Box 6-3). It is known, however,

---

BOX 6-3
Nutrition and HIV/AIDS: Addressing Knowledge Gaps

Questions to be addressed by research on nutrition and HIV/AIDS include the following:

• What is the impact of ART in malnourished populations?
• Does nutritional status affect the efficacy of therapy and the risk or severity of associated adverse events?
• Would nutrition interventions—particularly in undernourished populations and lactating mothers—provided concurrently with ART result in better health outcomes?
• Should there be a different mix of lifestyle change strategies (e.g., for dietary intake and physical activity) in resource-limited settings, where undernutrition is prevalent, than in developed countries?

SOURCE: WHO, 2003b.

that micro- and macronutrients affect the progression of HIV and the bioavailability and efficacy of particular drugs. Therefore, food and nutrition assistance programs should be a resource available to those using ART. Additional nutrition-related research questions include the following:

- What are the benefits of nutritional supplementation?
- What are the pharmacokinetics of ARVs in populations with poor nutrition?

BEHAVIORAL RESEARCH

Implementing ART in resource-poor settings poses difficult, complex medical, technical, and logistical questions, many of which have yet to be addressed through operations research programs. Yet many would argue that the social and behavioral dimensions of scaling up ART programs raise equally, if not more, challenging questions. HIV is as much a psychosocial as a biomedical phenomenon. A behavioral science research agenda is critical to elucidating underlying factors and achieving a better understanding with regard to improving adherence to ARVs, reducing risk behaviors associated with transmission of HIV, improving the accessibility of ARVs and treatment and prevention programs, and reducing the stigma associated with being at risk and living with HIV/AIDS.

Improving Adherence

Given the high degree of susceptibility to resistance of some of the less expensive, WHO-recommended NNRTI-based ARV regimens in resource-constrained settings, adherence will be a critically important factor in preventing or reducing treatment failure and the consequences of such failure for both patients and the population at large (see Chapter 3). Thus one of the most urgent behavioral research needs is to identify and better understand the underlying factors that contribute to poor adherence, as well as ways to improve adherence. While adherence has been determined in a variety of ways among persons living with HIV/AIDS in wealthy countries, it remains to be determined which measurement approaches are culturally best suited to resource-poor countries and whether innovative alternatives have the potential to serve as more accurate and acceptable measures.

According to a recent assessment of available evidence for HIV/AIDS interventions performed by the Cochrane Collaborative Review Group on HIV Infection and AIDS (2004), controlled trials are urgently needed to determine which interventions can improve adherence to highly active antiretroviral therapy (HAART) and whether those interventions also suppress viral load and improve clinical outcome. More research is also needed on interventions that support or foster adherence, as well as on personal triggers for nonadherence. This research should encompass the provider and the provider–patient relationship, variables related to the treatment regimen (e.g., FDCs), and contextual factors. Specific behaviors to be better understood include the seeking of help from family and friends; the seeking of health care from traditional healers through primary care clinics; the seeking of treatment for a diagnosis; behaviors involved in obtaining and using medications correctly; supportive behaviors of partners, parents, and others; and coping behaviors in the face of stigma. More research is needed as well on the timing of adherence interventions and strategies focused on particular groups of patients (e.g., children and drug users).

Changing Behaviors That Place People at Risk

As ART scale-up proceeds, the intimate relationship between treatment and prevention must be recognized. The HIV/AIDS pandemic demands intensive prevention campaigns, along with accelerated ARV coverage. Short of a cure or highly effective vaccine, the adoption of informed and safe behavior in the entire population at risk of acquiring and transmitting HIV will remain critical to slowing the epidemic.

A crucial focus for the behavioral science research agenda should be discovering ways to change the behaviors and conditions that lead to HIV transmission (Eaton et al., 2003; Reddy and Meyer-Weitz, 1999; Reddy et al., 2003). It will be important to identify what determinants (knowledge, attitudes, and beliefs), processes, and cultural and other contextual factors are keeping people from utilizing prevention and treatment services and from changing their behavior in ways that will reduce the transmission of HIV. Although the increased availability and accessibility of ARVs and ART programs may make the HIV/AIDS pandemic more visible and infection with HIV more accepted, thus reducing some of the stigma associated with being infected or sick (see below) and encouraging more people to seek counseling and ART, it cannot be assumed that this will inevitably happen.

Since prevention and treatment programs must be intertwined for optimal synergy, behavioral research is needed to better understand how not only to foster adherence to ARV regimens, but also to improve primary prevention. Specific objectives should be to understand how to:

- Increase a person's knowledge about HIV risk reduction and HIV treatment.
- Increase perceptions of personal risk for HIV.
- Enhance motivations for behavioral change.
- Identify personal triggers for engaging in risky behaviors.

- Teach people how to communicate to their partners about the need to use condoms.
- Motivate people to use condoms correctly when appropriate.
- Teach proper condom use.
- Increase access to voluntary counseling and testing.

Research is needed as well to understand and improve the organization, management, accessibility, delivery, cost-effectiveness, and cost-utility of each of the following services with regard to reducing HIV risk behaviors and transmission:

- Health care
- Family planning
- Social services
- Drug treatment services
- Alcoholism treatment centers

Addressing the Familial and Social Context of HIV/AIDS

Designing interventions that help partners improve their communication skills and foster safer sex norms within relationships is critical to controlling the HIV/AIDS pandemic. There has been growing recognition of the importance of family, community, and society at large in the adoption and utilization of HIV prevention efforts. Strategies in this area encompass creating settings that support testing and counseling and encouraging practices that prevent transmission between HIV positive and negative persons, such as delaying the onset of sexual activity in young people and encouraging proper use of condoms when serostatus is unknown. Using the family to foster norms supportive of safer sexual practices and therapeutic adherence, providing HIV/AIDS education within the context of the family, and enhancing communication skills between parents and their children can be effective strategies for reducing detrimental behaviors. Effective interventions at the community level (e.g., neighborhoods, social network members, organizations, institutions) involve enhancing community norms that favor safer sex practices and adherence to therapeutic regimens. Societal-level interventions involve modifying economic, legal, policy, and regulatory practices such that they foster safer sex and support therapeutic efforts.

Given this familial and community context of HIV/AIDS, research should be directed toward identifying family- and community-level behavioral intervention strategies that promote prevention among both infected and uninfected individuals, as well as adherence among individuals under treatment. The engagement of families and communities in providing palliative care as AIDS patients approach the end of life is another worthy research focus. How can family providers best be supported at this stressful time? How can they be prepared most effectively to support the medical, emotional, and spiritual needs of the dying?

Treating Women with HIV/AIDS

Women experience HIV/AIDS differently from men in a number of important respects, both physiological and social (see also Chapter 4). They are more vulnerable to HIV infection as a result of cultural attitudes and their general social and economic position. Within the context of heterosexual relationships and social arrangements, they often have less power than men, which further exacerbates their risk of contracting HIV (Dunkle et al., 2004). It is crucial to understand these socially constructed aspects of male and female relationships, including the economic dependence of women, their role in political decision making, and the resulting impacts on access to health services and education, all of which may influence access to ART and the practice of safer sex. Domestic and sexual violence are common additional obstacles to the ability of women and girls to protect themselves even if they are well informed. Although HIV-infected pregnant women have received a great deal of attention, the focus has been primarily on preventing transmission to their offspring (as discussed in Chapter 4). Greater attention must be given to women, particularly since they are often infected earlier and at higher rates: the HIV prevalence among those aged 15–24 is 2.5 times higher among women than men in some African communities (UNAIDS, 2003).

Accordingly, a priority research objective is to better understand how to design effective HIV prevention and treatment interventions for women and girls, including how to improve adherence. Interventions should be gender-specific, as well as involve couples and be culturally appropriate and acceptable. Box 6-4 summarizes key points to be considered in addressing this research objective.

Reducing Stigma

Research is needed on how to develop, evaluate, and encourage the adoption of strategies to prevent or minimize the negative physical, psychological, cognitive, and social consequences of HIV, including the stigmatization of persons with or at risk for HIV infection (see Chapter 4). An important issue to be investigated is how to promote modifications in the health care delivery system that lead to more effective, culturally sensitive treatment of infected individuals. For example, what can be done to modify the behavior of health care providers in ways that will enhance health care

---

BOX 6-4
Women and HIV/AIDS: Implications for Treatment

Women play a central role in family life and in the provision of care for children, spouses, and other relatives with HIV infection. This role highlights the familial impact associated with the fact that women represent 50 percent of the victims of the global AIDS pandemic. In the worst-affected region of the world, sub-Saharan Africa, this figure is 58 percent. As a result of disparities linked to sexual abuse, coercion, discrimination, and poverty, teenage girls in sub-Saharan Africa are infected at rates four to seven times those of their male counterparts. Moreover, while women are more likely to become infected, they may be less likely to get tested or to seek and receive treatment because of gender-based inequalities.

Factors affecting access to and use of ART by women include the following:

• Level of recognition of the need to treat women with HIV outside of the context of preventing perinatal transmission
• Household and childrearing responsibilities affecting the priority accorded to a woman obtaining health care
• The need to pay for therapy when women are not in control of financial resources
• The threat of violence as a disincentive for women to get tested
• Pressure women may feel to share ARVs with infected children, spouses, and other family members

HIV treatment programs should be sensitive to the roles in which women find themselves as both patients and providers. Factors that pose additional barriers to their accessing needed HIV-related care deserve specific attention by program managers, especially given the importance of supporting the role of women in family life.

SOURCES: Fleischman, 2004; Gruskin and Maluwa, 2002; Tlou, 2002.

---

utilization; improve screening, counseling, and testing services; and decrease the stigma associated with seeking preventive care and treatment for HIV/AIDS? What can be done to improve providers' communication skills and ability to make shared decisions with their patients about how and when to initiate therapy?

Improving Methodological Tools

To address the above behavioral research needs rapidly and in a meaningful manner, the qualitative and quantitative methodological tools used in behavioral research, including those for evaluating HIV prevention interventions, need to be strengthened and expanded. New and rigorous methodological and statistical techniques should be encouraged.

More-effective methods are needed to increase recruitment, retention, and compliance with protocols for research on interventions aimed at HIV prevention and adherence to treatment. The efficacy of such interventions should be evaluated using rigorous research methods, including randomized controlled behavioral trials. Evaluations of behavioral interventions should use behavioral self-reports as outcome measures, as well as HIV seroincidence data and other biological markers. In addition to assessing efficacy, researchers should assess the cost-effectiveness of interventions. Finally, more research and debate are needed to address the pressing ethical issues involved in the conduct of such research.

Addressing Comorbidity and Poverty

It is increasingly being recognized that many individuals who are at risk of and become infected with HIV are also impoverished and afflicted with a number of comorbid conditions, including other infectious diseases (hepatitis, sexually transmitted diseases, TB, malaria, and other endemic diseases), substance abuse, and mental illness. The potential for negatively synergistic interactions between comorbidities and poverty is obvious. Research is needed to test the efficacy of interventions that simultaneously address multiple diagnoses and risks, including how to improve adherence to ART among those suffering from any number of other diseases and substance abuse problems. Means of mitigating the complications imposed by coexistent poverty should also be investigated.

Research is needed as well to better understand the underlying factors that contribute to the co-occurrence of HIV/AIDS and the progression of AIDS with other infectious diseases, substance abuse, alcohol abuse, and mental illness. Such research should encompass how to design efficacious and cost-effective strategies for addressing such comorbid conditions. It will be essential to better understand the intersection of HIV/AIDS with these related conditions if the treatment and prevention programs now being implemented are to be sustained for the decades that will be necessary to bring the pandemic under control.

ENSURING SUSTAINABILITY ALONG THE PATH FORWARD

Sustained action along the path forward presumes solutions to numerous discrete scientific and management challenges. At the same time, as wealthy, middle-income, and poor nations join together in perhaps an unprecedented way to tackle the overarching challenge of bringing the pandemic under control, it bears emphasizing that the global problem of HIV/AIDS will likely be present for decades despite research findings and optimized interventions. In a few years, when it may be hoped that the initial objectives of WHO's 3-by-5 campaign and the U.S. Emergency Plan will have been met, we must not abandon the millions started on therapy or ignore the pleas of the tens of millions more who will soon need these medicines and subsequently make a claim on our humanity. Even short-term interruptions in support could be clinically disastrous and ethically problematic by allowing successfully suppressed HIV infections to emerge in drug-resistant forms. Thus, ART must not be seen simply as a short-term goal or the end point of a 5-year plan. The world is indeed at the beginning of a very long path forward.

The role of donors, whether they be funders from government, foundations, or international banks or individuals and organizational partners providing care-related services, will steadily increase for decades to come. The legacy of the United States and its international partners, and indeed of the entire global community in the early twenty-first century, will be measured against how we respond to the challenges of the day with the resources at our disposal. The response to the global HIV/AIDS pandemic must be a sustained claim on those resources. Lifetime ART for 30–40 million people will likely require annual investments of at least US$9–12 billion (Council on Foreign Relations, 2004). In parallel, sufficient funding must be sustained for prevention activities to curb the emergence of new cases that will demand therapy. Considering the familial, political, economic, and institutional destabilization that could well occur without these infusions of assistance, as well as the costly international military responses that could be required to restore and maintain peace (and ensure access to important natural resources) as a result of such breakdowns, ongoing support for ART programs may well be more economically prudent than the alternative. Indeed, the ongoing erosion of state capacity in sub-Saharan Africa associated with uncontrolled HIV/AIDS contributed to the Bush Administration's assertion in the current National Security Strategy that "America is now threatened less by conquering states than we are by failing ones," and the will to sustain investments for HIV/AIDS prevention and treatment will be threatened for states that appear to be failing (White House, 2004).

Ensuring the sustainability of political will, funding, and service will be a challenge even if initial scale-up activities are deemed generally successful. The measure of success in the intermediate term will be treatment outcomes (measured by decreased morbidity and mortality and durable suppression of viral loads). To achieve these objectives will require unprecedented attention to quality of care in resource-constrained settings, along with constant learning. Quality needs to be viewed as a necessity, not a luxury, because only quality programs will be able to sustain favorable treatment effects for a decade or more. The potential for negative collateral effects of scale-up programs, such as the diversion of workers and resources from other critical health programs, must also be anticipated and dealt with in a preventive fashion. Because success is the best justification for sustained and increasing investments, the lessons learned that are documented in this report and the management and clinical principles that are recommended must not be ignored in the urgency to move forward. The path forward has been illuminated. It is imperative to act now, but also to act well.

REFERENCES

Brown A. 2001. *Integrating Vertical Health Programs into Sector Wide Approaches: Experiences and Lessons.* [Online]. Available: http://www.ihsd.org [accessed June 5, 2004].

Cochrane Collaborative Review Group on HIV Infection and AIDS. 2004. *Evidence Assessment: Strategies of HIV/AIDS Prevention, Treatment, and Care.* [Online]. Available: http://www.igh.org/Cochrane/pdfs/EvidenceAssessment.pdf [accessed August 31, 2004].

Council on Foreign Relations. 2004. *Addressing the HIV/AIDS Pandemic: A U.S. Global AIDS Strategy for the Long Term.* New York: Council on Foreign Relations and Milbank Memorial Fund.

Dunkle K, Jewkes R, Brown H, Gray G, McIntryre J, Harlow S. 2004. Gender-based violence, relationship power, and risk of HIV infection in women attending antenatal clinics in South Africa. *Lancet* 363(9419):1415–1421.

Eaton L, Flisher AJ, Aaro LE. 2003. Unsafe sexual behaviour in South African youth. *Social Science and Medicine* 56:149–165.

Fisher A, Foreit J. 2002. *Designing HIV/AIDS Intervention Studies: An Operations Research Handbook.* New York: The Population Council, Inc.

Fleischman J. 2004. *Breaking the Cycle: Ensuring Equitable Access to HIV Treatment for Women and Girls.* Center for Strategic and International Studies. [Online]. Available: http://www.csis.org/africa/0402_breakingcycle.pdf [accessed August 24, 2004].

Gilks C, Abouzhar C, Turmen T. 2001. HAART in Haiti: Evidence needed. *Bulletin of the World Health Organization* 79(12):1154–1155.

Gruskin S, Maluwa M. 2002. Human Rights and HIV/AIDS. In: Essex M, Mboup S, Kanki P, Marlink R, Tlou S, eds. *AIDS in Africa.* 2nd Edition. New York: Kluwer Academic/Plenum Publishers. Pp. 641–651.

Reddy SP, Meyer-Weitz A. 1999. *Sense and Sensibilities: The Psychosocial and Contextual Determinants of STD Related Behaviours.* Cape Town, South Africa: South African Medical Research Council.

Reddy SP, Panday S, Swart D, Jinabhai CC, Amosun SL, James S, Monyeki KD, Stevens G, Morejele N, Kambaran NS, Omardien RG, Van den Borne RG. 2003. *UmthembtheUhlaba Usamila: The South African Youth Risk Behaviour Survey 2002.* Cape Town, South Africa: South African Medical Research Council.

The HIV Netherlands Australia Thailand Research Collaboration. 2004. *The HIV Netherlands Australia Thailand Research Collaboration Homepage.* [Online]. Available: http://www.hivnat.org/ [accessed January 5, 2004].

Tlou SD. 2002. Gender and HIV/AIDS. In: Essex M, Mboup S, Kanki P, Marlink R, Tlou S, eds. *AIDS in Africa.* 2nd Edition. New York: Kluwer Academic/Plenum Publishers. Pp. 654–663.

UNAIDS (Joint United Nations Programme on HIV/AIDS). 2003. *AIDS Epidemic Update 2003.* [Online]. Available: http://www.unaids.org/EN/other/functionalities/document.asp?href=http%3A%2F%2Fwww%2Eunaids%2Eorg%2Fhtml%2Fpub%2FPublications%2FFIR%2Dpub06%2FEpi03%5F00%5Fen%5Fhtml%2Ehtm&PDFHref=&FileSize=120 [accessed August 24, 2004].

Vermund SH, Powderly WG. 2003. Developing a human immunodeficiency virus/acquired immunodeficiency syndrome therapeutic research agenda for resource-limited countries: A consensus statement. *Clinical Infectious Diseases* 37(Suppl 1):S4–S12.

White House. 2004. *Overview of America's International Strategy*. [Online]. Available: http://www.whitehouse.gov/nsc/nss1.html [accessed April 2, 2004].

WHO (World Health Organization). 2003a. *Scaling up Antiretroviral Therapy in Resource-Limited Settings: Treatment Guidelines for a Public Health Approach, 2003 Revision*. [Online]. Available: http://www.siecus.org/inter/WHO_ARV_Guidelines2003.pdf [accessed August 24, 2004].

WHO. 2003b. *Nutrient Requirements for People Living with HIV/AIDS: Report of a Technical Consultation*. Geneva: WHO.

WHO. 2004. *Operational Research for the 3 by 5 Initiative*. [Online]. Available: http://www.who.int/3by5/publications/briefs/operational_research/en/ [accessed August 24, 2004].

Appendix
A

Information Gathering Workshop Agenda

Committee on Examining the Probable Consequences of
Alternative Patterns of Widespread Antiretroviral Drug Use in
Resource-Constrained Settings

Tuesday, January 27, 2004
Room 100, Keck Building
500 5th Street, NW
Washington, DC 2001

8:00-8:20   Welcome, Introduction of Committee, and
              Statement of Charge
                  Dr. James Curran and Dr. Haile Debas
                  Committee Cochairs

The Opportunity

8:20-8:45   The Challenge of HIV/AIDS in 2004 and the
              WHO 3 × 5 Program
                  Dr. Jim Kim
                  Advisor to the Director-General
                  World Health Organization
                  Geneva, Switzerland

8:45-9:10   The Global Funds' Lessons Learned Regarding ARV
Drug Scale-up in Resource-Constrained Settings
Dr. Bernhard Schwartlander
Director
Strategic Information and Measurement
Global Fund to Fight AIDS, TB, and Malaria
Geneva, Switzerland

9:10-9:35   The U.S. Emergency Plan for Antiretroviral Scale-up:
The Latest Programmatic Developments
Dr. Joe O'Neil
Deputy Coordinator
Office of the Global AIDS Coordinator
Department of State
Washington, DC

9:35-9:55   General Discussion

9:55-10:15   BREAK

Antecedents

10:15-10:40   Durability of ARV Therapy: U.S. Experience and Its
Implications for Resource-Constrained Settings
Dr. Robert Redfield
Cofounder and Director of Clinical Care and
   Research Division, Institute of Human Virology
University of Maryland
Baltimore, MD

10:40-11:05   A U.S. Clinical Perspective on the Implications of ARV
Resistance for Resource-Constrained Settings
Dr. Steven Deeks
Associate Clinical Professor of Clinical Medicine
University of California, San Francisco
San Francisco, CA

11:05-11:30   Lessons Learned from the Scale-up of ARV
Treatment in Brazil
Dr. Mauro Schechter
Professor of Infectious Diseases
Universidade Federal do Rio de Janeiro, Brazil

11:30-11:55   Lessons Learned from the Use of ARVs in Very
Low-Resource Settings: The Haiti Experience
Dr. Daniel Fitzgerald
Groupe Haitien d'Étude du Sarcome de Kaposi et des
infections Opportunistes (GHESKIO)
Port-au-Prince, Haiti, and
Division of International Medicine and
Infectious Diseases
Cornell University Medical College
New York, NY

11:55-12:20   MSF Perspectives on ARV Administration:
Experiences from 20 countries and 10,000 Patients
Ms. Rachel Cohen
U.S. Director, Campaign for Access to
Essential Medicines
Médecins sans Frontières
New York, NY

12:20-12:50   General Discussion

12:50-1:50   LUNCH

Clinical Principles for ARV Scale-up Programs

1:50-2:15   The 2003 WHO Guidelines for ARV Use:
Perspectives from a User
Dr. John Idoko
Professor
Jos University Teaching Hospital
Jos, Nigeria

2:15-2:40   MTCT-Plus Initiative: Perspectives from a
Multicountry Comprehensive HIV Care and
Treatment Program
Dr. Wafaa El-Sadr
Professor
Mailman School of Public Health
Columbia University and Harlem Hospital
New York, NY

2:40-3:05   The Role of the Laboratory in Managing ARV Care
              in a Country with Highly Limited Resources
                  Dr. Brooks Jackson
                  Baxley Professor and Director of Pathology
                  Johns Hopkins University School of Medicine
                  Baltimore, MD

3:05-3:30   The Social and Behavioral Dimensions of Adherence:
              Implications for Patient Education
                  Dr. Carla Makhlouf Obermeyer
                  Scientist
                  Department of HIV/AIDS
                  World Health Organization
                  Geneva, Switzerland

3:30-3:50   General Discussion

3:50-4:10   BREAK

4:10-4:35   Preventing Mother-to-Child Transmission:
              Issues of Therapy and Resistance
                  Dr. Lynne Mofenson
                  Pediatric, Adolescent and Maternal AIDS Branch
                  Center for Research for Mothers and Children
                  National Institute of Child Health and
                      Human Development
                  National Institutes of Health
                  Bethesda, MD

4:35-5:00   Pediatric Considerations for ARV Programs in
              Resource-Constrained Settings
                  Dr. Mark Kline
                  Chief, Retrovirology Clinic
                  Professor of Pediatrics
                  Director, Baylor International Pediatric AIDS
                      Initiative
                  Baylor College of Medicine/Texas Children's Hospital
                  Houston, TX

5:00-5:25   The Integration of Counseling, Prevention, and
             ARV Programs
                Dr. Sam Dooley
                Division of HIV/AIDS Prevention
                Centers for Disease Control and Prevention
                Atlanta, GA

5:25-6:00   Wrap-up Comments and Discussion

Wednesday, January 28, 2004

Management Principles for Scale-up of ARV Programs

8:00-8:05   Opening Comments
                Dr. James Curran and Dr. Haile Debas
                Committee Cochairs

8:05-8:30   Principles of Design and Scale-up for National
             Clinical Care Programs and Applications to the
             WHO 3 × 5 Targets
                Dr. M. Rashad Massoud
                Vice President and Director
                Quality and Performance Institute
                University Research Co., LLC
                Bethesda, MD

8:30-8:55   An Overview of Health Care Manpower, Health Care
             Infrastructure, and Economics in Select Resource-Poor
             Countries
                Mr. Mead Over
                Lead Economist
                Development Research Group
                World Bank
                Washington, DC

8:55-9:20   The Role of Community Mobilization in the Scale-up
             of ARV programs
                Ms. Emi MacLean
                Médecins sans Frontières
                New York, NY

9:20-9:45   Distribution of ARVs: Issues of Security, Logistics, and Quality
                 Ms. Yasmin Chandani
                 HIV/AIDS Advisor for DELIVER
                 John Snow, Inc.
                 Arlington, VA

9:45-10:10   Large Scale Training for ARV Providers: Observations from the United States
                 Dr. John McNeil
                 Chief, Infectious Diseases
                 Howard University
                 PI, National Minority AIDS Education and
                     Training Center
                 Washington, DC

10:10-10:30   General Discussion

10:30-10:50   BREAK

10:50-11:15   Perspectives on Purchasing First and Second Line ARVs
                 Ms. Lynn Margherio
                 Executive Vice President
                 The Clinton Foundation HIV/AIDS Initiative

11:15-11:40   Delivering ARVs: The Economic Consequences of Resistance
                 Dr. Stefano Bertozzi
                 Director
                 Economics and Policy
                 Center of Research on Health Systems
                 National Institute of Public Health
                 Cuernavaca, Mexico

11:40-12:00   General Discussion

12:00-1:00   LUNCH

The Path Forward

1:00-1:25   Assessing Readiness for ARV Program Implementation
             Dr. Eric Goosby
             Chief Executive Officer
             Pangea Global AIDS Foundation
             San Francisco, CA

1:25-1:50   Specific Questions for Operations Research in the
             Scale-up of ARV Treatment Programs in Low-Resource
             Settings
             Dr. Tom Quinn
             Professor of Medicine
             Johns Hopkins University School of Medicine
             Baltimore, MD

1:50-2:15   The Role of Statistical Prediction Methods for
             Managing ARV Scale-up Programs
             Dr. Victor De Gruttola
             Professor of Biostatistics
             Harvard School of Public Health
             Boston, MA

2:15-2:40   Ethical Issues in the Scale-up of ARV Programs in
             Resource-Poor Settings
             Ms. Angela Wasunna
             Lawyer/Bioethicist
             Associate for International Programs
             The Hastings Center
             Garrison, NY

2:40-3:05   Discussion

3:05-3:30   BREAK

3:30-3:55   Information Management Considerations in
             Managing ARV Programs
             Mr. Ronaldo Lima
             International AIDS Vaccine Initiative
             New York, New York

3:55-4:20   ARV Resistance: Epidemiologic Implications and
              Public Health Surveillance
                   Dr. Diane Bennett
                   World Health Organization
                   Geneva, Switzerland

4:20-4:45   Monitoring and Evaluation for ARV Programs in
              Resource-Poor Settings
                   Dr. Paul DeLay
                   UNAIDS
                   Geneva, Switzerland

4:45-5:10   The South African Plan for ARV Scale-up
                   Dr. Tony Mbewu,
                   Executive Director
                   Medical Research Council of South Africa
                   Capetown, South Africa

5:10-6:00   Discussion and Wrap-up

Appendix
B

Primer on Human Immunodeficiency Virus, Acquired Immune Deficiency Syndrome, and Antiretroviral Therapy

This primer is intended to provide the reader with a broad overview of HIV, AIDS, and antiretroviral therapy and guidelines for adults and adolescents in the United States. For a more complete review of antiretroviral therapy and guidelines, including for pregnant women and children, the reader is directed to the U.S. Department of Health and Human Services November 2003 *Guidelines for the Use of Antiretroviral Agents in HIV-1-Infected Adults and Adolescents* and the January 2004 *Guidelines for the Use of Antiretroviral Agents in Pediatric HIV Infection*. Both documents are available at: http://aidsinfo.nih.gov/.

HUMAN IMMUNODEFICIENCY VIRUS AND THE ACQUIRED IMMUNE DEFICIENCY SYNDROME

Human immunodeficiency virus (HIV) is a single-stranded RNA virus of the *Retroviridae* family. When a person becomes infected with this virus, that person develops a lifelong condition resulting from this virus' ability to integrate its genome into the genome of certain human cells. Without treatment, this virus causes a progressive weakening in the host's immune system, culminating in the acquired immune deficiency syndrome (AIDS), and death over a period of years.

The virus consists of a core and an envelope. The core contains two copies of single stranded RNA. The virus particle also contains several viral (and host cell) proteins that assist with replication. The three main enzymes are reverse transcriptase, protease, and integrase. The envelope contains proteins that allow the virus to attach to and enter its main target cells in the body: the CD4+ T lymphocyte (also known as CD4+ T cell or CD4 cell) and the macrophage. The CD4+ T lymphocyte is a critical element in orchestrating the normal immune response to a wide range of infectious agents. Once inside the CD4+ cell, the virus replicates. Early in this process, HIV viral RNA is transcribed to double stranded DNA by the virus' reverse transcriptase enzyme. This newly produced viral DNA is integrated into the DNA of the host's CD4+ T lymphocyte and becomes known as "proviral DNA." As infection depletes CD4+ cells, the immune system becomes compromised and the person develops AIDS; this process typically occurs over the course of years in an otherwise normal adult. When the immune system becomes debilitated to the point of the AIDS, the person can develop a range of opportunistic infections (OI), like tuberculosis, pneumocystosis, cryptococcus, toxoplasmosis, and certain cancers, like Kaposi's sarcoma and lymphoma.

An HIV-infected person is categorized as having AIDS when the CD4+ white blood cell count drops to below 200 cells/mm^3 (normal counts vary significantly but typically range between around 500 and 1500 cells/mm^3) or when he or she develops opportunistic infections or cancers. The complete criteria for diagnosing AIDS may be found in the December 1992 Morbidity and Mortality Weekly Report article (Centers for Disease Control and Prevention, 1992).

While there is no cure for HIV or AIDS, treatment is now available. This includes antibiotics to prevent and treat OIs and specific antiretroviral (ARV) therapy to control HIV viral replication itself. In resource-rich countries where ARVs have been available and affordable for several years, HIV infection has ceased to be considered an automatic death sentence. With carefully managed therapy and a motivated patient, HIV infection is a serious but treatable chronic disease that does not necessarily preclude additional decades of good quality life.

The Goals of Antiretroviral Therapy

The use of antiretroviral therapy for HIV infection has become complex as more has been learned about the virus and its ever-changing response to therapeutics and about patient factors affecting therapy. The goals of therapy are to inhibit viral replication while minimizing toxicities and side effects associated with the available drugs. This inhibition of virus replication permits restoration of the immune system. Viral eradication from the host genome is not achievable; thus a cure for HIV is not yet possible. By using an appropriate antiretroviral treatment regimen it is possible to minimize the morbidity and mortality associated with HIV, to delay or prevent the onset of AIDS, and to allow those infected to lead a productive life.

Goals of Antiretroviral Therapy

- viral load suppression
- restoration or preservation of immunologic function
- quality of life improvement
- reduction in HIV related morbidity and mortality

SOURCE: U.S. DHHS, 2003.

Restoration of immune function and suppression of viral replication have been assessed largely by laboratory criteria. The goal of therapy is to achieve a CD4 cell count of greater than 200 copies/mm^3 and an "undetectable" viral load (less than < 50 copies/mL). Within 4–6 months of starting antiretroviral therapy, these goals should be achieved. Failure is multifactorial; some issues will be highlighted in this report.

The Four Classes of Therapy: Mechanisms of Action

Drugs used to treat HIV principally belong to hree main classes, each based on a different mechanism of action; a fourth class was recently added. Three of the classes affect viral enzymes. The fourth class affects the ability of the virus to enter target cells in the body. The first class developed was the nucleoside analogue reverse transcriptase inhibitors (NRTIs). The first drug in this class (zidovudine [AZT or ZDV]) was introduced in 1987. The NRTIs compete with physiologic nucleosides—the building blocks of host and viral DNA—for binding to the reverse transcriptase enzyme. This has the effect of interrupting viral DNA chain elongation. There are eight FDA approved drugs in this class. The next two classes of drugs were introduced in late 1995 to mid-1996. One of these is the nonnucleoside reverse transcriptase inhibitors (NNRTIs). The NNRTIs bind to the reverse transcriptase enzyme and change the "shape" of the enzyme thereby preventing the enzyme's action of transcribing viral RNA into viral DNA. There are three FDA-approved drugs in this class. The other class of drugs that was introduced is the protease inhibitors (PIs). The PIs work at a later stage of new virus production. The PIs inhibit the viral enzyme that cleaves a polypeptide protein necessary to produce new mature infectious virus particles. Virions treated with PI's do not become infectious. There are eight

FDA-approved drugs in this class. The fourth and newest class of drugs available for HIV treatment is the entry inhibitors (also known as fusion inhibitors). The sole FDA-approved fusion inhibitor, enfuvirtide (T-20), has generated the most limited experience in treatment of HIV since it was only approved for use in 2003. Unlike the other classes of drugs that work by affecting viral enzymes, this class of drugs prohibits the entry of HIV into the host target cell, like the CD4+ lymphocyte. Also, unlike the traditional drugs used to treat HIV, this drug is not available in oral form. It requires twice-daily subcutaneous injection. When added to regimens containing the other classes of drugs taken by treatment-experienced patients with advanced disease with resistant virus, this therapy was shown to reduce viral load and increase CD4 counts after 6 months of observation (Kilby and Eron, 2003; Lalezari et al., 2003).

Lessons Learned: More Is Better Than One

Over the past 20 years, many lessons have been learned in the developed world about the selection, timing, and combination of drugs used to treat HIV. The first medication used to treat HIV was (AZT, ZDV, a NRTI approved for use in 1987. This drug was used as monotherapy for HIV and, during initial years of use, allowed for increases in CD4 cell counts (or delays in decreases in CD4 counts) and prolonged survival. It was soon learned that these effects were transient, with benefits not lasting much longer than 2 years. Nearly 10 years after the introduction of AZT, the PIs and NNRTIs were approved. Based on clinical trials using these newer drug classes, it was quickly learned that combination therapy was superior in reducing viral load, delaying the emergence of HIV drug resistance, slowing the rate of immune destruction (i.e., CD4 cell decline), and slowing the rate of disease progression. By 1997, there was a 47 percent decrease in HIV-related mortality rates and a 60–80 percent reduction in AIDS-defining diagnoses and hospitalizations for patients using combination therapy (Bartlett, 2004).

It is now known that the most effective and recommended way to use the drugs to treat HIV is in at least triple combination. Mono- or dual-therapy, which was used at the start of the epidemic, has now been proven to be less effective and have limited long-term durability and, therefore, should be avoided. Highly active antiretroviral therapy (HAART) refers to the use of three or more drugs in a daily regimen. The three drugs used in a HAART-based regimen should come from at least two different classes. Of note, while there are 20 FDA-approved drugs, not all combinations that could be formed result in an effective regimen. In fact, certain combinations of drugs are antagonistic and must be avoided. See "Selecting a Regimen" for guidance on HAART design.

Balancing the Risks and Benefits

Lifelong Treatment

While curing HIV with antiretroviral therapy is not yet possible, halting further viral replication and production and restoring immune function remain the goals of therapy. These goals must be balanced with the consequences of receiving antiretroviral therapy: toxicities, side effects, and viral resistance development limiting further therapy options. Furthermore, as morbidity and mortality have decreased with antiretroviral therapy, patients are living longer; HIV has thus become a chronic disease requiring lifelong treatment. With the experience of over a decade of use of these therapies, it has become clear that long-term use can result in metabolic derangements with potentially serious non-immunologic long term implications. This is particularly relevant with the PI class, which has been shown to cause hyperglycemia and hyperlipidemia (U.S. DHHS, 2003). Conflicting data exist associating these metabolic derangements with an increase in cardiovascular morbidity and mortality; longer observations may clarify this (Sklar and Masur, 2003). In recognition of long term adverse effects resulting from long-term treatment, clinicians are no longer encouraged to abide by the "hit early, hit hard" strategy; more thoughtful and thorough risk-benefit analyses between physician and patient should be addressed prior to therapy initiation (Sepkowitz, 2001).

Side Effects

There are class-specific toxicities and side effects, in addition to unique toxicities and side effects of individual antiretroviral drugs. Different drugs within the NRTI class are associated with lactic acidosis and hepatic steatosis, peripheral neuropathy, pancreatitis, and anemia. Of note, abacavir (ABC) has been associated with a life-threatening hypersensitivity reaction requiring immediate and permanent discontinuation of the drug. Drugs within the NNRTI class are associated with rash and hepatotoxicity. Of note, efavirenz has been associated with psychiatric side effects such as insomnia and vivid dreams and nevirapine has been associated with hepatotoxicity and the Stevens-Johnson syndrome. Drugs within the PI class are associated with nephrolithiasis and gastrointestinal side effects such as nausea and diarrhea. Metabolic derangements, as described above, also are more frequently associated with this class of drugs. Based on early clinical trial studies of the newest class of drugs, the fusion inhibitors, adverse events associated with the drug in this class include: local injection-site reactions such as the development of painful, pruritic subcutaneous nodules; eosinophilia (rarely associated with systemic hypersensitivity); and an increased incidence of bacterial pneumonia. For a more comprehensive listing of drug-specific side effects, see Table B-1.

Resistance and Its Determinants

In deciding to initiate or change antiretroviral drug therapy, an understanding of the concept of drug resistance is important, since the benefits of therapy can be compromised if drug resistance develops. Because HIV undergoes high rates of replication and turnover, there is potential for genetic variation leading to HIV variants that are no longer susceptible to the mechanisms of action of existing drugs. Resistance develops during drug therapy (Clavel and Hance, 2004). If virus continuously replicates in the presence of drug therapy (i.e., incomplete viral suppression in the presence of selective drug pressure), drug resistance will emerge (Deeks, 2002; Hirsch et al., 2003). Mutations conferring resistance are selected and maintained by drug pressure (Hirsch et al., 2003; Petrello et al., 2002; Richman et al., 2004).

There are two approaches to measuring HIV drug resistance. Phenotypic assays measure inhibition (or lack of it) of viral replication in presence of a given drug. Genotypic assays detect the presence of mutations in the viral genome previously determined to account for resistance with the phenotypic assay. Drug-resistant HIV can be resistant to individual drugs or to the whole class within a given class. As aforementioned, any regimen that does not completely inhibit viral replication can lead to the emergence of resistance (Bennett et al., 2000). It is estimated that 50 percent of patients receiving antiretroviral therapy in the United States have a virus that is resistant to at least one drug in the armamentarium (Richman et al., 2004).

There are many factors that can lead to the development of HIV resistance to antiretroviral therapy. As noted above, if complete suppression of viral replication is not achieved, resistance mutations will develop and the virus may become clinically resistant. Suboptimal exposure of the virus to the drug is an important mechanism by which drug resistance develops. Suboptimal exposure can result from underdosing, improper prescription of antiretroviral regimens, poor adherence, altered drug metabolism, and the presence of tissue sanctuaries where virions "hide" from the action of drug therapy (Deeks, 2002). While all mechanisms operate, the one factor that most critically depends on the patient is adherence. If at least 95 percent of doses are taken, there is a greater than 80 percent probability of achieving a viral load of less than 500 copies/mL; if less than 95 percent of doses are taken, less than 50 percent achieve this goal (Bartlett, 2004).

TABLE B-1 Antiretroviral Drugs and Selected Side Effects

Generic Name	Trade Name	Comments and Common Side Effects
Nucleoside Reverse Transcriptase Inhibitors (NRTIs)		
Abacavir (ABC)	Ziagen	rash with or without hypersensitivity reaction; those that develop hypersensitivity reactions must not be rechallenged
Didanosine (ddI)	Videx EC	peripheral neuropathy; pancreatitis; avoid alcohol
Emtricitabine (FTC)	Emtriva	active against hepatitis B
Lamivudine (3TC)	Epivir	active against hepatitis B
Stavudine (d4T)	Zerit	peripheral neuropathy; lipodystrophy
Zalcitabine (ddC)	Hivid	peripheral neuropathy; oral ulcers
Zidovudine (ZDV, AZT)	Retrovir	initial "flu-like" symptoms; anemia; myopathy
Tenofovir[a]	Viread	renal insufficiency (rare)
Protease Inhibitors (PIs)		
Amprenavir	Agenerase	rash; diarrhea; perioral paresthesia; hyperlipidemia
Fosamprenavir	Lexiva	similar to amprenavir
Indinavir	Crixivan	nephrolithiasis; nausea; hyperlipidemia
Atazanavir	Reyataz	hyperbilirubinemia, nausea, diarrhea
Lopinavir		gastrointenstinal intolerance; hyperlipidemia
Ritonavir	Norvir	nausea; diarrhea; numb lips; hyperlipidemia
Nelfinavir	Viracept	diarrhea; hyperlipidemia
Saquinavir (soft gel) (hard gel)	Fortovase Invirase	Gastrointestinal intolerance; hyperlipidemia
Nonnucleoside Reverse Transcriptase Inhibitors (NNRTIs)		
Delavirdine	Rescriptor	transient rash; increase in liver enzymes
Efavirenz	Sustiva	transient rash; insomnia; vivid dreams; rare suicidal/homicidal ideation
Nevirapine	Viramune	transient rash; hepatitis
Fusion Inhibitors		
Enfuvirtide (T-20)	Fuzeon	injection-site reactions; eosinophilia; rare hypersensitivity reaction

[a]Tenofovir is a nucleotide reverse transcriptase inhibitor.
SOURCES: Schutz and Wendrow, 2001; U.S. DHHS, 2003.

THE ART OF MEDICINE:
DESIGNING AND STARTING A REGIMEN

The goal in selecting a treatment regimen is to select a combination of drugs that will have additive or synergetic effects in viral suppression and immune stabilization or reconstitution. An overlying goal is to select a regimen that will minimize the development of drug resistance—especially to an entire class of drugs—thus leading to limited future treatment options. Other factors that are to be considered include: pharmokinetic and toxicity profiles and characteristics that favor adherence. There are many considerations in selecting a regimen. The text below will highlight examples of such considerations based largely on research endeavors from the developed world. *For a more thorough review of regimen options and associated advantages and disadvantages, the reader is directed to the U.S. Department of Health and Human Services November 2003 "Guidelines for the Use of Antiretroviral Agents in HIV-1-Infected Adults and Adolescents" available at http://AIDSinfo.nih.gov.*

What Not to Do

The first principle in designing a regimen is knowing what to avoid. Mono or dual therapy combinations should be avoided because of their inferior antiretroviral activity and high risk of fostering resistance. A combination therapy with three or more drugs—from different classes—is the recommended treatment regimen. There are certain combinations of antiretroviral drugs that are antagonistic and, therefore, should be avoided. The most notable combination to be avoided is zidovudine (ZDV, AZT) with stavudine (d4T) (Bennett et al., 2000; U.S. DHHS, 2003). Other combinations should be avoided because of pharmokinetic interactions. Didanosine cannot be taken with antiretrovirals requiring an acidic milieu for absorption; therefore, didanosine should not be combined with indinavir (Bennett et al., 2000). Didanosine also should also not be taken at full dosage with tenofovir. Toxicity profiles also should be considered when selecting a regimen. For example, didanosine, stavudine, and zalcitabine used in various combinations increase the risk of peripheral neuropathy (U.S. DHHS, 2003). As adherence to antiretroviral therapy can affect clinical outcome, thought should be given to the number of pills prescribed per day, food requirements, and to side effects. (There are many psychosocial determinants of adherence that are outside the scope of this review.) The combination formulation containing zidovudine with lamivudine (Combivir) allows two pills to be simplified to one pill. Indinavir and nelfinavir have fluid or food requirements that may need to be taken into account when using either of these in a regimen (U.S. DHHS, 2003).

What to Do

As previously noted, HAART—a three or more drug combination—should be used with the goal of suppressing viral replication, restoring immune function, and delaying morbidity and mortality. Based on regimens for which the most extensive clinical trial data are available, the U.S. Department of Health and Human Services recommends three categories of regimens for first-line therapy use (U.S. DHHS, 2003):

1 NNRTI + 2 NRTIs	(PI-sparing regimen)
1-2 PIs + 2 NRTIs	(NNRTI-sparing regimen)
3 NRTIs	(PI and NNRTI-sparing regimen)

The objective is to select a combination that is potent, tolerable, and to which the patient is mostly likely to adhere. Clinical studies have found that using one of these combinations of drugs can result in viral suppression in 80–95 percent of patients.

When to Start

As described throughout this report, there are many considerations in selecting a regimen and many possible complications that can arise with any given regimen. The "hit hard and hit early" approach that was used when HAART became available in the mid-1990s has been replaced by an approach that takes into account the many lessons learned about antiretroviral therapy use in the developed world (see Box B-1).

At this time, based on clinical trials and prospective studies, U.S. recommendations for starting therapy based on laboratory criteria are (U.S. DHHS, 2003):

CD4 ≤ 200 mm^3	Start therapy
CD4 > 200 mm^3 but < 350 mm^3	Offer therapy, weigh risks or benefits
CD4 > 350 mm^3 and viral load > 55,000	Consider therapy
CD4 > 350 mm^3 and viral load < 55,000	Defer therapy and follow CD4 count
Any values and patient with symptomatic AIDS	Start therapy

These laboratory parameters should be used as a guide. Ultimately, the decision should be made by the clinician and the patient after discussion of the goals of treatment and the risks and benefits associated with it.

BOX B-1
Factors for Consideration by Clinicians and Patients
When Deciding to Start Antiretroviral Therapy:
Lessons Learned from the United States

- Clinical criteria: CD4 count and viral load
- Patient acceptance and readiness
- Recognition of long-term nonimmunologic health risks: lipodystrophy, hyperlipidemia, diabetes, osteonecrosis
- Side effects affecting morbidity and quality of life (e.g., diarrhea, nephrolithiasis, rash, insomnia)
- No cure possible
- Demands of adherence
- Possible decrease in viral transmission if viral load is reduced

SOURCES: Bartlett, 2004; U.S. DHHS, 2003.

ANTIRETROVIRAL THERAPY IN RESOURCE-CONSTRAINED SETTINGS: OPPORTUNITIES AND CHALLENGES

The developed world experience with treatment for HIV/AIDS has helped guide other nations in developing treatment plans and goals. While many of the considerations in initiating and selecting therapy have no borders, there are certain issues that developing nations must weigh more heavily in the treatment of HIV/AIDS. As the treatment for HIV/AIDS can be lifelong, continuous access to drug therapy is one such issue. In developing nations, access can be hindered by cost; drug delivery, supply, and storage; counterfeiting; and infrastructure to administer the therapy. Fortunately, many pharmaceutical manufacturers have lowered the prices of ARV drugs for the developing world. Some drugs may require a cold chain, which is not be available in parts of the developing world. Resistance profiles vary across borders and this also has an impact on regimens of therapy that may be selected. Factors affecting adherence may be affected by culture and, therefore, differ among communities and nations. The stigma associated with having HIV/AIDS may hinder adherence to therapy. The ability to use laboratory testing to monitor toxicities may influence the regimens chosen in the developing world where technological infrastructure may be limited. Finally, pharmacological interactions between antiretroviral and antituberculosis drugs is a more common concern in resource constrained settings.

Recognizing the many barriers the developing world may face as ARV treatment is made available to millions across the globe, the World Health Organization (WHO), in its ambitious "3 by 5" initiative has recommended four first-line regimens. (For the WHO's recommended criteria for when to initiate therapy, see Appendix C.) The WHO has decided upon these regimens based on clinical trial and observational study data, experience with use of ART in resource constrained settings—including efficacy and side effect information, and cost and availability of drugs (WHO, 2003a). The four regimens are all PI-sparing.[1] The WHO decided to spare PIs in their first-line recommendations for several reasons which include: higher cost, higher pill burden, food and water needs, cold chain requirements, and short- and long-term side effects that may require more intensive monitoring (WHO, 2003a). The four regimens recommended as first-line therapy in resource limited settings are:

> stavudine + lamivudine + nevirapine
> zidovudine + lamivudine + nevirapine
> stavudine + lamivudine + efavirenz
> zidovudine + lamivudine + efavirenz

The first two regimens listed are available as fixed dose combinations (FDCs) in which all three drugs are combined into one tablet. FDCs have several advantages and disadvantages (MSF, 2004; WHO, 2003a,b). Advantages include: promoting patient adherence; improving health care worker adherence to treatment standards; minimizing prescription errors; and simplifying drug supply, management, and distribution. Disadvantages include: addressing the need to individualize the dosing of individual drug components and the differential half-life of the drugs and allergies to a component.

While the United States relies heavily on laboratory criteria to determine when to start and how to monitor therapy, limited infrastructure in resource-constrained settings may preclude this. The WHO recognizes this fact and recommends using clinical criteria and, when available, laboratory criteria to initiate and monitor therapy for HIV-infected persons in these constrained settings.

For further information regarding the advantages and disadvantages of the WHO-recommended regimens and the criteria used to start therapy, the reader is directed to the *WHO 2003 Revision of Scaling Up Antiretroviral Therapy in Resource-Limited Setting: Treatment Guidelines for a Public Health Approach available at http://www.who.int/3by5/publications/documents/arv_guidelines/en/.*

---

[1] If NNRTI resistance is expected to be 5–10 percent, PIs may be considered in first-line regimens.

CONCLUSION

Over the past two decades much has been learned about the virus that causes AIDS and the natural history of the disease. Much research that guided success in treating HIV has been done in the developed world. The virus's pathogenic mechanisms are still being investigated. Research continues to develop improved and additional therapeutics to combat HIV and AIDS. As the epidemic knows no borders, it will be important that research on antiretroviral therapies and their advantages and disadvantage continue to be conducted around the globe.

REFERENCES

Bartlett J. 2004. Antiretroviral treatment. In: Gorbach SL, Bartlett JG, Blacklow NR, eds. *Infectious Diseases*. 3rd Edition. Philadelphia, PA: Lippincott, Williams & Wilkins. Pp. 1028–1038.

Bennett JE, Dolin R, Mandell GL. 2000. *Mandell, Douglas and Bennett's Principles and Practice of Infectious Diseases*. 5th Edition. Philadelphia, PA: Churchill Livingstone.

Centers for Disease Control and Prevention. 1992. 1993 revised classification system for HIV infection and expanded surveillance case definition for AIDS among adolescents and adults. *Morbidity and Mortality Weekly Review Weekly* 41(51):961–962.

Clavel F, Hance A. 2004. HIV drug resistance. *New England Journal of Medicine* 350(10): 1023–1035.

Deeks S. 2002. Treatment of antiretroviral-drug-resistant HIV-1 infection. *Lancet* 362(9400): 2002–2011.

Hirsch MS, Brun-Vezinet F, Clotet B, Conway B, Kuritzkes DR, D'Aquila RT, Demeter LM, Hammer SM, Johnson VA, Loveday C, Mellors JW, Jacobsen DM, Richman DD. 2003. Antiretroviral drug resistance testing in adults infected with human immunodeficiency virus type 1: 2003 recommendations of an international AIDS society-USA panel. *Clinical Infectious Diseases* 37:113–128.

Kilby JM, Eron JJ. 2003. Mechanisms of disease: Novel therapies based on mechanisms of HIV-1 cell entry. *New England Journal of Medicine* 348(22).

Lalezari JP, Henry K, O'Hearn M, Montaner JS, Piliero PJ, Trottier B, Walmsley S, Cohen C, Kuritzkes DR, Eron JJ Jr, Chung J, DeMasi R, Donatacci L, Drobnes C, Delehanty J, Salgo M; TORO 1 Study Group. 2003. Enfuvirtide, an HIV-1 fusion inhibitor, for drug-resistant HIV Infection in North and South America. *New England Journal of Medicine* 348(22):2175–2185.

Lazzarin A, Clotet B, Cooper D, Reynes J, Arasteh K, Nelson M, Katlama C, Stellbrink HJ, Delfraissy JF, Lange J, Huson L, DeMasi R, Wat C, Delehanty J, Drobnes C, Salgo M; TORO 2 Study Group. 2003. Efficacy of Enfuvirtide in Patients Infected with Drug-Resistant HIV-1 in Europe and Australia. *New England Journal of Medicine* 348(22): 2228–2238.

MSF (Médecins sans Frontières). 2004. *Two Pills a Day Saving Lives: Fixed-Dose Combinations (FDCs) of Antiretroviral Drugs*. Geneva: Médecins sans Frontières.

Petrello M, Brenner B, Loemba H, Wainberg MA. 2002. HIV drug resistance implications for the introduction of antiretroviral therapy in resource-poor countries. *Drug Resistance Updates* 4:339–346.

Richman DD, Morton SC, Wrin T, Hellmann N, Berry S, Shapiro M, Bozzette S. 2004. The prevalence of antiretroviral drug resistance in the United States. *AIDS* 18:1–7.

Schutz M, Wendrow A. 2001. Adapted from "Quick Reference Guide to Antiretrovirals." [Online]. Available: http://www.law.duke.edu/aidsProject/400_01/GuideAntriRetros.pdf [accessed September 2, 2004].

Sepkowitz KA. 2001. AIDS: The first 20 years. *New England Journal of Medicine* 344(23):1764–1772.

Sklar P, Masur H. 2003. HIV infection and cardiovascular disease: Is there really a link? *New England Journal of Medicine* 349(21):2065–2067.

U.S. DHHS (United States Department of Health and Human Services). 2003. *Guidelines for the Use of Antiretroviral Agents in HIV-1-Infected Adults and Adolescents.* [Online]. Available: http://AIDSinfo.nih.gov [accessed August 23, 2004].

WHO (World Health Organization). 2003a. *Scaling Up Antiretroviral Therapy in Resource-Limited Settings: Treatment Guidelines for a Public Health Approach.* [Online]. Available: http://www.who.int/3by5/publications/documents/arv_guidelines/en/ [accessed August 23, 2004].

WHO. 2003b. *Emergency Scale-up of Antiretroviral Therapy in Resource-Limited Settings: Technical and Operational Recommendations to Achieve 3 by 5.* [Online]. Available: http://www.who.int/3by5/publications/briefs/arv_guidelines/en/ [accessed August 23, 2004].

Appendix C

Scaling Up Antiretroviral Therapy in Resource-Limited Settings: Treatment Guidelines for a Public Health Approach

2003 REVISION

The creation of the present guidelines would not have been possible without the participation of numerous experts.

The World Health Organization wishes to express special gratitude to the Writing Committee that developed this document. This Committee was chaired by Professor Scott Hammer of Columbia University *(New York City, USA)* and its other members were Diane Havlir *(University of California at San Francisco, USA)*, Elise Klement *(Médecins sans Frontières, France)*, Fabio Scano *(WHO/ HTM/STB, Switzerland)*, Jean-Ellie Malkin *(ESTHER, France)*, Jean-François Delfraissy *(CHU BICETRE, ANRS, Paris, France)*, Joep Lange *(International AIDS Society, Sweden)*, Lydia Mungherera *(GNP+, Uganda)*, Lynne Mofenson *(National Institute of Health, NICHD, USA)*, Mark Harrington *(Treatment Action Group, New York, USA)*, Mauro Schechter *(Universidade Federal do Rio de Janeiro, Brazil)*, N. Kumarasamy *(YRG Centre for AIDS Research and Education, India)*, Nicolas Durier *(Médecins sans Frontières, Thailand)*, Papa Salif Sow *(University of Dakar, Senegal)*, Shabir Banoo *(Medicines Control Council, South Africa)* and Thomas Macharia *(Nazareth Hospital, Kenya)*.

This document was developed through an expert consultation process in which account was taken of current scientific evidence and the state of the art in the treatment of HIV infection. The primary focus was the context of resource-limited settings. After the production of draft guidelines by the Writing Committee in October 2003, the document was sent to more than 200 institutional and organizational partners worldwide and made available for public consultation from 28 October to 14 November 2003 on the WHO and ITAC websites. WHO wishes to acknowledge comments and contributions by Alexandra Calmy *(Switzerland)*, Andrew Hill *(USA)*, Annabel Kanabus *(United Kingdom)*, Anthony Amoroso *(USA)*, Anthony Harries *(Malawi)*, Artur Kalichman *(Brazil)*, Bernard Taverne *(Senegal)*, Beverley Snell *(Australia)*, Bess Miller *(USA)*, Brian Eley *(South Africa)*, Carrie Jeffries (USA), Charles Gilks *(WHO, Switzerland)*, Chris Duncombe *(Thailand)*, Chris Green *(Indonesia)*, Clement Malau *(Australia)*, David Cohn *(USA)*, Diana Gibb *(United Kingdom)*, Emanuele Pontali *(Italy)*, Emilia Rivadeneira *(USA)*, Eric Van Praag *(USA)*, Fionuala Mcculagh *(Cameroon)*, Francis Onyango *(WHO, AFRO)*, François Dabis (France), Gray Sattler *(Philippines)*, Guido Levi *(Brazil)*, Heloisa Marques *(Brazil)*, Herbert Peterson *(WHO, Switzerland)*, Isabelle Girault *(United Kingdom)*, Jaime Uhrig *(Myanmar)*, Jeffrey Sturchio *(USA)*, Joia Mukherjee *(Haiti)*, Jonathan Cohn *(USA)*, Jose Zuniga *(USA)*, Karin Timmermans *(Indonesia)*, Karyaija Barigye *(USA)*, Keith Alcorn *(United Kingdom)*, Kenji Tamura *(WHO, Switzerland)*, Kulkanaya Chokephaibulkit *(Thailand)*, Lali Khotenashvilli *(WHO, EURO)*, Leon Levin *(South Africa)*, Márcia Dal Fabbro *(Brazil)*, Marcia Rachid *(Brazil)*, Marga Vitgnes *(South Africa)*, Maria Vigneau *(WHO, Switzerland)*, Marinella de la Negra *(Brazil)*, Marta Segu *(Spain)*, Monica Beg *(WHO, Switzerland)*, Mukadi Ya-Diul *(USA)*, Olavo Munhoz *(Brazil)*, Paul Jareg *(Norway)*, Paula Fujiwara *(IUATLD, France)*, Peter Anton *(South Africa)*, Peter Godfrey-Faussett *(United Kingdom)*, Pier Angelo Todo *(Italy)*, Praphan Pranuphak *(Thailand)*, Ricardo Marins *(Brazil)*, Richard Laing *(WHO, Switzerland)*, Robin Gray *(WHO, Switzerland)*, Rosana Del Bianco *(Brazil)*, Sailesh Upadhyay *(Nepal)*, Stephen Spector *(USA)*, Sudarshan Kumari *(India)*, Taimor Nawaz *(Bangladesh)*, Thurma Goldman *(USA)*, Vincent Habiyambere *(WHO, Switzerland)*, William Burman *(Denver, USA)* and Wladimir Queiroz *(Brazil)* during the public consultation process. Their contributions were discussed by the Writing Committee on 26 October 2003 and, where appropriate, the draft guidelines were amended to take their suggestions into account.

WHO also wishes to thank the Agence Nationale de Recherche contre le SIDA, Paris, for hosting the meeting of the Writing Committee on 15–17 October 2003.

This work was coordinated by Marco Vitória and Jos Perriëns of WHO/HTM/HIV, Geneva, Switzerland.

ABBREVIATIONS

ABC abacavir
ACTG AIDS Clinical Trials Group
AIDS acquired immunodeficiency syndrome
ALT alanine aminotransferase
ART antiretroviral therapy
ARV antiretroviral
ATV atazanavir
bid twice daily
CD4 T-lymphocyte CD4+
CNS central nervous system
d4T stavudine
DART development of antiretroviral therapy in Africa
ddI didanosine
DOT directly observed therapy
EFV efavirenz
ENF (T-20) enfuvirtide
FBC full blood count
FDC fixed-dose combination
FTC emtricitabine
GI gastrointestinal
HAART highly active antiretroviral therapy
Hgb haemoglobin
HIV human immunodeficiency virus
HIVab human immunodeficiency virus antibody
IDU injecting drug user
IDV indinavir
LPV lopinavir
MTCT mother-to-child transmission (of HIV)
NAM nucleoside analogue mutation
NFV nelfinavir
NGO nongovernmental organization
NNRTI non-nucleoside reverse transcriptase inhibitor
NsRTI nucleoside analogue reverse transcriptase inhibitor
NtRTI nucleotide analogue reverse transcriptase inhibitor
NVP nevirapine
PCR polymerase chain reaction
PI protease inhibitor
qd once daily
RT reverse transcriptase
RTI reverse transcriptase inhibitor
RTV ritonavir

RTV-PI ritonavir-boosted protease inhibitor
sgc soft gel capsule
SQV saquinavir
TB tuberculosis
TDF tenofovir disoproxil fumarate
TLC total lymphocyte count
UN United Nations
UNAIDS Joint United Nations Programme on HIV/AIDS
WBC white blood cell
WHO World Health Organization
ZDV zidovudine (also known as AZT)
/r low dose ritonavir

INTRODUCTION

The advent of potent antiretroviral therapy (ART) in 1996 led to a revolution in the care of patients with HIV/AIDS in the developed world. Although the treatments are not a cure and present new challenges with respect to side-effects and drug resistance, they have dramatically reduced rates of mortality and morbidity, have improved the quality of life of people with HIV/ AIDS, and have revitalized communities. Moreover, HIV/AIDS is now perceived as a manageable chronic illness rather than as a plague (Palella et al., 2003).

Unfortunately, most of the 40 million people currently living with HIV/ AIDS reside in developing countries and do not share this vastly improved prognosis (Joint United Nations Programme on HIV/AIDS and World Health Organization, 2003). WHO conservatively estimated that, at the end of 2003, some 6 million people in developing countries were in immediate need of life-sustaining ART. However, only about 400 000 persons were being treated, over a third of them in Brazil. At the UN General Assembly High-Level Meeting on HIV/AIDS on 22 September 2003, WHO declared that the lack of access to HIV treatment was a global health emergency. WHO calls for unprecedented action to ensure that by the end of 2005 at least 3 million people in need of ART will have access to it.

In order to achieve this target, WHO will develop a strategic framework with the following pillars:

- global leadership, strong partnership and advocacy;
- urgent sustained country support;
- simplified standardized tools for the delivery of ART;
- an effective and reliable supply of medicines and diagnostics;
- rapid identification and reapplication of new knowledge and success.

The present updated and simplified treatment guidelines are a cornerstone of the WHO 3-by-5 Plan and are more directive than its predecessor with respect to first-line and second-line therapies. They take into account not only the evidence generated by clinical trials and observational studies on the efficacy and side-effects of the treatment regimens discussed, but also the experience gained with ART by programmes in resource-limited settings and the cost and availability of drugs in those settings. By taking this approach, WHO seeks to assist countries and regions in providing effective antiretroviral therapy to the millions of individuals in immediate or imminent need of treatment. This document, dealing with recommendations for ARV treatment and monitoring, is intended to be a component of a comprehensive package of care at the country level, including the prevention and treatment of opportunistic infections, nutritional programmes and psychosocial support for infected persons. Treatment for HIV, facilitated by these guidelines, complements the full range of HIV prevention efforts for uninfected people at the country level.

The following recent advances in the ART field have been considered in the preparation of this revision:

- clinical trial data, including those suggesting the inferior virological efficacy of the triple nucleoside combination, ZDV/3TC/abacavir (ABC) in comparison with a three-drug or four-drug efavirenz-based regimen;
- the availability of the nucleotide analogue, tenofovir disoproxil fumarate (TDF);
- toxicity concerns regarding the dual nucleoside component of stavudine (d4T)/didanosine (ddI);
- increasing recognition of the extent of drug class cross-resistance among the nucleoside and nucleotide analogues;
- the approval of a new nucleoside analogue, emtricitabine (FTC), a protease inhibitor, atazanavir (ATV), the fusion inhibitor, enfuvirtide (ENF, T-20) and increasing availability and clinical experience with generic ARV preparations, particularly in fixed-dose combinations and blister packs (ENF will not be considered further in this document because of the requirement for parenteral administration and the cost of the drug, making it impractical for use in resource-limited settings). These treatment guidelines are part of WHO's commitment to the treatment of persons living with HIV/AIDS. The first edition of these recommendations, published in April 2002, reflected the best practices at that time on the basis of a review of evidence. In this rapidly evolving field, WHO recognized at the outset that the recommendations would have to be regularly updated. The present revision has been brought forward as a result of new scientific data and the increasing reality of ART scale-up in many countries.

DOCUMENT OBJECTIVES

Currently, fewer than 5% of people in developing countries who need ART can access the medicines in question. WHO believes that at least 3 million people needing care should be able to get the medicines by 2005. This represents almost a tenfold increase. These treatment guidelines are intended to support and facilitate the proper management and scale-up of ART in the years to come by proposing a public health approach to achieve the goals. The key tenets of this approach are as follows.

1.   Scaling-up of antiretroviral treatment programmes with a view to universal access, i.e. all persons requiring treatment as indicated by medical criteria should have access to it.

2.   Standardization and simplification of ARV regimens so as to support the efficient implementation of treatment programmes in resource-limited settings.

3.   Ensuring that ARV treatment programmes are based on scientific evidence in order to avoid the use of substandard protocols that compromise the outcomes of individual patients and create a potential for the emergence of drug-resistant virus. However, it is also important to consider the realities with respect to the availability of human resources, health system infrastructures and socioeconomic contexts so that clear and realistic recommendations can be made.

While it is hoped that this document will be useful to clinicians in resource-limited settings, it is primarily intended for use by treatment advisory boards, national AIDS programme managers and other senior policy-makers who are involved in the planning of national and international HIV care strategies in developing countries. The treatment guidelines serve as a framework for selecting the most potent and feasible ARV regimens as components of expanded national responses for the care of HIV-infected individuals. The framework aims to standardize and simplify antiretroviral therapy, as with tuberculosis (TB) treatment in national TB control programmes, while acknowledging the relative complexity of HIV treatment. Accordingly, options for first-line and secondline regimens are presented, bearing in mind the need to strengthen health systems that often lack staffing power and monitoring facilities, with a view to maximizing the quality and outcomes of the treatments offered.

The guidelines consider when ART should begin, which ARV regimens should be introduced, the reasons for changing ART and the regimens that should be continued if treatment has to be changed. They also address how treatment should be monitored, with specific reference to the side-effects of ART and drug adherence, and make specific recommendations for certain subgroups of patients.

WHEN TO START ARV THERAPY IN
ADULTS AND ADOLESCENTS

WHO recommends that, in resource-limited settings, HIV-infected adults and adolescents should start ARV therapy when the infection has been confirmed and one of the following conditions is present.
- Clinically advanced HIV disease:
- WHO Stage IV HIV disease, irrespective of the CD4 cell count;
- WHO Stage III disease with consideration of using CD4 cell counts <350/mm^3 to assist decision-making.
- WHO Stage I or II HIV disease with CD4 cell counts <200/mm^3 (Table A).

The rationale for these recommendations is as follows. The treatment of patients with WHO Stage IV disease (clinical AIDS) should not be dependent on a CD4 cell count determination. However, where available, this test can be helpful in categorizing patients with Stage III conditions with respect to their need for immediate therapy. For example, pulmonary TB can occur at any CD4 count level and, if the CD4 cell count level is well maintained (i.e. >350/mm^3), it is reasonable to defer therapy and continue to monitor the patient. For Stage III conditions a threshold of 350/mm^3 has been chosen as the level below which immune deficiency is clearly present such that patients are eligible for treatment when their clinical condition portends rapid clinical progression. A level of 350/mm^3 is also in line with other consensus guideline documents (DHHS; Yeni et al., 2002). For patients with Stage I or Stage II HIV disease the presence of a CD4 cell count <200/mm^3 is an indication for treatment. In cases where CD4 cell counts cannot be assessed the presence of a total lymphocyte count of 1200/mm^3 or below can be used as a substitute indication for treatment in the presence of symptomatic HIV disease. While the total lymphocyte count correlates relatively poorly with the CD4 cell count in asymptomatic persons, in combination with clinical staging it is a useful marker of prognosis and survival (Badri and Wood, 2003; Beck et al., 1996; Brettle, 1997; Fournier and Sosenko, 1992; Kumarasamy et al., 2002; van der Ryst et al., 1998). An assessment of viral load (e.g. using plasma HIV-1 RNA levels) is not considered necessary before starting therapy. Because of the cost and complexity of viral load testing, WHO does not currently recommend its routine use in order to assist with decisions on when to start therapy in severely resource-constrained settings. It is hoped, however, that increasingly affordable methods of determining viral load will become available so that this adjunct to treatment monitoring can be more widely employed. It should be noted that the current WHO Staging System for HIV Infection and Disease for Adults and Adolescents was developed several years ago

TABLE A. Recommendations for Initiating Antiretroviraltherapy in Adults and Adolescents with Docummented HIV Infection

If CD4 testing available, it is recommended to document baseline CD4 counts and to offer ART to patients with:

- WHO Stage IV disease, irrespective of CD4 cell count
- WHO Stage III disease (including but not restricted to HIV wasting, chronic diarrhoea of unknown etiology, prolonged fever of unknown etiology, pulmonary TB, recurrent invasive bacterial infections or recurrent/persistent mucosal candidiasis), with consideration of using CD4 cell counts <350/mm^3 to assist decision-making[a]
- WHO Stage I or II disease with CD4 cell counts ≤ 200/mm^{3b}

If CD4 testing unavailable, it is recommended to offer ART to patients with:

- WHO Stage IV disease, irrespective of total lymphocyte count
- WHO Stage III disease (including but not restricted to HIV wasting, chronic diarrhoea of unknown etiology, prolonged fever of unknown etiology, pulmonary TB, recurrent invasive bacterial infections or recurrent/persistent mucosal candidiasis), irrespective of the total lymphocyte count[c]
- WHO Stage II disease with a total lymphocyte count ≤ 1200/mm^{3d}

---

[a]CD4 count advisable to assist with determining need for immediate therapy. For example, pulmonary TB may occur at any CD4 level and other conditions may be mimicked by non-HIV etiologies (e.g. chronic diarrhoea, prolonged fever).

[b]The precise CD4 level above 200/mm^3 at which ARV treatment should start has not been established.

[c]The recommendation to start ART in all patients with stage III disease, without reference to total lymphocyte counts reflects consensus of expert opinion. It took into account the need of a practical recommendation that allows clinical services and TB programmes in severely resource constrained settings to offer access to ART to their patients. As some adults and adolescents with stage III disease will be presenting with CD4 counts above 200, some of them will receive antiretroviral treatment before the CD4 < 200 threshold is reached. However, if CD4 counts cannot be determined, starting ART earlier in these patients was not considered problematic.

[d]A total lymphocyte count of ≤ 1200/mm^3 can be substituted for the CD4 count when the latter is unavailable and HIV-related symptoms exist. It is not useful in the asymptomatic patient. Thus, in the absence of CD4 cell testing, asymptomatic HIV-infected patients (WHO Stage I) should not be treated because there is currently no other reliable marker available in severely resourceconstrained settings.

and has consequent limitations. Adaptations at the level of national programmes may therefore be appropriate. Nevertheless, it remains a useful tool for assisting in defining parameters for initiating therapy in resource-limited settings and thus has continued to be applied in this revision.

RECOMMENDED FIRST-LINE ARV REGIMENS
IN ADULTS AND ADOLESCENTS

Countries are encouraged to use a public health approach to facilitate the scale-up of ARV use in resource-limited settings as delineated in the WHO 3-by-5 Plan. This means that ART programmes should be developed which can reach as many people as possible who are in need of therapy and requires that ARV treatment be standardized. In particular, it is suggested that countries select a first-line regimen and a limited number of second-line regimens, recognizing that individuals who cannot tolerate or fail the first-line and second-line regimens will be referred for individualized care by specialist physicians. The use of standardized regimens is an essential component of the 3-by-5 Plan and will facilitate WHO's efforts to assist Member States with achieving this goal. This is the approach to ARV regimen selection taken in the present document. Among the factors that should be considered in the selection of ART regimens at both the programme level and the level of the individual patient are:

- potency;
- side-effect profile;
- laboratory monitoring requirements;
- potential for maintenance of future treatment options;
- anticipated patient adherence;
- coexistent conditions (e.g. coinfections, metabolic abnormalities);
- pregnancy or the risk thereof;
- use of concomitant medications (i.e. potential drug interactions);
- potential for infection with a virus strain with diminished susceptibility to one or more ARVs, including that resulting from prior exposure to ARVs given for prophylaxis or treatment;
- very importantly, availability and cost.

The use of quality-assured[1] antiretrovirals in fixed-dose combinations (FDCs)[2] or as blister packs[3] is another important consideration as this pro-

---

[1] Quality-assured medicines assembled in fixed-dose combinations (FDCs), in the context of this document, include individual products which have been deemed to meet or exceed international standards for quality, safety and efficacy. In the case of drug combinations whose components are from different manufacturers the international standards include a requirement for clinical bioequivalence studies to establish therapeutic interchangeability of the components. For WHO's work on prequalification of ARVs see: http://www.who.int/medicines/ organization\qsm/activities/pilotproc/proc.shtml

[2] Fixed-dose combinations are based on the principle of inclusion of two or more active pharmacological products in the same pill, capsule, tablet or solution.

[3] A blister pack is a plastic or aluminum blister containing two or more pills, capsules or tablets.

motes better adherence and, in turn, limits the emergence of drug resistance. It also facilitates ARV storage and distribution logistics. Additional considerations relevant to the developing world include access to a limited number of ARV drugs, limited health service infrastructures (including human resources), the need to deliver drugs to rural areas, high incidences of TB and hepatitis B and/or C in populations and the presence of varied HIV types, groups and subtypes. The previous (April 2002) version of these treatment guidelines recommended that countries should select a first-line treatment regimen and identified regimens composed of two nucleosides plus either a non-nucleoside, or abacavir, or a protease inhibitor as possible choices. Since that version was published, many countries have started ARV treatment programmes and have chosen their first-line treatment regimens, taking into account how the above factors would come into play in the different settings. The majority of treatment programmes in developing countries have opted for a regimen composed of two nucleosides and a non-nucleoside RT inhibitor. Triple nucleoside regimens including abacavir were almost never selected because of their cost and concerns over hypersensitivity reactions, and regimens containing a protease inhibitor became secondary options, mainly because of their cost, notwithstanding price decreases. However, high pill counts, their side-effect profile and more difficult logistics (some requiring a cold chain) were probably also considerations.

The Writing Committee examined non-nucleoside-based regimens and took account of clinical experience with the efficacy and toxicity of the nucleoside reverse transcriptase inhibitor (NRTI) and non-nucleoside reverse transcriptase inhibitor (NNRTI) components, the availability of fixed-dose combinations (Annex D), the lack of a requirement for a cold chain, and drug availability and cost. On this basis the Committee concluded that the four first-line ARV regimens listed in Table B were appropriate for adults and adolescents. These regimens consist of a thymidine analogue NRTI, i.e. stavudine (d4T) or zidovudine (ZDV), a thiacytidine NRTI, i.e. lamivudine (3TC), and an NNRTI, i.e. nevirapine (NVP) or efavirenz (EFV).

The choice between d4T and ZDV should be made at the country level on the basis of local considerations but it is recommended that both drugs be available. d4T is initially better tolerated than ZDV and does not require haemoglobin monitoring. However, among the NRTIs, it has been consistently most associated in developed countries with lipoatrophy and other metabolic abnormalities, including lactic acidosis, particularly when combined with didanosine (ddI). It can also cause peripheral neuropathy and pancreatitis. ZDV has also been implicated in metabolic complications of therapy but to a lesser extent than d4T. Initial drug-related side-effects (headache, nausea) are more frequent with ZDV and the drug can cause severe anaemia and neutropenia, which, at the very least, requires that haemoglobin should be monitored before and during treatment with ZDV. d4T can be substituted for ZDV in the event of intolerance to the latter and vice versa (except in cases of suspected lactic acidosis, in which instance neither drug should be prescribed). However, the initial need for less laboratory monitoring might, at present, favour d4T as the nucleoside of choice for the majority of patients in ART programmes in settings with severe resource limitations where rapid scaling-up is intended.

3TC is a potent NRTI with an excellent record of efficacy, safety and tolerability. It can be given once or twice daily and has been incorporated into a number of fixed-dose combinations. Emtricitabine (FTC) is a recently approved nucleoside analogue that is structurally related to 3TC, shares its resistance profile and can be given once daily (Bang and Scott, 2003). It is currently being tested as a coformulated product with tenofovir disoproxil fumarate (TDF). Because of the relatively recent approval of FTC in a limited number of countries it is not included in WHO's recommended first-line regimens but this may change in the light of future experience with the drug and its availability and cost.

The dual nucleoside component of d4T/ddI is no longer recommended as part of first-line regimens because of its toxicity profile, particularly in pregnant women (Boubaker et al., 2001). It is also worth emphasizing that ZDV and d4T should never be used together because of proven antagonism between them (Pollard et al., 2002).

TDF has a long intracellular half-life and can therefore be used as part of once-daily triple-drug regimens. It has been shown that TDF is an effective component of first-line regimens in combination with 3TC and efavirenz (EFV) (Gallant and Deresinski, 2003; Staszewski et al., 2003). It is generally well tolerated although there have been reports of renal insufficiency in patients receiving TDF (Karras et al., 2003; Schaaf et al., 2003; Verhelst et al., 2002). However, worldwide experience with the drug is still relatively limited. In addition, its limited availability and relatively high cost in developing countries continue to be significant factors. For the purposes of the present treatment guidelines, therefore, discussion of its use will be restricted to second-line therapy. As experience, availability and cost issues in resource-limited settings become clarified the inclusion of TDF in WHO-recommended first-line regimens should be reconsidered.

Globally, NNRTI-based regimens are now the most widely prescribed combinations for initial therapy. They are potent and relatively simple but are inactive in respect of HIV-2 and group O of HIV-1. EFV and NVP are both potent NNRTIs with demonstrated clinical efficacy when administered in appropriate combination regimens. However, differences in toxicity profile, a potential for interaction with other treatments, and cost, allow the formulation of both positive and negative recommendations on their use (Staszewski et al., 2003; Ena et al., 2003; Keiser et al., 2002; Law et al., 2003; Martin-Carbonero et al., 2003; Moyle, 2003; van Leth et al., 2003). NVP has a higher incidence of rash, which may be severe and life-threatening, and a greater risk of hepatotoxicity, which may also be life-threatening. This makes the drug less suitable for treating patients who use other hepatotoxic medications, or drugs that can cause rash, or both, such as rifampicin. The major toxicities associated with EFV are related to the central nervous system (CNS), teratogenicity and rash. (Rash is more frequent in children than adults, is generally mild, and usually does not require discontinuation of therapy.) The CNS symptoms typically abate after 10 to 14 days in most, but not all, patients. EFV should be avoided in persons with a history of severe psychiatric illness, when there is a potential for pregnancy, and during pregnancy. EFV may be considered to be the NNRTI of choice in patients with TB coinfection, and NVP may be the best choice in women of childbearing potential or who are pregnant. EFV should not be given to women of childbearing potential unless effective contraception can be assured. However, it is important to emphasize that EFV and NVP may interact with estrogen-based contraceptive pills. NVP is available as part of three-drug FDC which could be used when assured-quality formulations of proven bioequivalence are available.

The use of the five-drug formulary approach (d4T or ZDV) + 3TC + (NVP or EFV) translates practically into four possible regimens (Table B) and provides options for drug substitutions in respect of toxicity (Table C). Because each is considered an appropriately potent, standard-of-care regimen with respect to efficacy, other factors should determine what a country chooses as a lead regimen.

Table B lists some of the factors that should be taken into account in making this decision. ARVs in FDCs and blister packs have potential advantages over conventional drug packaging: they are helpful tools for simplifying treatment and promote adherence. Moreover, they can minimize prescription errors, improve adherence of health care workers to treatment standards, decrease errors in drug administration, improve drug management (because of fewer items and a single expiration date), simplify drug forecasting, procurement, distribution and stocking because fewer items and lower volumes are necessary, and reduce the risk of misuse of single drugs. FDCs also present challenges with respect to the individualization of dosing of individual components, the treatment of children and the differential half-lives of drugs when treatment is interrupted. Laboratory monitoring requirements should also be taken into account.

When d4T/3TC/NVP or ZDV/3TC/NVP is chosen as the first-line regimen the availability of the two-drug combination (d4T/3TC or ZDV/3TC) is also important for use with NVP lead-in dosing during the first two weeks of treatment and for managing some toxicities associated with NVP (Annex D). Additional drugs should be available in districts (level 2) or regional hospitals (level 3). This tiered approach to ARV regimen availability can be paralleled by a tiered monitoring strategy for health care systems.

TABLE B. First-line ARV Regimens in Adults and Adolescents and Characteristics That Can Influence Choice

ARV regimen	Major potential toxicities	Usage in women (of childbearing age or pregnant)
d4T/3TC/NVP	d4T-related neuropathy, pancreatitis and lipoatrophy; NVP-related hepatotoxicity and severe rash	Yes
ZDV/3TC/NVP	ZDV-related GI intolerance, anaemia, and neutropenia; NVP-related hepatotoxicity and severe rash	Yes
d4T/3TC/EFV	d4T-related neuropathy, pancreatitis and lipoatrophy; EFV-related CNS toxicity and potential for teratogenicity	No[b]
ZDV/3TC/EFV	ZDV-related GI intolerance, anaemia and neutropenia; EFV-related CNS toxicity and potential for teratogenicity	No[b]

[a]People with TB disease and HIV coinfection.

[b]Women of childbearing potential or who are pregnant.

[c]These combinations have not been prequalified by WHO but could be used if assured-quality formulations of proven bioequivalence were available.

[d]Obtained from: *Sources and prices of selected medicines and diagnostics for people living with HIV/AIDS,* June 2003 (www.who.int/HIV_AIDS).

Additional Considerations for First-line Therapy Including Treatment of HIV-2 and Group O HIV-1 Infections

PI-based Regimens

While PI-based regimens remain an accepted standard of care for initial regimens, their high cost relative to NNRTI-based regimens makes their use problematic in resource-limited countries seeking to achieve rapid scale-up of therapy. Advantages of PI-based regimens (e.g. PI plus two NRTIs), however, are proven clinical efficacy and well-described toxicities. Disadvantages are higher pill counts, food and water requirements in some cases,

TABLE B. Continued

Usage in TB coinfection[a]	Availability as three-drug fixed-dose combination	Laboratory monitoring requirements	Price for least-developed countries, June 2003 (US$/year)[d]
Yes, in rifampicin-free continuation phase of TB treatment. Use with caution in rifampicin-based regimens[a]	Yes	No	281-358
Yes, in rifampicin-free continuation phase of TB treatment. Use with caution in rifampicin-based regimens[a]	Yes[c]	Yes	383-418
Yes, but EFV should not be given to pregnant women or women of childbearing potential, unless effective contraception can be assured	No. EFV not available as part of FDC; however, partial FDC available for d4T/3TC[c]	No	350-1086
Yes, but EFV should not be given to pregnant women or women of childbearing potential unless effective contraception can be assured	No. EFV not available as part of FDC; however, partial FDC available for ZDV/3TC	Yes	611-986

significant interactions with other drugs that preclude or complicate their use during TB treatment regimens using rifampicin, metabolic abnormalities and the need for a functioning cold chain for ritonavir-boosted regimens. Consequently, in these treatment guidelines, PI-based regimens are primarily reserved for second-line therapy. They should be considered as first-line regimens, however, in circumstances where there is concern for the presence of NNRTI resistance (e.g. prevalence in the community exceeding 5-10%) (Hirsch et al., 2003), where there are viral types with known insensitivity to NNRTIs (e.g. HIV-2 or HIV-1 group O) or where there is intolerance of the NNRTI class of agents. Considerations include (d4T or ZDV) + 3TC combined with either lopinavir/ritonavir (LPV/r), saquinavir/

ritonavir (SQV/r), indinavir/ritonavir (IDV/r), or nelfinavir (NFV), the choice(s) being dictated by national programme priorities. Ritonavir-boosted PIs are becoming preferred because of their high potency (Walmsley et al., 2002) and relatively lower pill burden, but the requirement for a cold chain and the support of frequent laboratory monitoring present problems for many low-resource countries. LPV/r is administered as a twice-daily regimen and is relatively well tolerated, but frequently causes elevations in plasma lipid levels. SQV/r can be administered once daily is known to achieve adequate blood levels in pregnancy and is compatible with rifampicin coadministration. However the pill burden with currently available formulations is high and gastrointestinal side-effects are frequent. NFV, although considered less potent than LPV/r, is an acceptable alternative, has been used extensively in pregnancy and does not require cold chain facilities. However, it is less effective against HIV-2 infection than other PIs (Adje-Toure et al., 2003; van der Ende et al., 2003; Smith et al., 2001). IDV/r also can be considered an alternative but is associated with a moderate incidence of renal adverse effects, particularly nephrolithiasis, and requires vigorous hydration.

The role of the recently approved protease inhibitor, atazanavir (ATV) in resource limited settings is currently unclear. The drug has the advantage of once-daily administration and does not induce hyperlipidaemia when administered without ritonavir boosting. It can also be given with low-dose ritonavir to enhance its potency (Haas et al., 2003; Piliero, 2002; Sanne et al., 2003). It is a reasonable alternative but much greater experience has been gained with the other PIs listed. Firmer recommendations will be made as the cost and availability of ATV, and experience with the drug, become clearer.

Triple NRTI-based Regimens

In the 2002 edition of these guidelines the ZDV/3TC/abacavir (ABC) regimen was considered the most user-friendly with respect to both patients and programmes (two pills per day and absence of significant drug interactions). The main disadvantages noted were uncertainty about its potency when the viral load was very high in patients with advanced disease, uncertainty as to whether the drugs, particularly ABC, would become available at an affordable cost, and the potential for fatal ABC hypersensitivity reactions. Recently released data from ACTG A5095 Study demonstrate that ZDV/3TC/ABC had a significantly higher virological failure rate than the other two study arms combined (ZDV/3TC/EFV or ZDV/3TC/ABC/EFV), 21% vs. 10% respectively, with a median follow-up of 32 weeks (Gulick et al., 2003). Importantly, significant differences in virological outcome were seen in persons with viral loads above and below 100 000 HIV RNA copies/ml. The study remains blinded with respect to the two EFV-containing arms. The incorporation of these findings into clinical practice and guidelines policy presents challenges because of the perceived advantages of triple nucleoside regimens, especially their attractiveness in the setting of coinfection with TB. It is important to note that the efficacy of ZDV/3TC/ABC in ACTG A5095 was comparable to that reported in previously reported studies of this regimen in the treatment of naive persons (Ibbotson and Perry, 2003; Staszewski et al., 2001). Moreover, in ACTG A5095 the CD4 cell responses were comparable to those of the combined EFV-containing arms. Thus, its virological inferiority to EFV-based regimens in a directly comparative trial moves this triple NRTI combination to a lower tier of consideration but does not, and should not, remove it from serious consideration. It may be useful, for example, when NNRTIs cannot be used because of intolerance or drug resistance and when PI-based regimens are not available. In particular, this regimen is a viable alternative for the management of patients coinfected with TB when antiretroviral and anti-TB therapy are coadministered. For the purposes of these guidelines it is considered to be a secondary alternative for initial therapy in specific situations (e.g. active TB coinfection, HIV-2 infection). It is also important to note that the ongoing DART trial will provide crucial additional information on the safety of ZDV/3TC/ABC in comparison with ZDV/3TC/TDF and ZDV/3TC/NVP in 3000 treatment-naïve patients in Africa (Kityo, 2003).

It should not be assumed that any triple NRTI regimen is comparable to any other: each triple NRTI combination needs to be evaluated on its own merits. Illustrative of this is the recently presented study of the combination of TDF/ 3TC/ABC administered once daily, in which there was a high virological failure rate (49%) and a high incidence of the K65R mutation, which confers crossresistance to non-ZDV nucleoside analogues (Gallant et al., 2003). This specific combination should be avoided in the light of these data. Similarly, in a 24-patient pilot study, TDF/ddI/3TC dosed once daily resulted in a 91% virological failure rate and a high incidence of the K65R mutation (Gilead, 2003). Another recent study reported low efficacy and a high frequency of adverse events with d4T/ddI/ABC (Gerstoft et al., 2003). These combinations should be avoided.

REASONS FOR CHANGING ART IN ADULTS AND ADOLESCENTS

It may be necessary to change ART because of either toxicity or treatment failure.

Toxicity

Toxicity is related to the inability to tolerate the side-effects of medication and to the significant organ dysfunction that may result. This can be monitored clinically on the basis of patient reporting and physical examination, and there may also be a limited number of laboratory tests, depending on the specific combination regimen that is utilized and the health care setting.

If a change in regimen is needed because of treatment failure, a new second-line regimen becomes necessary. When the toxicity is related to an identifiable drug in the regimen, the offending drug can be replaced with another drug that does not have the same side-effects, e.g. substitution of d4T for ZDV (for anaemia) or NVP for EFV (for CNS toxicity or pregnancy). Given the limited number of ARV combination options available in resource-limited settings, it is preferable to pursue drug substitutions where feasible so that premature switching to completely new alternative regimens is minimized. Table C lists the first-level medication switch options for toxicity for the four combination regimens listed in Table B. For life-threatening or more complex clinical situations, referral to district or regional hospital centres is recommended.

Treatment Failure

Treatment failure can be defined clinically as assessed by disease progression, immunologically using measurement of the CD4 counts, and/or virologically by measuring viral loads. Clinical disease progression should be differentiated from the immune reconstitution syndrome, an entity that can be seen early after ARV is introduced. This syndrome is characterized by the appearance of signs and symptoms of an opportunistic disease a few weeks after the start of potent ARV therapy in the setting of advanced immunodeficiency, as an inflammatory response to previously subclinical opportunistic infection. It is also possible that this immunological reconstitution may lead to the development of atypical presentations of some opportunistic infections.

Definitions of clinical and CD4-related treatment failure are listed in Table D. As viral loads are not normally available in resource-limited settings it is recommended that programmes primarily use clinical, and, where possible, CD4 count criteria, in order to define treatment failure. Similarly, drug resistance testing will not become a routine part of clinical care in resource-limited settings in the foreseeable future and so is not considered in these recommendations. However, it should be recognized that, in the developing world, treatment failure will be recognized later solely on the basis of clinical and/or CD4 criteria, thus providing a greater opportunity for drug resistance mutations to evolve before regimen change. This can

TABLE C. Major Potential Toxicities of First-line ARV Regimens and Recommended Substitutions

Regimen	Toxicity	Drug substitution
d4T/3TC/NVP	• d4T-related neuropathy or pancreatitis	• Switch d4T ZDV
	• d4T-related lipoatrophy	• Switch d4T TDF or ABC[a]
	• NVP-related severe hepatotoxicity	• Switch NVP EFV (except in pregnancy)
	• NVP-related severe rash	• Switch NVP EFV (but not life- threatening)
	• NVP-related life-threatening rash (Stevens-Johnson syndrome)	• Switch NVP PI[b]
ZDV/3TC/NVP	• ZDV-related persistent GI intolerance or severe haematological toxicity	• Switch ZDV d4T
	• NVP-related severe hepatotoxicity	• Switch NVP EFV (except in pregnancy; in this situation switch to NFV, LPV/r or ABC)
	• NVP-related severe rash (but not life-threatening)	• Switch NVP EFV
	• NVP-related life-threatening rash (Stevens-Johnson syndrome)	• Switch NVP PI[b]
d4T/3TC/EFV	• d4T-related neuropathy or pancreatitis	• Switch d4T ZDV
	• d4T-related lipoatrophy	• Switch d4T TDF or ABC[a]
	• EFV-related persistent CNS toxicity	• Switch EFV NVP
ZDV/3TC/EFV	• ZDV-related persistent GI intolerance or severe haematological toxicity	• Switch ZDV d4T
	• EFV-related persistent CNS toxicity	• Switch EFV NVP

[a]Switching off d4T typically does not reverse lipoatrophy but may slow its progression. TDF and ABC can be considered as alternatives but availability is currently limited in resource constrained settings. In the absence of TDF or ABC availability, ddI or ZDV are additional alternatives to consider.

[b]PI can be LPV/r or SQV/r. IDV/r or NFV can be considered as alternatives (see text).

compromise the NRTI component of the alternative regimen through drug class cross-resistance.

CLINICAL AND LABORATORY MONITORING

WHO recommends that in resource-limited settings the basic clinical assessment before the initiation of ART include documentation of past

TABLE D. Clinical and CD4+ Cell Count Definitions of Treatment Failure in HIV+ Adults and Adolescents

Clinical signs of treatment failure	CD4 cell criteria for treatment failure
• Occurrence of new opportunistic infection or malignancy signifying clinical disease progression. This must be differentiated from the immune reconstitution syndrome which can occur in the first three months following the initiation of ART.[a] The latter does not signify treatment failure and the opportunistic infection should be treated as usual, without changes in the antiretroviral regimen.	• Return of CD4 cell to pretherapy baseline below without other concomitant infection to explain transient CD4 cell decrease[c] • >50% fall from therapy CD4 peak level without other concomitant infection to explain transient CD4 cell decrease[c]
• Recurrence of previous opportunistic infection.[b]	
• Onset or recurrence of WHO Stage III conditions (including but not restricted to HIV wasting, chronic diarrhoea of unknown etiology, prolonged fever of unknown etiology, recurrent invasive bacterial infections, or recurrent/persistent mucosal candidiasis).	

[a]Immune reconstitution syndrome (IRS) is characterized by the appearance of signs and symptoms of an opportunistic disease a few weeks after the start of potent antiretroviral therapy in the setting of advanced immunodeficiency, as an inflammatory response to previously subclinical opportunistic infection. It is also possible that this immunological reconstitution may lead to the development of atypical presentations of some opportunistic infections.

[b]Recurrence of TB may not represent HIV disease progression, as reinfection may occur. Clinical evaluation is necessary.

[c]If patient is asymptomatic and treatment failure is being defined by CD4 cell criteria alone, consideration should be given to performing a confirmatory CD4 cell count if resources permit.

medical history, identification of current and past HIV-related illnesses, identification of coexisting medical conditions that may influence the timing of initiation and choice of ART (such as TB or pregnancy), and current symptoms and physical signs. Active TB should be managed in accordance with national TB control programmes.

In order to facilitate the scale-up of ARV use in resource-limited settings, WHO has tiered its monitoring recommendations to primary health

TABLE E. Recommended Tiered Laboratory Capabilities for ARV Monitoring in Limited-Resource Settings[a]

Primary health care centres (level 1)	District hospitals (level 2)	Regional referral centres (level 3)
Rapid HIV[ab] testing	Rapid HIV[ab] testing	Rapid HIV[ab] testing
Haemoglobin (if ZDV is being considered for use)[b]	Capability to resolve indeterminant rapid HIV[ab] test by second serological method	FBC and differential
		CD4+ cell count[c]
Pregnancy testing[d]		Full serum chemistries including (but not restricted to electrolytes, renal function, liver enzymes, lipids)[d]
Referral for sputum smear for TB (if microscopy not available)	FBC and differential	
	CD4+ cell count[c]	
	ALT	Pregnancy testing[d]
	Pregnancy testing[d]	Sputum smear for TB
	Sputum smear for TB	Viral load testing[e]

[a]This table only considers testing that is desirable for proper monitoring of ARV toxicity, efficacy and two prominent concomitant conditions (pregnancy and TB). It is not meant to be comprehensive with respect to other diagnostic capabilities that are important in the comprehensive care of HIV-infected persons. Other resources are available for these considerations.

[b]In primary health care centres where laboratory facilities are not available or in the absence of laboratory-based haemoglobinometry, the WHO haemoglobin colour scale can be used together with clinical signs to evaluate anaemia (more details at www.who.int/bct/).

[c]Scale-up of ART under the 3-by-5 Plan does not require uniform CD4 testing availability but, because of the value of this test in patient monitoring, WHO will work with Member States to make this a reality.

[d]EFV should not be given to women of childbearing potential unless adequate contraception is assured, not to women in the first trimester of pregnancy.

[e]Because of the cost and technical issues associated with viral load testing, this test is not currently recommended as part of the present treatment guidelines. However, it is hoped that more cost-effective technologies will allow regional referral centres to acquire this capability, given its utility in assessing treatment failure.

care centres (level 1), district hospitals (level 2) and regional referral centres (level 3) (Table E). WHO recognizes the importance of laboratory monitoring for efficacy and safety but does not want restricted infrastructure for these tests to place undue limitations on the scale-up effort.

This section concentrates on the basic clinical and laboratory monitoring indicated for the WHO-recommended first-line regimens outlined in Table B. These recommendations are designed to be implemented at the level of community health centres and/or that of district hospitals, working in concert, with backup from regional referral centres. National programme managers, working with WHO to implement the 3-by-5 Plan, should determine country-specific policies on how and where decisions about initiating therapy for individual patients are to be made. Similarly, the specific interactions of the health care delivery system levels for maximizing ART efficacy and safety require decisions to be made at the national programme level.

Clinical and laboratory assessments are considerations at baseline (pre-ART) and on treatment. Many studies conducted in developed and developing countries have demonstrated a reasonable correlation between TLC with CD4 levels in symptomatic patients (Badri and Wood, 2003; Beck et al., 1996; Brettle, 1997; Fournier and Sosenko, 1992; Kumarasamy et al., 2002; van der Ryst et al., 1998). This means that even if CD4 cell count testing is unavailable, simple tools such as haemoglobin measurement and TLC can be used as laboratory markers to initiate HAART in resource-poor settings. The baseline clinical assessment is the same for all four recommended first-line regimens. It should include:

- staging of HIV disease;
- determination of concomitant medical conditions (e.g. TB, pregnancy, major psychiatric illness);
- detailing of concomitant medications, including traditional therapies;
- assessment of patients' readiness for therapy.

Once therapy has begun, clinical assessment should cover

- signs/symptoms of potential drug toxicities (Table D);
- adherence;
- response to therapy;
- weight;
- basic laboratory monitoring considerations as listed in Table F.

Need for Scale-up of Laboratory Capacity

WHO recognizes the current limitations on laboratory capacity in resource limited settings. The 3-by-5 Plan is designed to move forward with current realities in place. WHO will work with Member countries and diagnostic manufacturers to scale up laboratory infrastructure at the country level so as to permit the uniform availability of CD4 testing, wider availability of automated haematology and chemistry testing, and regional availability of viral load testing. This will require choosing uniform, cost-

TABLE F. Basic Laboratory Monitoring for Recommended First-line ARV Regimens at Primary Health Care Centres (Level 1) and District Hospitals (Level 2)

Regimen	Laboratory assessment at baseline (pretherapy)	Laboratory assessment on therapy
d4T/3TC/NVP	Desirable but not required: CD4	Symptom-directed determination of ALT for toxicity CD4 q6-12 months, if available, for efficacy
ZDV/3TC/NVP	Recommended: Hgb Desirable but not required: FBC, CD4	Symptom-directed determination of Hgb, WBC, ALT for toxicity CD4 q6-12 months, if available, for efficacy
d4T/3TC/EFV	Pregnancy test (mandatory) Desirable but not required: CD4	Symptom-directed testing but none routinely required for toxicity CD4 q6-12 months, if available, for efficacy
ZDV/3TC/EFV	Pregnancy test (mandatory) Recommended: Hgb Desirable but not required: FBC, CD4	Symptom-directed determination of Hgb, WBC for toxicity CD4 q6-12 months, if available, for efficacy

effective methodologies at the country level and ensuring supplies of reagents and the maintenance of equipment.

CHOICE OF ARV REGIMENS IN THE EVENT OF TREATMENT FAILURE OF FIRST-LINE COMBINATIONS IN ADULTS AND ADOLESCENTS

WHO recommends that the entire regimen be changed from a first-line to a second-line combination in the setting of treatment failure. The new second-line regimen should involve drugs that retain activity against the patient's virus strain and should preferably include at least three new drugs, one or more of them from a new class, in order to increase the likelihood of treatment success and minimize the risk of cross-resistance.

Figure 1 lists the second-line regimens that might be considered in

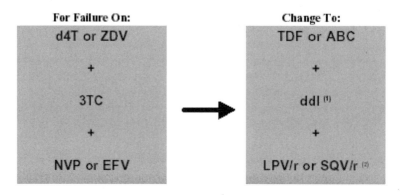

FIGURE 1. Recommended second-line regimens in adults and adolescents in the event of treatment failure of first-line ARV regimens.

adults and adolescents for the first-line regimens identified in Table B. When (d4T or ZDV) + 3TC are used as part of the first-line regimen, nucleoside cross-resistance may compromise the potency of alternative dual nucleoside components in the second-line regimen, especially in the presence of long-standing virological failure. In this situation it is necessary to make empirical alternative choices with a view to providing as much antiviral activity as possible. Given the cross-resistance that exists between d4T and ZDV, second-line regimens that might offer more activity include TDF/ddI or ABC/ddI. The issues of cost and drug hypersensitivity with ABC remain. Furthermore, high-level ZDV/3TC coresistance confers diminished susceptibility to ABC. TDF can be compromised by multiple nucleoside analogue mutations (NAMs) but often retains activity against nucleoside-resistant viral strains. It is attractive in that, like ddI, it is administered once daily. TDF raises the level of ddI and the dose of the latter should therefore be reduced when the two drugs are given together, in order to reduce the chance of ddI-associated toxicity (e.g. neuropathy and pancreatitis).

Because of the diminished potential of almost any second-line nucleoside component, a ritonavir-enhanced PI (RTV-PI) component, i.e. lopinavir (LPV)/r, saquinavir (SQV)/r or indinavir (IDV)/r, is preferable to nelfinavir (NFV) in second-line regimens, given their potency (Walmsley et al., 2002). NFV can be considered as an alternative for the PI component if a ritonavir-enhanced PI is not available, if a cold chain is not secure or if there is a clinical contraindication to the use of another PI.

Despite being considered a potent option, IDV/r is associated with substantial renal side-effects and should also be considered as an alternative. As noted above, the role and availability of ATV/r in the developing world cannot be fully specified at present.

For treatment failure with a first-line PI-based regimen, the choice of an alternative regimen depends on the reason for the initial choice of a PI-based, rather than an NNRTI-based, regimen. If the reason was suspected NNRTI resistance or HIV-2 infection the choice of the alternative regimen is not straightforward. In these situations the options depend on the constraints imposed by the circumstances of individual patients, the capabilities of individual managements to test for resistance to drugs, and the limited ARV formulary that may exist in particular country programmes.

Treatment failure on a triple NRTI regimen is more easily managed because two important drug classes (NNRTIs and PIs) will have been spared. Thus a RTV-PI + NNRTI +/- alternative NRTIs (e.g. ddI and/or TDF) can be considered if drug availability permits.

CONSIDERATIONS FOR SPECIFIC CATEGORIES OF PATIENTS

Women of Childbearing Potential or Pregnant Women

The guiding principle for the treatment of women of childbearing potential or pregnant women is that therapeutic decisions should be based solely on their need and eligibility for ART as outlined in Section III. The special circumstances of pregnancy or breast-feeding raise additional issues concerning toxicity to mothers and children, the choice of ARV drugs, and the prevention of HIV transmission from mothers to infants. These matters should be dealt with in the context of assuring optimal treatment to preserve the health of the mothers. Consequently, the recommended WHO first-line regimen for this patient subgroup is:

$$(d4T \text{ or } ZDV) + 3TC + NVP.$$

The choice of ART for women with the potential to become pregnant must involve a consideration of the possibility that the ARV drugs may be received early in the first trimester, before the recognition of pregnancy and during the primary period of fetal organ development. EFV should be avoided in such women because of its potential for teratogenicity. Women who are receiving ART and do not wish to become pregnant should have effective and appropriate contraceptive methods available to them in order to reduce the likelihood of unintended pregnancy. In those women for whom effective contraception can be assured, EFV remains a viable option for the NNRTI component of the regimen. Women who are receiving ART and become pregnant should continue their treatment unless they are in the first trimester of pregnancy and EFV has been part of the regimen, in which circumstances EFV should be discontinued and replaced by NVP.

For pregnant women it may be desirable to initiate ART after the first trimester, although for such women who are severely ill the benefit of early therapy clearly outweighs any potential fetal risks, and therapy should be initiated in these cases. Additionally, the dual NRTI combination of d4T/ddI should be avoided in pregnancy and only used when no other alternatives exist, because of the potential increased risk of lactic acidosis with this combination in pregnant women.

Symptomatic NVP-associated hepatic or serious rash toxicity, although uncommon, is more frequent in women than in men and is more likely to be seen in women with comparatively elevated CD4 cell counts ($>250/mm^3$) (Boehringer-Ingleheim Pharmaceuticals, 2003; Imperiale et al., 2002; Stern et al., 2002, 2003). It is not known if pregnancy further predisposes women to such toxicities but cases have been reported in pregnant women (Langlet et al., 2000; Lyons et al., 2003).

An important issue is the potential impact of NVP prophylaxis for the prevention of MTCT on the subsequent treatment of mothers and their infected infants. This question has arisen in the past two years because a single point mutation is associated with resistance for NVP. Mutations associated with NNRTI drug resistance have been detected in plasma virus in approximately 20% of women following single-dose NVP prophylaxis at six weeks postpartum; higher rates of mutant virus (67%) have been detected at six weeks postpartum where women have received two doses instead of a single intrapartum dose of NVP for the prevention of transmission (Eshleman et al., 2001; Sullivan, 2002). Additionally, NVP resistance can develop even among women receiving additional antiretroviral drugs if they have detectable viral replication at the time of administration of single-dose NVP; genotypic NVP resistance was detected at six weeks postpartum in 15% of women who received single-dose NVP and who had received ZDV alone or combination antiretroviral drugs during pregnancy and intrapartum (Chaowanachan et al., 2003; Cunningham et al., 2002). Resistance to 3TC is also associated with a single mutation. In a study in which 3TC was added to ZDV therapy at 32 weeks of gestation in pregnant women in France, the 3TC resistance mutation M184V was observed at six weeks postpartum in 39% of women (Mandelbrot et al., 2001); 3TC resistance was also detected at one week postpartum in 12% of women receiving ZDV/3TC for four weeks for the prevention of MTCT in the PETRA study (Giuliano et al., 2003). No ZDV or 3TC resistance was observed with intrapartum/oneweek-postpartum ZDV/3TC in the SAINT study in South Africa (Giuliano et al., 2003; Sullivan, 2002).

There is no information about the clinical consequences of the selection of these resistance mutations for responses to future antiretroviral therapy in women or infected infants. The mutations fade with time but doubtless remain archived in minor viral subpopulations and have the potential to re-emerge when a subsequent regimen containing NNRTI or 3TC is intro-duced. Studies are in progress and others are planned with a view to deter-mining whether single-dose NVP prophylaxis compromises subsequent HAART with NNRTI-based regimens. This is one of the most pressing operational research questions in the field.

Until definitive data are available on this matter, women who have received single-dose NVP prophylaxis or 3TC prophylaxis for the preven-tion of MTCT should be considered eligible for NNRTI-based regimens and should not be denied access to life-sustaining therapy.

Several country programmes are already considering the use of short-course triple combination therapy for the prevention of MTCT in women who are not yet in need of treatment for their own HIV infection, and the cessation of therapy postpartum if the women do not require its continua-tion for their own health. The use of highly active combination therapy in such situations should prevent the emergence of resistance to the drugs and should also be highly effective in reducing perinatal HIV transmission to infants. However, this intervention also exposes both mother and fetus to potential drug toxicities in situations where therapy is not required for maternal health. Studies are in progress with a view to assessing the safety and efficacy of this approach for women and their infants, particularly for the prevention of MTCT in breast-feeding women.

When a PI-based option is preferred to an NNRTI-based regimen dur-ing pregnancy, SQV/r or NFV are reasonable choices, given the safety experience in pregnancy.

It is important to note that ARV drugs have the potential to either decrease or increase the bioavailability of steroid hormones in hormonal contraceptives. The limited data available suggest that potential drug inter-actions between many ARVs (particularly some NNRTIs and PIs) and hor-monal contraceptives may alter safety and effectiveness of both the hor-monal contraceptives and the ARVs. It is not known whether the contraceptive effectiveness of progestogen-only injectable contraceptives (such as depot medroxyprogesterone acetate and norethisterone enantate) would be compromised, as these methods provide higher blood hormone levels than other progestogen-only hormonal contraceptives, as well as than combined oral contraceptives. Studies are underway to evaluate potential interactions between depot medroxyprogesterone acetate and selected PI and NNRTI drugs. Thus, if a woman on ARV treatment decides to initiate or continue hormonal contraceptive use, the consistent use of condoms must be recommended for preventing HIV transmission and may also com-pensate for any possible reduction in the effectiveness of the hormonal contraceptive.

Children

When to Start ARV Therapy in Infants and Children

The laboratory diagnosis of HIV infection in infants aged under 18 months is difficult because of the persistence of maternal antibody. Virological tests are required in order to make definitive diagnoses of HIV infection in this age group. WHO recommendations for the initiation of ARV therapy in children are therefore divided into categories related to age and the availability of virological diagnostic tests (Table G). When CD4 cell assays are available the use of the CD4 cell percentage is recommended for decision-making on ARV treatment rather than of the absolute CD4 cell count, because the former varies less with age (Annex B) (Embree et al., 2001; Shearer et al., 2003; Wade and Ades, 1994). WHO strongly encourages the development of tests applicable to resource-limited settings which would allow early diagnosis of HIV infection in infants. The availability of such tests is critical to the development of improved recommendations for the initiation of therapy in infants aged under 18 months.

• For HIV-seropositive infants aged under 18 months, WHO recommends the initiation of ARV therapy in the following circumstances:
• The infant has virologically proven infection (using either HIV DNA PCR, HIV RNA assay, or immune-complex dissociated p24 antigen) and has:
  • WHO Paediatric Stage III HIV disease (i.e. clinical AIDS) (Annex E), irrespective of CD4%; or
  • WHO Paediatric Stage II disease (Annex E), with consideration of using CD4 <20% to assist in decision-making; or
  • WHO Paediatric Stage I (i.e. asymptomatic) (Annex E) and CD4 <20% (asymptomatic children, i.e. WHO Stage I, should only be treated when there is access to CD4 assays).
• If virological tests to confirm HIV infection status are not available but CD4 cell assays are available, WHO recommends that ARV therapy can be initiated in HIV-seropositive infants who have WHO Stage II or III disease and a CD4 percentage below 20%. In such cases, HIV antibody testing must be repeated at the age of 18 months in order to definitively confirm that the children are HIV-infected; ARV therapy should only be continued in infants with confirmed infection.
• For HIV-seropositive children aged 18 months or over, WHO recommends initiation of ARV therapy in the following circumstances:
  • WHO Paediatric Stage III HIV disease (i.e. clinical AIDS) (Annex E), irrespective of CD4 %; or

- WHO Paediatric Stage II disease (Annex E), with consideration of using CD4 <15% to assist decision-making; or
- WHO Paediatric Stage I (i.e. asymptomatic) (Annex E) and CD4 <15%.

It should be noted that breast-feeding infants are at risk of HIV infection during the entire period of breast-feeding, and that a negative virological or antibody test at one age does not exclude the possibility of infection occurring subsequently if breast-feeding continues.

As in HIV-infected adults, the total lymphocyte count significantly correlates with the risk of mortality in HIV-infected children (European Collaborative Study, 2004; Mofenson et al., 2003). The 12-month risk of mortality is >20% for children aged under 18 months with a total lymphocyte count of <2500/mm^3 and for children aged 18 months or more with a total lymphocyte count of <1500/mm^3. In cases where the CD4 cell count cannot be assessed, therefore, the total lymphocyte count may be used as a substitute indication for the treatment of infants or children with documented HIV infection in the presence of symptomatic disease (WHO Paediatric Stage II or III). It is preferable that an abnormal total lymphocyte count or CD4 cell count/percentage be confirmed with a second test before therapeutic decisions are made but it is recognized that this may not always be possible.

WHO recognizes that the current staging system for HIV infection in children was developed several years ago and that many of the clinical symptoms in Paediatric Stage II and III are not specific for HIV infection and may significantly overlap with those seen in children without HIV infection in resource-limited settings. Recognizing this limitation, WHO is planning a consultation with paediatric experts in order to revise the classification system in 2004. In the interim, however, the use of this WHO disease classification (Annex F) can be of value in assisting to define parameters for the initiation of therapy in resource-limited settings, although individual adaptation at the country programme level may be appropriate.

The penetration of ARVs into human breast milk in lactating women has not been quantified for most ARVs. Although some ARVs, such as nevirapine, are known to be present in breast milk, the concentration and quantity of drug ingested by infants would be less than those needed to achieve therapeutic levels. Consequently, if a breast-feeding infant is ill enough to require ARV treatment (Table G), the administration of ARVs at standard paediatric doses should be initiated regardless of whether the mother is receiving ARV therapy. Infected breast-feeding infants whose mothers are receiving ARV therapy may ingest subtherapeutic levels of some ARVs, and this could lead to the development of drug resistance in the infant's virus. It is not known whether ARVs should be administered

TABLE G. Recommendations for Initiating ART in Infants and Children

CD4 testing	Age	HIV diagnostic testing	Treatment recommendation
If CD4 testing is available	< 18 months	HIV virological testing not available but infant is HIV antibody-seropositive (Note: HIV antibody test must be repeated at age 18 months to obtain definitive diagnosis of HIV infection)	WHO Paediatric Stages II and III disease with CD4 < 20%[a]
		Positive HIV virological test[b]	WHO Paediatric Stage III (i.e. AIDS) (Annex F) irrespective of CD4% WHO Paediatric Stage II disease (Annex F), with consideration of using CD4 <20% to assist in decision-making[a,c] WHO Paediatric Stage I disease (i.e. asymptomatic) (Annex F), CD4 <20%[a,d]
	≥ 18 months	HIV antibody-seropositive	WHO Paediatric Stage III disease, irrespective of CD4% WHO Paediatric Stage II disease, with consideration of using CD4 <15% to assist in decisionmaking[a, c] WHO Paediatric Stage I disease with CD4 < 15%[a,d]

If CD4 testing is not available			Treatment not recommended[d,e]
	< 18 months	HIV virological testing not available but infant HIV antibody-seropositive	WHO Paediatric Stage III, irrespective of total lymphocyte count
		Positive HIV virological test	WHO Paediatric Stage II disease, with consideration of using total lymphocyte count <2500/mm³ to assist in decision-making[f]
	≥ 18 months	HIV antibody-seropositive	WHO Paediatric Stage III irrespective of total lymphocyte count
			WHO Paediatric Stage II disease, with consideration of using total lymphocyte count <1500/mm³ to assist in decision-making[f]

[a] A CD4 cell percentage <20% corresponds to an absolute CD4 count of approximately <1000/mm³ for children aged <12 months and <750/mm³ for children aged 12-18 months; CD4 <15% corresponds to <500/mm³ for children aged 1-5 years and to <200/mm³ for children aged > 6 years.

[b] HIV DNA PCR or HIV RNA amplification assays or immune complex dissociated p24 antigen assays.

[c] CD4 cell percentage is advisable to assist with determining the need for immediate therapy.

[d] If a child is asymptomatic and treatment is being initiated on basis of CD4 criteria, consideration should be given to performing a confirmatory CD4 assay if resources permit.

[e] Many of the clinical symptoms in the WHO Paediatric Stage II and III disease classification are not specific for HIV infection and significantly overlap those seen in children without HIV infection in resource-limited settings; thus, in the absence virological testing and CD4 cell assay availability, symptomatic HIV-seropositive infants <18 months of age should only be considered for ARV therapy in exceptional circumstances (e.g. a child with a classic AIDS-defining opportunistic infection such as Kaposi's sarcoma, Pneumocystis carinii pneumonia or cryptococcal meningitis). If ARVs are given to a symptomatic HIV-seropositive infant in the absence of a definitive virological diagnosis, HIV antibody testing should be repeated at the age 18 months to confirm infection status; ARV therapy should only be continued in infants with confirmed HIV infection.

[f] A total lymphocyte count of <2500/mm³ for children aged <18 months or of <1500/mm³ for children aged ≥18 months can be substituted for CD4% when the latter is unavailable and HIV-related symptoms exist. Its utility in asymptomatic children is unknown. In the absence of CD4 cell testing, therefore, asymptomatic HIV-infected children (WHO Paediatric Stage I) should not be treated because no other reliable marker is currently available in severely resource-constrained settings.

during the breast-feeding period to infants with documented HIV infection who do not require ARV therapy themselves but whose mothers are receiving ARV treatment, and further research is needed on this matter.

Recommended First-line ARV Regimens in Infants and Children

Studies of HAART in children demonstrate that similar improvements are seen in morbidity, mortality and surrogate markers with many different potent ARV regimens (De Martino et al., 2000; Gortmaker et al., 2001). Drug doses must be adjusted as a child grows in order to avoid the risk of underdosage and the development of resistance; dosing in children is therefore based on either body surface area or weight. Standardization is important so that non-expert personnel can safely dispense correct doses, and consequently it is desirable to provide health care workers with a table of drug doses that can be administered according to weight bands. Such tables may vary between localities in accordance with the availability of ARV drugs and formulations in the country concerned. In order to improve adherence, regimens chosen for children should take account of those that may be used by their parents in order to avoid different timings, and, if possible, to permit the use of the same drugs. WHO recognizes the need to provide assistance to countries in the development of such tables for training manuals so that ARV programmes can be implemented. Pending the development of a consensus on such tables in the course of 2004, samples of tables used by some paediatricians will be made available on request.

Some ARVs available for adults are also available in formulations specifically designed for children. However, formulations appropriate for use by young children who cannot swallow whole tablets or capsules are not widely available in resource-limited settings. For some ARVs, capsules and tablets are available in sufficiently low doses to enable accurate dosing for children (e.g. d4T capsules of 15, 20 and 30 mg, or NFV scored tablets that can be halved and crushed), and the pharmacokinetics of crushed tablets or sprinkled capsule contents in children have been evaluated. However, many drugs do not have solid formulations in doses appropriate for paediatric use and some solid formulations do not have all drug components evenly distributed in the tablets (e.g. fixed-dose ZDV/3TC). The use of tablets that require cutting up, particularly unscored tablets, can result in the underdosing or overdosing of children, which can lead to an increased risk of resistance or toxicity. Moreover, the doses cannot easily be adjusted as the children grow. However, WHO recognizes that until appropriate formulations can be made more widely available the splitting of adult-dose solid formulation ARVs, while suboptimal, may be the only way a severely ill child can receive therapy, and should be considered when no alternatives are available. Health care providers should be aware that current fixed-dose combination formulations may not contain the appropriate doses of each of the component drugs for children on a weight basis. This is a specific problem for the NVP component of the fixed-dose formulation of ZDV/3TC/NVP, for which additional NVP may be necessary if tablets are used to treat younger children (Annex F). WHO strongly encourages the development of formulations appropriate for paediatric use, particularly solid formulations in doses that can be used by paediatric patients (e.g. crushable tablets or openable capsules), as liquid formulations may have a more limited shelf-life than solid formulations, they may be more expensive, they may be difficult to store and they may require the use of syringes for accurate administration.

The preferred first-line treatment option for children includes (d4T or ZDV) + 3TC plus an NNRTI (NVP or EFV) (Table H), for the same reasons as discussed for adult initial ARV regimens. A caveat is that EFV cannot be used currently in children under 3 years of age because of a lack of appropriate formulation and dosing information, although these matters are under study. Consequently, for children aged under 3 years or weighing under 10 kg, NVP should be the NNRTI of choice. The use of ZDV/3TC/ABC as first-line therapy is now considered a secondary alternative because of the results obtained with ACTG A5095 in adults; further data are awaited.

EFV would be the NNRTI of choice for children who require ARV therapy but need or are receiving anti-TB therapy containing rifampicin. For children under 3 years of age who require ARV therapy while receiving anti-TB therapy, the use of ZDV/3TC/ABC should be considered while the TB therapy is being administered, as SQV/r is not available in a formulation that is appropriate for children of this age. Monitoring for possible ABC hypersensitivity should be assured. SQV/r may also be considered for older children who can receive adult doses of the drugs (i.e. children weighing ≥25 kg).

TABLE H. Recommended First-line ARV Regimens for Infants and Children

First-line regimen	Comment
d4T or ZDV	
plus 3TC	
plus N VP or EF V	NNRTI choice: • If age < 3 years or weight <10 kg, NVP • If age > 3 years or weight >10 kg, NVP or EFV

If a mother has received ARV during pregnancy, either to reduce MTCT or for her own disease, there is a possibility that the baby may become infected with drug-resistant virus. Additionally, resistance could be induced de novo in an infected infant who is exposed to an ARV drug being used for prophylaxis before the infection status of the infant is known. This is a particular problem if NVP or 3TC has been used, either alone or as a component of a two-drug regimen, for prophylaxis of MTCT, because a single point mutation is associated with resistance to these two drugs (Eshleman et al., 2001; Mandelbrot et al., 2001). Following single-dose NVP, 46% of infants have NNRTI-associated mutations (primarily the Y181C mutation, which may not always be associated with cross-resistance to EFV). As has been observed in mothers, these mutations fade with time but probably remain as minor viral subpopulations (Eshleman et al., 2001). It is not known whether ARV choices should be modified for infants who have been exposed to ARVs used for the prevention of MTCT. Studies in children are in progress or are planned, as they are in mothers, to investigate whether single-dose NVP prophylaxis compromises subsequent HAART with NNRTI-based regimens. WHO recognizes the urgency of such research. However, until there are data allowing these questions to be definitively answered, children who require ARV therapy and who have previously received single-dose NVP or 3TC as part of MCTC prophylaxis should be considered eligible for NNRTI-based regimens and should not be denied access to life-sustaining therapy.

Clinical Assessment of Infants and Children Receiving ARV Therapy

Important clinical signs of response to ARV therapy in children include: improvement in growth in children who have been failing to grow; improvement in neurological symptoms and development in children who have been demonstrating delay in the achievement of developmental milestones or encephalopathy; and/or decreased frequency of infections (bacterial infections, oral thrush, and/or other opportunistic infections).

Laboratory assessments for children on ARV therapy are the same as those recommended for adults (Table G). In addition to the clinical assessments recommended for adults, the clinical monitoring of ARV treatment in children should cover:

- nutrition and nutritional status;
- weight and height growth;
- developmental milestones;
- neurological symptoms.

Reasons for Changing ARV Therapy in Infants and Children

The principles on which to base changes in therapy for children are similar to those applied for adults, and the management of drug toxicity is the same. If toxicity is related to an identifiable drug in the regimen, the offending drug can be replaced with one that does not have the same side-effects. In children, important clinical signs of drug failure include: a lack of growth in children who show an initial response to treatment, or a decline in growth among children who show an initial growth response to therapy; a loss of neurodevelopment milestones or the development of encephalopathy; and the recurrence of infections, such as oral candidiasis that is refractory to treatment (Lindsey et al., 2000; Verweel et al., 2002; Saulsbury, 2001; McCoig et al., 2002) (Table I). It should not be concluded, on the basis of clinical criteria, that an ARV regimen is failing until the child in question has had a reasonable trial on the therapy (e.g. the child should have received the regimen for at least 24 weeks).

TABLE I. Clinical and CD4 Count Definitions of Treatment Failure in Infants and Children

Clinical signs of treatment failure	CD4 cell criteria for treatment failure[a]
• Lack of growth among children who show an initial response to treatment, or decline in growth among children who show an initial growth response to therapy.	• Return of CD4 cell percentage (or for children > 6 years of age, of absolute CD4 cell count) to pretherapy baseline or below, in absence of other concurrent infection explaining transient CD4 decrease
• Loss of neurodevelopmental milestones or development of encephalopathy.	• ≥ 50% fall from peak level on therapy of CD4 cell percentage (or for children > 6 years of age, of absolute CD4 cell count) in absence of other concurrent infection explaining transient CD4 decrease.
• Occurrence of new opportunistic infection or malignancy signifying clinical disease progression.[b]	
• Recurrence of prior opportunistic infections, such as oral candidiasis that is refractory to treatment.	

[a]If a child is asymptomatic and treatment failure is being defined by CD4 cell criteria alone, consideration should be given to performing a confirmatory CD4 count if resources permit.

[b]This must be distinguished from immune reconstitution syndrome, which can occur in the first three months following the initiation of HAART and does not signify treatment failure.

Because of age-related declines in CD4 absolute cell counts until the age of 6 years, when near-adult levels are reached, it is difficult to use such counts for assessing therapy failure in younger children. However, for children aged 6 years or more, similar CD4 cell count criteria to those used for adults are appropriate (Table E). Because the CD4 cell percentage varies less with age it can be used to gauge treatment response regardless of age. No data are available on the use of total lymphocyte counts for the evaluation of response to ARV therapy.

Recommended Second-line ARV Therapy for Infants and Children

Second-line therapy for children in the event of failure of a first-line regimen includes a change in the nucleoside backbone, in accordance with the same principles as are applied for adults (e.g. from ZDV + 3TC to ABC + ddI), plus a protease inhibitor (Table J). The use of PIs other than LPV/r and NFV is more problematic in children because of a lack of suitable paediatric drug formulations for IDV and SQV and a lack of appropriate dosing information for ritonavir-boosted PIs other than LPV/r. However, the use of SQV/r can be considered as an alternative for children who are able to swallow capsules and who weigh 25 kg or more, and can therefore receive the adult dosage. TDF cannot be recommended for paediatric treatment at present because of limited data on appropriate dosing for children, particularly those aged under 8 years, and because of questions about bone toxicity, which may be of more concern and/or more frequent in growing children than in adults.

TABLE J. Recommended ARV Regimens for Infants and Children with Treatment Failure

First-line regimen	Second-line regimen
d4T or ZDV	ABC
plus	*plus*
3TC	ddI
plus	*plus*
NNRTI:	Protease inhibitor:
NVP or EFV	LPV/r or NFV, or SQV/r if weight ≥25 kg

People with Tuberculosis Disease and HIV Coinfection

Tuberculosis is an entry point for a significant proportion of patients eligible for ART. ART is recommended for all patients with TB who have CD4 counts below 200 cells/mm[3], and should be considered for patients with CD4 counts below 350 cells/mm[3]. In the absence of CD4 cell counts, ART is recommended for all patients with TB. It is acknowledged that this will result in the treatment of individuals with CD4 cell counts over 350 who otherwise would not receive ART. The treatment of TB remains a central priority for patient management and should not be compromised by ART (Santoro-Lopes et al., 2002; Giarardi et al., 2000; Badri et al., 2002; Harvard University, 2001).

Patients with TB merit special consideration because comanagement of HIV and TB is complicated by rifampicin drug interactions with NNRTIs and PIs, pill burden, adherence and drug toxicity. Data supporting specific treatment recommendations are incomplete and research is urgently needed in this area (Burman and Jones, 2001; Wagner and Bishai, 2001; Havlir and Barnes, 1999; Dean et al., 2002). Taking the available data into account, the first-line treatment recommendation for patients with TB and HIV coinfection is (ZDV or d4T) + 3TC + EFV (600 or 800 mg/day). The 800-mg dose of EFV achieves higher drug levels than those seen in the absence of rifampicin and thus may reduce the chance of HIV drug resistance. However, it can also increase the toxicity risk. SQV/RTV 400/400 mg bid, SQV/r 1600/200 mg qd (in soft gel formulation-sgc) or LPV/ RTV 400/400 mg bid in combination with the NRTI backbone are alternatives to EFV, although tolerability, clinical monitoring and risk of resistance may be problematic. Endorsement of these PI-based regimens requires further data. ABC is another alternative to EFV with the advantages of low pill burden, no interaction with rifampicin, and suitability for administration to children weighing 25 kg or less, for whom appropriate EFV dosing information is not yet available. Concerns about this regimen include ones relating to monitoring for hypersensitivity syndrome and virological potency. Data on the use of NVP + rifampicin are limited and conflicting. NVP levels are reduced in the presence of rifampicin, and higher NVP doses have not been evaluated. Although some clinical experience reports adequate viral and immunological response and acceptable toxicity, this regimen should only be considered when no other options are available. For women of child-bearing age (without effective contraception), pregnant women, and children with TB, either SQV/r or ABC + (d4T or ZDV) + 3TC is recommended. For children weighing 25 kg or less, (d4T or ZDV)/3TC/ABC is recommended as an alternative (Lopez-Cortes et al., 2002; Patel et al., 2003; Pedral-Samapio et al., 2003; Dean et al., 1999; Ribera et al., 2001, 2002; Oliva et al., 2003; la Porte et al., 2002).

TABLE L. ART Recommendations for Individuals with TB Disease and HIV Coinfection

CD4 cell count	Recommended regimen	Comments
CD4 <200 mm^3	Start TB treatment. Start ART as soon as TB treatment is tolerated (between 2 weeks and 2 months):[a] EFV-containing regimens[b,c,d]	Recommend ART. EFV is contraindicated in pregnant women or women of childbearing potential without effective contraception.
CD4 200-350/mm^3	Start TB treatment. Start one of the regimens below after the initiation phase (start earlier if severely compromised): EFV-containing regimens[b] or NVP-containing regimens in case of rifampicin-free continuation phase TB treatment regimen.	Consider ART.
CD4 >350 mm^3	Start TB treatment.	Defer ART.[e]
CD4 not available	Start TB treatment.	Consider ART.[a,f]

[a]Timing of ART initiation should be based on clinical judgement in relation to other signs of immunodeficiency (Table A). For extrapulmonary TB, ART should be started as soon as TB treatment is tolerated, irrespective of CD4 cell count

[b]Alternatives to the EFV portion of the regimen include: SQV/RTV (400/400 mg bid), SQV/r (1600/200 mg qd in sgc), LPV/RTV (400/400 mg bid) and ABC.

[c]NVP (200 mg qd for two weeks followed by 200 mg bid) may be used in place of EFV in absence of other options. NVP-containing regimens include: d4T/3TC/NVP or ZDV/3TC/NVP.

[d]EFV-containing regimens include d4T/3TC/EFV and ZDV/3TC/EFV.

[e]Unless non-TB Stage IV conditions are present (Table A). Otherwise start ART upon completion of TB treatment.

[f]If no other signs of immunodeficiency are present and patient is improving on TB treatment, ART should be started upon completion of TB treatment.

The optimal time to initiate ART in patients with TB is not known. Case-fatality rates in many patients with TB during the first two months of TB treatment are high, particularly when they present with advanced HIV disease, and ART in this setting might be life-saving. On the other hand, pill burden, drug-to-drug interaction, potential toxicity and immune reconstitution syndrome should be kept in mind when deciding on the best time to begin treatment (Burman and Jones, 2001; Wagner and Bishai, 2001; Narita et al., 1998; Harries et al., 2001). The management of patients with HIV and TB poses many challenges, including that of achieving patient acceptance of both diagnoses. Pending current studies, WHO recommends that ART in patients with CD4 cell counts below 200/mm3 be started between two weeks and two months after the start of TB therapy, when the patient has stabilized on this therapy. This provisional recommendation is meant to encourage rapid initiation of therapy in patients among whom there may be a high mortality rate. However, deferring the start of ART may be reasonable in a variety of clinical scenarios. For example, in patients with higher CD4 cell counts the commencement of ART may be delayed until after the induction phase of TB therapy is completed in order to simplify the management of treatment.

Injecting Drug Users

The clinical and immunological criteria for initiating HAART in substance dependent patients do not differ from those in the general recommendations. Injecting drug users who are eligible for ART should therefore be guaranteed access to this life-saving therapy. Special considerations for this population include dealing prospectively with lifestyle instability that challenges drug adherence and accounting for the potential drug interactions of ARVs with agents such as methadone. The development of programmes which integrate care of drug dependence (including drug substitution therapy) and HIV is encouraged. In such settings, approaches such as directly observed therapy can be implemented. Once-daily ARV regimens are being intensively explored in this arena and lend themselves to such approaches. The number of ARVs approved or being investigated for once-daily use is steadily increasing. They include 3TC, FTC, ddI, d4T, TDF, ABC, EFV, SQV/r, LPV/r and ATV.

The coadministration of methadone with EFV, NVP or RTV in HIV-infected individuals with a history of injecting drug use resulted in decreased plasma levels of methadone and signs of opiate withdrawal. Patients should be monitored for signs of withdrawal and their methadone dose should be increased in appropriate increments over time so as to alleviate withdrawal symptoms. An important option can thus be provided for treatment programmes directed at this vulnerable population.

ADHERENCE TO ANTIRETROVIRAL THERAPY

Adherence to ART is well recognized to be an essential component of individual and programmatic treatment success (Bang and Scott, 2003; Staszewski et al., 2003; Schaaf et al., 2003; Martin-Carbonero et al., 2003;

Adje-Toure et al., 2003; Piliero, 2002; Eshleman et al., 2001; Sullivan, 2002; Mandelbrot et al., 2001; Mofenson et al., 2003; Lindsey et al., 2000; Giarardi et al., 2000; Havlir et al., 2002). Studies of drug adherence in the developed world have suggested that higher levels of drug adherence are associated with improved virological and clinical outcomes and that rates exceeding 95% are desirable in order to maximize the benefits of ART. It is difficult to achieve rates this high over a long period of time. Numerous approaches to improving adherence have been investigated in the developed world and have begun to be explored in the developing world. Viral load testing will not be widely introduced in the developing world in the near future because of cost and technical considerations. Consequently, it is particularly important to focus on maximizing adherence in order to try to avoid drug resistance and ensure the durability of effect of ARV regimens.

The proper education of patients before the initiation of therapy is vital for the success of adherence strategies. Such education should cover basic information about HIV and its manifestations, the benefits and side-effects of ARV medications, how the medications should be taken and the importance of not missing any doses. Peer counsellors and visual materials can be particularly useful in this process. Keys to success once treatment has begun include trying to minimize the number of pills (in part through the use of FDCs), the packaging of pills (coblister packs when available), the frequency of dosing (no more than twice-daily regimens), avoidance of food precautions, fitting the ARVs into the patient's lifestyle, and the involvement of relatives, friends and/or community members in support of the patient's adherence.

After the initiation of therapy it is essential to maintain support for adherence. This should involve adherence assessments whenever there is a visit to a health centre, reinforcement of adherence principles to the patient by treatment supporters, and the continuous involvement of relatives, friends and/or community support personnel. Although the penetration of ART in the developing world has been low in relation to the burden of disease, important lessons have been learnt which can be incorporated into newly developing or expanding programmes. These lessons relate to the following measures.

• Provision of medications free of charge through subsidization or other financing strategies for people who can least afford treatment. It has been suggested that cost-sharing may assist adherence, although experiences can be expected to vary between countries. Recent data from Senegal and other African countries indicates that cost-sharing is detrimental to long-term adherence. These issues need further exploration (Desclaux et al., 2003; Laniece et al., 2003).

• Engagement of family or community members in adherence education and maintenance programmes. Home visits can be particularly useful. Minimizing stigma through psychosocial support is essential.

• Family-based care when more than one family member is HIV-infected. This is particularly important when both mother and child are infected.

• Use of pillboxes or blister packs.

• Directly observed therapy (DOT) or modified DOT programmes. This approach is resource-intensive and difficult to introduce on a large scale and for the lifelong duration of ART. However, it may be helpful for certain groups and for early patient training.

• Use of mobile vans to reach rural communities.

• At the programmatic level it is essential to ensure proper stock and storage of ARVs and the provision of necessary resources for culturally appropriate adherence programmes.

Adherence may be more difficult in pregnant women and immediately postpartum women than in non-pregnant individuals. Pregnancy-associated morning sickness and gastrointestinal upset may complicate ART and the situation may be exacerbated by ARV-associated side-effects or concern about the potential effects of drugs on the fetus. In the postpartum period, physical changes and the demands of caring for a neonate may compromise maternal drug adherence. Specific, culturally appropriate adherence supports should be developed at the country level in order to address the special problems associated with pregnant and postpartum women.

Adherence in children is a special challenge, particularly if the family unit is disrupted as a consequence of adverse health or economic conditions. Family-based HIV care programmes are one of the best approaches to ensuring children's health. Moreover, it is imperative that paediatric formulations be improved and made widely available. Where possible they should match the adult regimens so that that family-based care can be pursued effectively and so that children can be properly dosed.

DRUG RESISTANCE SURVEILLANCE

ARV drug resistance is a major challenge to treatment programmes for both developed and developing countries. Currently, approximately 10% of new HIV-1 infections in the USA and Europe involve viral strains exhibiting resistance to at least one drug. Scale-up programmes in the developing world can take advantage of the lessons learnt in developed countries through proper initiation of potent regimens, incorporation of culturally appropriate adherence training and maintenance programmes, and synchronization with drug resistance surveillance and monitoring initiatives.

Drug resistance genotyping is not on the near-term or mid-term horizon for individual patient management in resource-limited settings but country programmes are encouraged to develop or participate in drug resistance surveillance and monitoring programmes to assist with planning at the population level. This may involve developing or expanding genotypic capabilities at regional or national centres of excellence. Such capabilities can be considered an important public health tool that can be used to inform national, regional and global ARV scale-up programmes concerning trends in the prevalence of drug resistance so that decisions can be made to minimize its impact.

WHO recommends that countries planning to implement ART programmes should concurrently introduce HIV drug resistance sentinel surveillance systems. This will allow countries to detect potential drug resistance at the population level and to modify recommended treatment regimens accordingly. Initially, treatment-naive persons should be surveyed in order to establish prevalence rates of drug resistance in the infected population, and treatment-experienced persons should be monitored, particularly those diagnosed with their first episode of treatment failure. A Global HIV Drug Resistance Surveillance and Monitoring Network is being established by WHO in collaboration with partner organizations with a view to assisting Member States in this arena (Havlir et al., 2002).

CONCLUSIONS

Member States of WHO face both a great challenge and a great opportunity. The world community can confront the AIDS pandemic in developing countries with ART, the most effective life-sustaining tool in the HIV care package. The current nexus of political commitment, new sources of funding, ARV availability and lower drug prices have created this opportunity. WHO is committed to assisting resource-limited countries with the scale-up of ART through its comprehensive 3-by-5 Plan. The present updated ARV treatment guidelines are intended to help national programmes to provide ARV access for all infected adults and children in need of treatment.

ANNEX A. Dosages of Antiretroviral Drugs for Adults and Adolescents

Drug class/drug	Dose[a]
Nucleoside RTIs	
Abacavir (ABC)	300 mg twice daily
Didanosine (ddI)	400 mg once daily (250 mg once daily if <60 kg) (250 mg once daily if administered with TDF)
Lamivudine (3TC)	150 mg twice daily or 300 mg once daily
Stavudine (d4T)	40 mg twice daily (30 mg twice daily if <60 kg)
Zidovudine (ZDV)	300 mg twice daily
Nucleotide RTI	
Tenofovir (TDF)	300 mg once daily (Note: drug interaction with ddI necessitates dose reduction of latter)
Non-nucleoside RTIs	
Efavirenz (EFV)	600 mg once daily[b]
Nevirapine (NVP)	200 mg once daily for 14 days, then 200 mg twice daily
Protease inhibitors	
Indinavir/ritonavir (IDV/r)	800 mg/100 mg twice daily[c,d]
Lopinavir/ritonavir (LPV/r)	400 mg/100 mg twice dailyb (533 mg/133 mg twice daily when combined with EFV or NVP)
Nelfinavir (NFV)	1250 mg twice daily
Saquinavir/ritonavir (SQV/r)	1000 mg/100 mg twice daily or 1600 mg/200 mg once daily[b,d,e]

[a]These dosages are in common clinical use. The dosages featured in this table were selected on the basis of the best available clinical evidence. Dosages that can be given once daily or twice daily were preferred in order to enhance adherence to therapy. The doses listed are those for individuals with normal renal and hepatic function. Product-specific information should be consulted for dose adjustments that may be indicated with renal or hepatic dysfunction or for potential drug interactions with other HIV and non-HIV medications.

[b]See TB section for other specific TB dosing.

[c]This dosage regimen is in common clinical use. Other IDV/r dosage regimens that range from 800 mg/200 mg bid to 400 mg/100 mg bid are also in clinical use.

[d]Dosage adjustment when combined with an NNRTI is indicated but a formal recommendation cannot be made at this time. One consideration is to increase the RTV component to 200 mg bid when EFV or NVP is used concomitantly. More drug interaction data are needed.

[e]Both the hard-gel and soft-gel capsule formulations can be used when SQV is combined with RTV.

ANNEX B. Human Immunodeficiency Virus Paediatric Immune Category Classification System Based on Age-specific CD4+ T Cell Count and Percentage

Immune category	<12 months		1–5 years		6–12 years	
	No./mm^3	%	No./mm^3	%	No./mm^3	%
Category 1: No suppression	≥1500	≥25%	≥1000	≥25%	≥500	≥25%
Category 2: Moderate suppression	750–1499	15%–24%	500–999	15%–24%	200–499	15%–24%
Category 3: Severe suppression	<750	<15%	<500	<15%	<200	<15%

Modified from: Centers for Disease Control and Prevention. 1994 revised classification system for human immunodeficiency virus infection in children less than 13 years of age. MMWR 1994;43(No. RR-12):1-10.

continued

ANNEX C. Summary of Paediatric Drug Formulations and Doses

Name of drug	Formulations	Pharmaco-kinetic data available	Age (weight), dose and dose frequency	Other comments
Nucleoside analogue reverse transcriptase inhibitors				
Zidovudine (ZDV)	Syrup: 10 mg/ml Capsules: 100 mg; 250 mg Tablet: 300 mg	All ages	<4 weeks: 4 mg/kg/dose twice daily 4 weeks to 13 years: 180 mg/m^2/dose twice daily [a] Maximum dose: ≥13 years: 300 mg/dose twice daily	Large volume of syrup not well tolerated in older children Syrup needs storage in glass jars and is light-sensitive Can be given with food Doses of 600 mg/m^2/dose per day required for HIV encephalopathy Capsule can be opened and contents dispersed or tablet crushed and contents mixed with small amount of water or food and immediately taken (solution is stable at room temperature) Do not use with d4T (antagonistic antiretroviral effect)

ANNEX C. Continued

Name of drug	Formulations	Pharmaco-kinetic data available	Age (weight), dose and dose frequency	Other comments
Lamivudine (3TC)	Oral solution: 10 mg/ml Tablet: 150 mg	All ages	<30 days: 2 mg/kg/dose twice daily ≥30 days or <60 kg: 4 mg/kg/dose twice daily Maximum dose: >60 kg: 150 mg/dose twice daily	Well tolerated Can be given with food Store solution at room temperature (use within one month of opening) Tablet can be crushed and contents mixed with small amount water or food and immediately taken
Fixed-dose combination of ZDV plus 3TC	No liquid available Tablet: 300 mg ZDV plus 150 mg 3TC	Adolescents and adults	Maximum dose: >13 years or >60 kg: 1 tablet/dose twice daily (should not be given if weight <30 kg)	Preferably, tablet should not be split Tablet can be crushed and contents mixed with small amount of water or food and immediately taken At weight <30 kg, ZDV and 3TC cannot be dosed accurately in tablet form
Stavudine (d4T)	Oral solution: 1 mg/ml Capsules: 15 mg, 20 mg, 30 mg, 40 mg	All ages	<30 kg: 1 mg/kg/dose twice daily 30 to 60 kg: 30 mg/dose twice daily Maximum dose: >60 kg: 40 mg/dose twice daily	Large volume of solution Keep solution refrigerated; stable for 30 days; must be well shaken and stored in glass bottles Capsules can be opened and mixed with small amount of

Drug	Formulations	Ages	Dosing	Comments
				food or water (stable in solution for 24 hours if kept refrigerated) Do not use with AZT (antagonistic antiretroviral effect)
Fixed-dose combination of d4T plus 3TC	No liquid available Tablet: d4T 30 mg plus 3TC 150 mg; d4T 40 mg plus 3TC 150 mg	Adolescents and adults	Maximum dose: 30-60 kg: one 30-mg d4T-based tablet twice daily >60 kg: one 40-mg d4T-based tablet twice daily	Preferaby, tablet should not be split See comments under individual drug components
Didanosine (ddI, dideoxyinosine)	Oral suspension paediatric powder/water: 10 mg/ml; in many countries needs to be made up with additional antacid Chewable tablets: 25 mg; 50 mg; 100 mg; 150 mg; 200 mg Enteric-coated beadlets in capsules: 125 mg; 200 mg; 250 mg; 400 mg	All ages	<3 months: 50 mg/m^2/dose twice daily[a] 3 months to <13 years: 90-120 mg/m^2/dose twice daily or 240 mg/m^2/dose once daily Maximum dose: ≥13 years or >60 kg: 200 mg/dose twice daily or 400 mg once daily	Keep suspension refrigerated; stable for 30 days; must be well shaken Administer on empty stomach, at least 30 minutes before or 2 hours after eating If tablets dispersed in water, at least 2 tablets of appropriate strength should be dissolved for adequate buffering Enteric-coated beadlets in capsules can be opened and sprinkled on small amount of food

continued

266

ANNEX C. Continued

Name of drug	Formulations	Pharmaco-kinetic data available	Age (weight), dose and dose frequency	Other comments
Abacavir (ABC)	Oral solution: 20 mg/ml Tablet: 300 mg	Over age of 3 months	<16 years or <37.5 kg: 8 mg/kg/dose twice daily Maximum dose: >16 years or ≥37.5 kg: 300 mg/dose twice daily	Can be given with food Tablet can be crushed and contents mixed with small amount water or food and immediately ingested PARENTS MUST BE WARNED ABOUT HYPERSENSITIVITY REACTION ABC should be stopped permanently if hypersensitivity reaction occurs
Fixed-dose combination of ZDV plus 3TC plus ABC	No liquid available Tablet: ZDV 300 mg plus 3TC 150 mg plus ABC 300 mg	Adolescents and adults	Maximum dose: >40 kg: 1 tablet/dose twice daily	Preferably, tablet should not be split At weight <30 kg, ZDV/3TC/ABC cannot be dosed accurately in tablet form MUST WARN PARENTS ABOUT HYPERSENSITIVITY REACTION. ZDV/3TC/ABC should be stopped permanently if hypersensitivity reaction occurs

Non-nucleoside reverse transcriptase inhibitors

| Nevirapine (NVP) | All ages | Oral suspension: 10 mg/ml
Tablet: 200 mg | 15 to 30 days:
5 mg/kg/dose once daily × 2 weeks, then 120 mg/m^2/dose twice daily × 2 weeks, then 200 mg/m^2/dose twice daily[a]
>30 days to 13 years:
120 mg/m^2/dose once daily for 2 weeks, then 120-200 mg/m^2/dose twice daily[a]
Maximum dose:
>13 yrs: 200 mg/dose once daily for first 2 weeks, then 200 mg/dose twice daily | If rifampicin coadministration, avoid use (see TB section)
Store suspension at room temperature; must be well shaken
Can be given with food
Tablets are scored and can be divided into two equal parts to give a 100 mg dose; can be crushed and combined with a small amount of water or food and immediately administered
PARENTS MUST BE WARNED ABOUT RASH.
Do not escalate dose if rash occurs (if mild/moderate rash, hold drug; when rash has cleared, restart dosing from beginning of dose escalation; if severe rash, discontinue drug)
Drug interactions |

continued

ANNEX C. Continued

Name of drug	Formulations	Pharmaco-kinetic data available	Age (weight), dose and dose frequency	Other comments
Efavirenz (EFV)	Syrup: 30 mg/ml (note: syrup requires higher doses than capsules; see dosing chart) Capsules: 50 mg, 100 mg, 200 mg	Only for children over 3 years of age	Capsule (liquid) dose for >3 years: 10 to 15 kg: 200 mg (270 mg = 9 ml) once daily 15 to <20 kg: 250 mg (300 mg = 10 ml) once daily 20 to <25 kg: 300 mg (360 mg = 12 ml) once daily 25 to <33 kg: 350 mg (450 mg = 15 ml) once daily 33 to <40 kg: 400 mg (510 mg = 17 ml) once daily Maximum dose: ≥40 kg: 600 mg once daily	Capsules may be opened and added to food but have very peppery taste; however, can be mixed with sweet foods or jam to disguise taste Can be given with food (but avoid after high-fat meals, which increase absorption by 50%); best given at bedtime, especially first 2 weeks, to reduce CNS side-effects. Drug interactions
Fixed-dose combination of d4T plus 3TC plus NVP	No liquid available Tablet: 30 mg d4T/150 mg 3TC/200 mg NVP; 40 mg d4T/150 mg 3TC/200 mg NVP	Adults and adolescents	Maximum dose: 30-60 kg: one 30 mg d4T-based tablet twice daily ≥60 kg: one 40 mg d4T-based tablet twice daily	Preferably, tablet should not be split At weight <30 kg, d4T/3TC/ NVP cannot be dosed accurately in tablet form; if tablets are split, NVP dose requirements will be inadequate for very young children and additional NVP is needed to give total of 200 mg/m^2/dose twice daily

				Contains NVP, therefore dose escalation required (see NVP dosing recommendations) See comments under individual drug components
Protease inhibitors				
Nelfinavir (NFV)	Powder for oral suspension (mix with liquid): 200 mg per level teaspoon (50 mg per 1.25 ml scoop): 5 ml Tablet: 250 mg (tablets can be halved; can be crushed and added to food or dissolved in water)	All ages However, extensive pharmacokinetic variability in infants, with requirement for very high doses in infants <1 year	<1 year: 50 mg/kg/dose three times daily or 7 5 mg/kg/dose twice daily >1 year to <13 years: 55 to 65 mg/kg/ dose twice daily Maximum dose: ≥13 years: 1250 mg/dose twice daily	Powder is sweet, faintly bitter but gritty and hard to dissolve; must be reconstituted immediately before administration in water, milk, formula, pudding, etc.; do not use acidic food or juice (which increase bitter taste); solution stable for 6 hours Because of difficulties with use of powder, use of crushed tablets preferred (even for infants) if appropriate dose can be given Powder and tablets can be stored at room temperature Take with food Drug interactions (less than ritonavir-containing protease inhibitors)

continued

ANNEX C. Continued

Name of drug	Formulations	Pharmaco-kinetic data available	Age (weight), dose and dose frequency	Other comments
Lopinavir/ritonavir, (LPV/r)	Oral solution: 80mg/ml lopinavir plus 20 mg/ml ritonavir Capsules: 133.3 mg lopinavir plus 33.3 mg ritonavir	6 months of age or older	>6 months to 13 years: 225 mg/m² LPV/57.5 mg/m² ritonavir twice daily[a] or weight-based dosing: 7–15 kg: 12mg/kg LPV/3 mg/kg ritonavir/ dose twice daily 15–40 kg: 10 mg/kg lopinavir/2.5 mg/kg ritonavir twice daily Maximum dose: >40 kg: 400 mg LPV/100 mg ritonavir (3 capsules or 5 ml) twice daily	Preferably, oral solution and capsules should be refrigerated; however, can be stored at room temperature up to 25°C (77°F) for 2 months; at temperature >25°C (77°F) the drug degrades more rapidly Liquid formulation has low volume but bitter taste Capsules large Capsules should not be crushed or opened but must be swallowed whole Should be taken with food Drug interactions

[a]Metre 2 (m²) body surface area calculation: square root of (height in centimetres times weight in kilograms divided by 3600).

ANNEX D. Fixed-dose Combinations of ARVS Available on 1 December 2003

Three-drug fixed-dose combinations	d4T (40 mg) + 3TC (150 mg) + NVP (200 mg)
	d4T (30 mg) + 3TC (150 mg) + NVP (200 mg)
	ZDV (300 mg) + 3TC (150 mg) + ABC (300 mg)
	ZDV (300 mg) + 3TC (150 mg) + NVP (200 mg)
Two-drug fixed-dose combinations	d4T (30 mg) + 3TC (150 mg)
	d4T (40 mg) + 3TC (150 mg)
	ZDV (300 mg) + 3TC (150 mg)

NOTE: WHO encourages the use of fixed-dose combinations when formulations of assured quality and proven bioequivalence are available and offer operational advantages. Not all the FDCs in this table have been evaluated for prequalification by WHO. WHO operates a voluntary prequalification system, in which, as of 1 December 2003, three manufacturers prequalified ZDV/3TC combinations, two prequalified d4T/3TC/NVP combinations, and one prequalified ZDV/3TC/ABC. The list of WHO-prequalified manufacturers is continuously updated and is available at: http://www.who.int/ medicines

ANNEX E. WHO Staging System for HIV Infection and Disease and Disease in Adults and Adolescents

Clinical Stage I:
    4. Asymptomatic
    5. Generalized lymphadenopathy
Performance scale 1: asymptomatic, normal activity
Clinical Stage II:
    6. Weight loss <10% of body weight
    7. Minor mucocutaneous manifestations (seborrhoeic dermatitis, prurigo, fungal nail infections, recurrent oral ulcerations, angular cheilitis)
    8   Herpes zoster within the last five years
    9. Recurrent upper respiratory tract infections (i.e. bacterial sinusitis)
And/or performance scale 2: symptomatic, normal activity
Clinical Stage III:
  10. Weight loss >10% of body weight
  11. Unexplained chronic diarrhoea, >1 month
  12. Unexplained prolonged fever (intermittent or constant), >1 month
  13. Oral candidiasis (thrush)
  14. Oral hairy leucoplakia
  15. Pulmonary tuberculosis
  16. Severe bacterial infections (i.e. pneumonia, pyomyositis)
And/or performance scale 3: bedridden <50% of the day during last month
Clinical Stage IV:
  17. HIV wasting syndrome[a]
  18. Pneumocystic carinii pneumonia
  19. Toxoplasmosis of the brain
  20. Cryptosporidiosis with diarrhoea >1 month
  21. Cryptococcosis, extrapulmonary
  22. Cytomegalovirus disease of an organ other than liver, spleen or lymph node (e.g. retinitis)
  23. Herpes simplex virus infection, mucocutaneous (>1month) or visceral
  24. Progressive multifocal leucoencephalopathy
  25. Any disseminated endemic mycosis
  26. Candidiasis of oesophagus, trachea, bronchi
  27. Atypical mycobacteriosis, disseminated or pulmonary
  28. Non-typhoid Salmonella septicaemia
  29. Extrapulmonary tuberculosis
  30. Lymphoma
  31. Kaposi's sarcoma
  32. HIV encephalopathy[b]
And/or performance scale 4: bedridden >50% of the day during last month

---

[a]HIV wasting syndrome: weight loss of >10% of body weight, plus either unexplained chronic diarrhoea (>1 month) or chronic weakness and unexplained prolonged fever (>1 month).

[b]HIV encephalopathy: clinical findings of disabling cognitive and/or motor dysfunction interfering with activities of daily living, progressing over weeks to months, in the absence of a concurrent illness or condition, other than HIV infection, which could explain the findings.

ANNEX F. WHO Staging System for HIV Infection and Disease in Children

Clinical Stage I:
  1. Asymptomatic
  2. Generalized lymphadenopathy

Clinical Stage II:
  3. Chronic diarrhoea >30 days duration in absence of known etiology
  4. Severe persistent or recurrent candidiasis outside the neonatal period
  5. Weight loss or failure to thrive in the absence of known etiology
  6. Persistent fever >30 days duration in the absence of known etiology
  7. Recurrent severe bacterial infections other than septicaemia or meningitis (e.g. osteomyelitis, bacterial (non-TB) pneumonia, abscesses)

Clinical Stage III:
  8. AIDS-defining opportunistic infections
  9. Severe failure to thrive (wasting) in the absence of known etiology[a]
  10. Progressive encephalopathy
  11. Malignancy
  12. Recurrent septicaemia or meningitis

---

[a]Persistent weight loss >10% of baseline or less than 5th percentile on weight for height chart on 2 consecutive measurements more than 1 month apart in the absence of another etiology or concurrent illness.

REFERENCES

Adje-Toure CA, Cheingsong R, Garcia- Lerma JG, et al. Antiretroviral therapy in HIV- 2-infected patients: changes in plasma viral load, CD4+ cell counts, and drug resistance profiles of patients treated in Abidjan, Côte d'Ivoire. AIDS 2003; 17(Suppl 3):S49-S54.

Badri M, Wood R. Usefulness of total lymphocyte count in monitoring highly active antiretroviral therapy in resource-limited settings. AIDS 2003;17(4):541-545.

Badri M, Wilson D, Wood R. Effect of highly active antiretroviral therapy on incidence of tuberculosis in South Africa: a cohort study. Lancet 2002;359:2059-2064.

Bang LM, Scott LJ. Emtricitabine: an antiretroviral agent for HIV infection. Drugs 2003;63(22):2413-2424; discussion 2425-2426.

Beck EJ, Kupek EJ, Gompels MM, et al. Correlation between total and CD4 lymphocyte counts in HIV infection: not making the good an enemy of the not so perfect. Int J STD AIDS 1996;7(6):422-428.

Boehringer-Ingelheim Pharmaceuticals, Inc. Viramune drug label. Revised 20 June 2003.

Boubaker K, Flepp M, Sudre P, et al. Hyperlactatemia and antiretroviral therapy: the Swiss HIV Cohort Study. Clin Infect Dis 2001;33(11):1931-1937.

Brettle RP. Correlation between total and CD4 lymphocyte counts in HIV infection. Int J STD AIDS. 1997;8(9):597.

Burman WJ, Jones BE. Treatment of HIVrelated tuberculosis in the era of effective antiretroviral therapy. Am J Respir Crit Care Med 2001; 164(1):7-12.

Chaowanachan T, Chotpitayasunondh T, Vanprapar N, et al. Resistance mutations following a single-dose intrapartum administration of nevirapine to HIV-infected Thai women and their infants receiving short-course zidovudine. 10th Conference on Retroviruses and Opportunistic Infections; 2003 Feb 10-14; Boston, Massachusetts (Abstract 855).

Cunningham CK, Chaix ML, Rackacewicz C, et al. Development of resistance mutations in women receiving standard antiretroviral therapy who received intrapartum nevirapine to prevent perinatal human immunodeficiency virus type 1 transmission: a substudy of Pediatric AIDS Clinical Trials Group protocol 316. J Infect Dis 2002;186:181-188.

De Martino M, Tovo P-A, Balducci M, et al. Reduction in mortality with availability of antiretroviral therapy for children with perinatal HIV-1 infection. JAMA 2000;284:190-197.

Dean G, Back D, de Ruiter A. Effect of tuberculosis therapy on nevirapine trough plasma concentration. AIDS 1999;13:2489-2490.

Dean GL, Edwards SG, Ives NJ, et al. Treatment of tuberculosis in HIV-infected persons in the era of highly active antiretroviral therapy. AIDS 2002; 16(1):75-83.

Desclaux A, Ciss M, Taverne B, et al. Access to antiretroviral drugs and AIDS management in Senegal. AIDS 2003;17(Suppl 3):S95-S101.

DHHS. Guidelines for the use of antiretroviral agents in HIV-1 infected adults and adolescents. Available from: URL: http://AIDSInfo.nih.gov/ guidelines

Embree J, Bwayo J, Nagelkerke N, et al. Lymphocyte subsets in human immunodeficiency virus type 1-infected and uninfected children in Nairobi. Pediatr Infect Dis J 2001;20:397-403.

Ena J, Amador C, Benito C, et al. Risk and determinants of developing severe liver toxicity during therapy with nevirapine- and efavirenz-containing regimens in HIV-infected patients. Int J STD AIDS 2003;14(11):776-781.

Eshleman SH, Mracna M, Guay LA, et al. Selection and fading of resistance mutations in women and infants receiving nevirapine to prevent HIV-1 vertical transmission (HIVNET 012). AIDS 2001;184:914-917.

European Collaborative Study. Gender and race do not alter early-life determinants of clinical disease progression in HIV-1 vertically infected children. AIDS 2004 (in press).

Fournier AM, Sosenko JM. The relationship of total lymphocyte count to CD4 lymphocyte counts in patients infected with human immunodeficiency virus. Am J Med Sci. 1992;304(2):79-82.

Gallant JE, Deresinski S. Tenofovir disoproxil fumarate. Clin Infect Dis 2003;37(7):944-950.

Gallant JERA, Weinberg W, Young B, et al. Early non-response to tenofovir DF and abacavir and lamivudine in a randomized trial compared to efavirenz + ABC and 3TC: ESS30009 unplanned interim analysis. 43rd Interscience Conference on Antimicrobial Agents and Chemotherapy; 2003 Sep 14-17; Chicago, Illinois.

Gerstoft J, Kirk O, Obel N, et al. Low efficacy and high frequency of adverse events in a randomized trial of the triple nucleoside regimen abacavir, stavudine and didanosine. AIDS 2003;17(14):2045-2052.

Giarardi E, Antonucci G, Vanacore P, et al. Impact of combination antireteroviral therapy on the risk of tuberculosis among persons with HIV infection. AIDS 2000;14:1985-1991.

Gilead. High rate of virologic failure in patients with HIV infection treated with once daily triple NRTI regimen containing didanosine, lamivudine, and tenofovir; 2003 (Letter).

Giuliano M, Palmisano L, Galluzzo CM, et al. Selection of resistance mutations in pregnant women receiving zidovudine and lamivudine to prevent HIV perinatal transmission. AIDS 2003;17:1570-1571.

Gortmaker SL, Hughes M, Cervia J, et al. Effect of combination therapy including protease inhibitors on mortality among children and adolescents infected with HIV-1. N Engl J Med 2001;345:1522-1528.

Gulick RMRH, Shikuma CM, Lustgarten S, et al. ACTG 5095: a comparative study of 3 protease inhibitor-sparing antiretroviral regimens for the initial treatment of HIV infection. 2nd IAS Conference on HIV Pathogenesis and Treatment; 2003 Jul 13-16; Paris.

Haas DW, Zala C, Schrader S, et al. Therapy with atazanavir plus saquinavir in patients failing highly active antiretroviral therapy: a randomized comparative pilot trial. AIDS 2003;17(9):1339-1349.

Harries AD, Hargreaves NJ, Kemp J, et al. Deaths from tuberculosis in sub-Saharan African countries with a high prevalence of HIV-1. Lancet 2001;357(9267):1519-1523.

Harvard University. Consensus statement on antiretroviral treatment for AIDS in poor countries. Boston: Harvard University; 2001.

Havlir D, Vella S, Hammer S. The Global HIV Drug Resistance Surveillance Program: a partnership between WHO and IAS. AIDS 2002;16(10):7-9.

Havlir DV, Barnes PF. Tuberculosis in patients with human immunodeficiency virus infection. N Eng J Med 1999;340(5):367-373.

Hirsch MS, Brun-Vezinet F, Clotet B, et al. Antiretroviral drug resistance testing in adults infected with human immunodeficiency virus type 1: 2003 recommendations of an International AIDS Society-USA Panel. Clin Infect Dis 2003;37(1):113-128.

Ibbotson T, Perry CM. Lamivudine/ zidovudine/abacavir: triple combination tablet. Drugs 2003; 63(11):1089-1098; discussion 1099-1100.

Imperiale SM, Stern JO, Love JT, et al. The VIRAMUNE (nevirapine) hepatic safety project: analysis of symptomatic hepatic events. 4th International Workshop on Adverse Events and Lipodystrophy in HIV; 2002 Sep 22-25; San Diego, California (Abstract 87).

Joint United Nations Programme on HIV/ AIDS (UNAIDS) and World Health Organization (WHO). AIDS epidemic update: 2003. Geneva.UNAIDS. Available from: URL: http://www.who.int/hiv/pub/epidemiology/epi2003/en/

Karras A, Lafaurie M, Furco A, et al. Tenofovir-related nephrotoxicity in human immunodeficiency virus-infected patients: three cases of renal failure, Fanconi syndrome, and nephrogenic diabetes insipidus. Clin Infect Dis 2003;36(8):1070-1073.

Keiser P, Nassar N, White C, et al. Comparison of nevirapine- and efavirenz-containing antiretroviral regimens in antiretroviral-naive patients: a cohort study. HIV Clin Trials 2002;3(4):296-303.

Keiser P, Nassar N, Yazdani B, et al. Comparison of efficacy of efavirenz and nevirapine: lessons learned for cohort analysis in light of the 2NN Study. HIV Clin Trials 2003;4(5):358-360.

Kityo C. A randomised trial of monitoring practice and structured treatment interruptions in the management of antiretroviral therapy in adults with HIV infection in Africa: the DART trial. 13th International Conference on AIDS and STIs in Africa (ICASA); 2003; Nairobi (Abstract 1098933).

Kumarasamy N, Mahajan AP, Flanigan TP, et al. Total lymphocyte count (TLC) is a useful tool for the timing of opportunistic infection prophylaxis in India and other resource constrained countries. J Acquir Immune Defic Syndr 2002;31(4):378-383.

la Porte C, Colbers E, Bertz R, et al. Pharmacokinetics of two adjusted dose regimens of lopinavir/ritonavir in combination with rifampin in healthy volunteers. 42nd Interscience Conference on Antimicrobial Agents and Chemotherapy; 2002; San Diego, California (Abstract A-1823).

Laniece I, Ciss M, Desclaux A, et al.Adherence to HAART and its principal determinants in a cohort of Senegalese adults. AIDS 2003;17(Suppl 3):S103-S108.

Langlet P, Guillaume M-P, Devriendt J, et al. Fatal liver failure associated with nevirapine in a pregnant HIV patient: the first reported case. Gastroenterol 2000;118(Suppl 2):Abstract 6623 (101st Annual Meeting of the American Gastroenterological Association; 2000 May 21-24; San Diego, California).

Law WP, Dore GJ, Duncombe CJ, et al. Risk of severe hepatotoxicity associated with antiretroviral therapy in the HIV-NAT Cohort, Thailand, 1996-2001. AIDS 2003; 17(15):2191-2199.

Lindsey JC, Hughes MD, McKinney RE, et al. Treatment mediated changes in human immunodeficiency virus (HIV) type 1 RNA and CD4 cell counts as predictors of weight growth failure, cognitive decline, and survival in HIVinfected children. J Infect Dis 2000;182:1385-1393.

Lopez-Cortes L, Ruiz-Valderas R, Viciana P, et al. Pharmacokinetic interactions between efavirenz and rifampin in HIV-infected patients with tuberculosis. Clin Pharmacokinet 2002;41:681-690.

Lyons F, Hopkins S, McGeary A, et al. Nevirapine tolerability in HIV infected women in pregnancy – A word of caution (late breaker). 2nd IAS Conference on HIV Pathogenesis and Treatment; 2003 Jul 13-16; Paris.

Mandelbrot L, Landreau-Mascaro A, Rekacewicz C, et al. Lamivudine-zidovudine combination for prevention of maternal-infant transmission of HIV-1. JAMA 2001;285:2083-2093.

Martin-Carbonero L, Nunez M, Gonzalez-Lahoz J, et al. Incidence of liver injury after beginning antiretroviral therapy with efavirenz or nevirapine. HIV Clin Trials 2003;4(2):115-120.

McCoig C, Castrejon MM, Castano E, et al. Effect of combination antiretroviral therapy on cerebrospinal fluid HIV RNA, HIV resistance, and clinical manifestations of encephalopathy. J Pediatr 2002;141:36-44.

Mofenson LM, Harris DR, Moye J, et al. Alternatives to HIV-1 RNA concentration and CD4 count to predict mortality in HIV-1-infected children in resource-poor settings. Lancet 2003; 362 (9396):1625-1627.

Moyle GJ. NNRTI choice: has 2NN changed our practice? AIDS Read 2003;13(7):325-328.

Narita M, Ashkin D, Hollander E, et al. Paradoxical worsening of tuberculosis following antiretroviral therapy in patients with AIDS. Am J Respir Crit Care Med 1998;158:157-161.

Olivia J, Moreno S, Sanz J, et al. Coadministration of rifampin and nevirapine in HIV-infected patients with tuberculosis. AIDS 2003;17:637-642.

Palella FJ, Jr., Deloria-Knoll M, Chmiel JS, et al. Survival benefit of initiating antiretroviral therapy in HIV-infected persons in different CD4+ cell strata. Ann Intern Med 2003; 138(8):620-626.

Patel A, Patel K, Patel J, et al. To study the safety and antiretroviral efficacy of rifampicin and efavirenz in antiretroviral-naïve tuberculosis coinfected HIV-1 patients in India. X Conference on Retroviruses and Opportunistic Infections; 2003; Boston, Massachusetts (Abstract 138).

Pedral-Samapio D, Alves C, Netto E, et al. Efficacy of efavirenz 600 mg dose in the ARV therapy regimen for HIV patients receiving rifampicin in the treatment of tuberculosis. 10th Conference on Retroviruses and Opportunistic Infections; 2003 Feb 10-14; Boston, Massachusetts (Abstract 784).

Piliero PJ. Atazanavir: a novel HIV-1 protease inhibitor. Expert Opin Investig Drugs 2002; 11(9):1295-1301.

Pollard RB, Tierney C, Havlir D, et al. A phase II randomized study of the virologic and immunologic effect of zidovudine + stavudine versus stavudine alone and zidovudine + lamivudine in patients with >300 CD4 cells who were antiretroviral naive (ACTG 298). AIDS Res Hum Retroviruses 2002;18(10):699-704.

Ribera E, Pou L, Lopez RM, et al. Pharmacokinetic interaction between nevaripine and rifampicin in HIV-infected patients with tuberculosis. J Acquir Immune Defic Syndr 2001;28:450-453.

Ribera E, Azuaje C, Montero F. Saquinavir, ritonavir, didanosine, and lamivudine in a once daily regimen for HIV infection in patients with rifampin-containing antituberculosis treatment. 14th International Conference on AIDS; 2002 Jul 7-12; Barcelona (Abstract ThPeB7280).

Sanne I, Piliero P, Squires K, et al. Results of a phase 2 clinical trial at 48 weeks (AI424-007): a dose-ranging, safety, and efficacy comparative trial of atazanavir at three doses in combination with didanosine and stavudine in antiretroviralnaive subjects. J Acquir Immune Defic Syndr 2003;32(1):18-29.

Santoro-Lopes G, de Pinho AM, Harrison LH, et al. Reduced risk of tuberculosis among Brazilian patients with advanced human immunodeficiency virus infection treated with highly active antiretroviral therapy. Clin Infect Dis 2002;34(4):543-546.

Saulsbury FT. Resolution of organ-specific complications of human immunodeficiency virus infection in children with use of highly active antiretroviral therapy. Clin Infect Dis 2001;32:464-468.

Schaaf B, Aries SP, Kramme E, et al. Acute renal failure associated with tenofovir treatment in a patient with acquired immunodeficiency syndrome. Clin Infect Dis 2003;37(3):41-43.

Shearer WT, Rosenblatt HM, Gelman RS, et al. Lymphocyte subsets in healthy children from birth through 18 years of age: the Pediatric AIDS Clinical Trials Group P1009 Study. J Allergy Clin Immunol 2003; 112(5):973-980.

Smith NA, Shaw T, Berry N, et al. Antiretroviral therapy for HIV-2-infected patients. J Infect Dis 2001;42:126-133.

Staszewski S, Keiser P, Montaner J, et al. Abacavir-lamivudine-zidovudine vs indinavirlami-vudine-zidovudine in antiretroviral-naïve HIV-infected adults: A randomized equivalence trial. JAMA. 2001;285 (9):1155-1163.

Staszewski SGJ, Pozniak AL, Suleiman JMAH, et al. Efficacy and safety of tenofovir DF versus stavudine when used in combination with lamivudine and efavirenz in antiretroviral naive patients: 96-week preliminary interim results. 10th Conference on Retroviruses and Opportunistic Infections; 2003 Feb 10-14; Boston, Massachusetts.

Stern JO, Love JT, Robinson, PA, et al. Hepatic safety of nevirapine: Results of the Boehringer Ingelheim Viramune Hepatic Safety Project. 14th International Conference on AIDS; 2002 Jul 7-12; Barcelona (Abstract LBOr15).

Stern JO, Robinson PA, Love JT, et al. A comprehensive hepatic safety analysis of nevirapine in different populations of HIV infected patients. J Acquired Immune Defic Syndr 2003;34, Supl 1:S21-S33.

Sullivan J. South African Intrapartum Nevirapine Trial: selection of resistance mutations. 14th International Conference on AIDS; 2002 Jul 7-12; Barcelona (Abstract LbPeB9024).

Van der Ende ME, Prins JM, Brinkman K, et al. Clinical, immunological and virological response to different antiretroviral regimens in a cohort of HIV-2-infected patients. AIDS 2003;17(Suppl 3):S55-S61.

van der Ryst E, Kotze M, Joubert G, et al. Correlation among total lymphocyte count, absolute CD4+ count, and CD4+ percentage in a group of HIV-1-infected South African patients. J Acquir Immune Defic Syndr Hum Retrovirol 1998;19(3):238-244.

van Leth FHE, Phanuphak P, Miller S, et al. Results of the 2NN study: a randomized comparative trial of first-line antiretroviral therapy with regimens containing either nevirapine alone, efavirenz alone, or both drugs combined, together with stavudine and lamivudine. 10th Conference on Retroviruses and Opportunistic Infections; 2003 Feb 10-14; Boston, Massachusetts.

Verhelst D, Monge M, Meynard JL, et al. Fanconi syndrome and renal failure induced by tenofovir: a first case report. Am J Kidney Dis 2002;40(6):1331-1333.

Verweel G, van Rossum AMC, Hartwig NG, et al. Treatment with highly active antiretroviral therapy in human immunodeficiency virus type 1-infected children is associated with a sustained effect on growth. Pediatrics 2002;109(2):E25 Available from: URL: http: //www.pediatrics.org/cgi/content/full/109/2/e25

Wade AM, Ades AE. Age-related reference ranges: significance tests for models and confidence intervals for centiles. Stat Med 1994;13:2359-2367.

Wagner KR, Bishai WR. Issues in the treatment of Mycobacterium tuberculosis in patients with human immunodeficiency virus infection. AIDS 2001;15(Suppl 5):S203-S212.

Walmsley S, Bernstein B, King M, et al. Lopinavir-ritonavir versus nelfinavir for the initial treatment of HIV infection. N Engl J Med 2002;346(26):2039-2046.

Yeni PG, Hammer SM, Carpenter CC, et al. Antiretroviral treatment for adult HIV infection in 2002: updated recommendations of the International AIDS Society-USA Panel. JAMA 2002;288(2):222-235.

Appendix
D

Human Ethical Issues Arising in ARV Scale-up in Resource-Constrained Settings[1]

INTRODUCTION

In their book, *Tragic Choices,* Guido Calabresi and Phillip Bobbit write:

> We cannot know why the world suffers. But we can know how the world decides that suffering shall come to some persons and not to others. In the distribution of scarce goods, society has to decide which methods of allotment to use . . . and when attention is riveted on such distributions they arouse emotions of compassion, outrage and terror. It is then that conflicts are laid bare between on the one hand, those values by which society determined the beneficiaries of the distributions and the perimeters of scarcity, and on the other hand, those humanistic moral values which prize life and well being. In such conflicts, at such junctures, societies confront the tragic choice (Calabresi and Bobbit, 1978).

Without a doubt, HIV/AIDS is the greatest health crisis in the world today. The demand for treatment for people living with HIV and AIDS worldwide cannot be ignored. At the same time, there are countless challenges to meeting this demand, not the least of which are the cost of drugs, the complexity of treatment regimens, the inadequacy of health and deliv-

---

[1]Commissioned paper, by Angela Amondi Wasunna, The Hastings Center.

ery systems, the lack of knowledge about treatment, and the threat of drug resistance (McCoy and Loewenson, 2004). In order to meet some of these challenges, several developing countries are engaged in efforts to create national HIV/AIDS programs that steadily expand their public health sector capacity with the long-term goal of providing universal HIV/AIDS treatment.

As countries start or continue to scale up their national antiretroviral (ARV) programs they will encounter difficult ethical decisions, including decisions about who should receive the limited available treatment. These choices will undoubtedly test their moral and ethical values. In the end, because not everyone will have immediate access to life-saving drugs, tragic choices will have to be made. However, if the scale-up programs are successful they will offer a world of hope to millions of people who are in dire need of treatment and have no other means of receiving effective therapy. Because there is a population in immediate and dire need of treatment, decisions must be made with a *degree of boldness*. But because the process is being scaled-up in an environment of great uncertainty, and because tragic choices will inevitably be made, these decisions must also be approached *with a level of humility*.

PROGRESS IN ARV SCALE-UP PROGRAMS

In the last two decades, over 30 million people have died of HIV/AIDS. Today, an estimated 40 million people live with HIV/AIDS—approximately 28.5 million of them in sub-Saharan Africa (WHO, 2003a). Outside of Africa, the Caribbean is the region hardest hit by HIV/AIDS (UNAIDS, 2003), but the HIV epidemic is also quickly growing in other areas such as India, Russia, and China. Unfortunately, of the 6 million people in developing countries who currently need ARV therapy, fewer than 8 percent are receiving it, and without rapid access to properly managed treatment these millions of women, children, and men will die (WHO, 2003a). ARVs, especially when used in combinations of three or more, can dramatically improve the health of people living with HIV/AIDS around the world (Wood et al., 2000). Unfortunately, for the vast majority of infected people in need, ARVs have been out of reach—until now.

In a span of about two years, mainly due to pressure from human rights and civil society organizations, we have seen the initiation of new programs such as The Global Fund to Fight AIDS, Tuberculosis, and Malaria, the United States Presidential Emergency Plan for AIDS Relief (United States Aid), and the World Health Organization's Three by Five Program, which aims to treat three million people in five years (WHO, 2003b). Global funding for HIV/AIDS in resource constrained countries has, as a result, increased from just over $300 million in 1999 to an unprecedented

$3 billion in 2002 and $4.7 billion in 2003, with additional funding promised by foreign governments and international donor agencies (WHO, 2003b). In less than a year, international discourse on HIV/AIDS in resource-constrained countries has changed from *"Is there a moral obligation on the part of industrialized nations to provide treatment?"* (there clearly is), to *"How can we best administer AIDS treatment programs?"* Unfortunately, managing patients with HIV/AIDS is not just about providing drugs. As succinctly put by Dr. Gordon Perkin:

> Even if we had free and unlimited supplies of ARVs and other essential HIV/AIDS commodities, they still would not be available to the majority of people who need them because of poor infrastructure (DELIVER, 2002).

Building capacity and mobilizing resources on the scale needed to meet national treatment targets is daunting for many countries. Most health systems in sub-Saharan Africa and other resource constrained regions are overstretched, underdeveloped and operate at suboptimal levels. There is a real danger that the benefits of drug availability could be undone by ineffective distribution and misuse, both of which could lead to the development of drug resistant viruses and the withdrawal of donor funding. In order for scale-up programs to be successful they must provide a package of services, including voluntary counseling and testing, monitoring of disease progression, prophylaxis, diagnosis and treatment of opportunistic infection, delay of viral replication with antiretrovirals, management of drug side effects, prevention of mother-to-child transmission, and provision of psychological and moral support to patients and their caregivers (WHO/UNAIDS, 2000). Therefore, to maximize the benefits of ARV drug regimens, countries have to urgently make concrete plans to scale up their treatment programs, establish or strengthen their national drug procurement and distribution policies, develop quality control mechanisms, and engage in the relevant operational research.

On average, the treatment targets set by countries remain cautious, amounting to a combined total in 52 countries of approximately 500,000 people on antiretroviral treatment by 2005, less than 10 percent of those currently in need (WHO/UNAIDS, 2003). Some countries are moving beyond pilot treatment programs to set targets that more accurately match feasibility with need. For example, Thailand is currently providing treatment to 13,000 people with HIV/AIDS and aims to provide universal access by 2005 (WHO/UNAIDS, 2003). The Economic Community of West African States (ECOWAS) is aiming to expand coverage to at least 400,000 people in 15 countries by 2005 (WHO/UNAIDS, 2003). In addition to these country programs, nongovernment organizations such as Médicins sans Frontièrs (MSF) are providing ARV treatment through small pilot schemes and community programs in several developing countries.[2] The general consensus emerging at the international platform is that the ethical and political battle to reduce drug prices and provide funding for treatment has largely been won; the next battle is to develop and implement fair, effective, and equitable national treatment plans.

ETHICAL CHALLENGES AHEAD

Ethical challenges are to be found at every level of the scale-up process, including in relationships between infected persons and their families/communities, between health care workers and patients, among institutions (both public and private), and among nations and/or international donor agencies. As scale-up programs progress, new ethical questions continue to emerge. This paper will focus on five major ethical problems that are of current concern, namely:

- The Allocation of Treatment
- Administration and Delivery of Care
- The Need for Operational Research
- Fairness across Disease Groups and Priority Setting
- Sustainability of Treatment Programs

ALLOCATION OF TREATMENT

Among the most difficult questions scale-up programs face are: Who should receive the limited supply of therapy? What is the legitimate authority to decide who gets treatment? Justice and equity are often, and rightly, invoked as the underlying values in the distribution of limited resources. In the human rights framework, justice is defined as the quality of *being fair*. Equity is an ethical and value-based concept that is grounded in the idea that people should be treated as having equal worth. How can the concept of justice be used to promote equitable distribution in an environment with limited resources?

There are several theories of justice that can be applied to the allocation of scarce resources. For example, some people believe that a just allocation is one that provides the greatest good to the greatest number of people.

---

[2]The countries where MSF is treating patients with ARVs are: Burkina Faso, Burundi, Cambodia, Cameroon, China, DR Congo, Guatemala, Honduras, Indonesia, Kenya, Laos, Malawi, Mozambique, Myanmar, Rwanda, South Africa, Thailand, Uganda, and Ukraine. See also Attawell and Mundy (2003).

They would therefore support the seeking of cures for more common (rather than rare) diseases, adopt programs that help many rather than few, and generally use funds where they will have the largest aggregate positive impact on the most people (Mill, 1863). Others attempt to solve allocation dilemmas by holding that access to the same benefits, goods, and services should be provided to everyone on the same basis. For expensive and scarce resources, lotteries might be used so that all similarly situated individuals have an equal opportunity and are recognized as of equal worth (and need) (Veatch, 1986).

Further, some believe that the primary responsibility for health care lies with private citizens and not with the state. They assert, therefore that market forces and personal choice should shape distribution of scarce resources (Nozick, 1974). Still others believe that distributions of social goods are fair when impartial people agree on the procedures that should be used for distribution. They contend that the way in which we form stable and just societies is through the process of building a consensus that merits endorsement by rational and informed people of good will (Daniels, 1985; Rawls, 1971). Finally, some argue that allocation is not primarily an ethical problem, but an economic one. That is, that the allocation of resources on the basis of efficiency would obviate the need for ethical principles.

What has become increasingly clear is that there is no consensus at the policy level on which principles should apply to resource allocation decisions. In addition, even if everyone agreed on certain principles, there would still be disagreement on how those principles should be translated into health policy. Having said that, it is important for countries to engage in a discussion on distributive justice because the very concept of justice is not a luxury in many countries and there is a real danger that some allocation programs may be manifestly unjust and unacceptable. I believe that it is possible (and necessary) for countries to make informed judgments on allocation methods that are ethically robust and better suited to them based on their own socioeconomic, political, and cultural circumstances.

In the real world, countries and institutions are already setting up treatment eligibility criteria based on a variety of factors and ethical principles. For example:

Technical Criteria: The World Health Organization has recommended using medical criteria (disease progression) as the way to select candidates for its Three by Five program (WHO, 2003b). Under this program, patients with CD4 counts that are 200 or below or those clinically diagnosed with AIDS (where CD4 testing is not possible) are given priority. This approach, although technical on its face, makes certain value judgments about those individuals who do not meet the set criteria. People with CD4 counts greater than 200 might argue that they stand to benefit more than those whose disease has progressed significantly if they are given early access to treatment. That is, they might argue that this particular technical criterion does not maximize the good that could result from the program.

Level of Health Care and Delivery Infrastructure: Some countries have decided to establish scale-up programs only where a certain level of basic health and delivery infrastructure already exists. In many developing countries, this limits the programs to urban areas. It can be argued that situating a treatment program in an existing health system that inherently favors the better-off (who generally live in urban areas) only serves to exacerbate existing inequities in health care systems that discriminate against the rural poor.

Social Worth and Other Value-Based Criteria: In Uganda some doctors have argued that priority for treatment must go to those with the greatest risk of transmitting infections, such as HIV-infected pregnant women (Ssmemakula, 2001). Other communities feel that every person suffering from HIV/AIDS ought to have an equal chance of receiving treatment and that a random, lottery type selection process is therefore the fairest procedure for distributing treatment. Yet others are making decisions on whom to treat on the basis of indicators like age, level of education, and vocation. For example, arguments are being made that the treatment of infected health care personnel should be prioritized in order to maintain the crucial health delivery infrastructure. Some countries ravaged by war and political instability might make the argument that, before any national treatment program can be implemented, infected military and security personnel should be treated so that they can maintain the civil order necessary for scale-up programs. Countries like Kenya argue that there are certain groups that merit special consideration for treatment, such as victims of rape, people who became infected during vaccine trials or through administration of infected blood, HIV/AIDS orphans, and infected pregnant women. In South Africa, MSF gives selection preference to patients on the basis of their number of dependents, health status, level of income, and the voluntary disclosure of their HIV status (McCoy, 2003a).

From the above, it is clear that different countries and communities will decide who receives treatment based on a variety of factors not limited to community values, local context, and/or the available health and delivery infrastructure. In the absence of established or structured decision-making processes, there is a real danger that some countries will determine who gets treatment in ethically questionable ways, or through processes that are likely to be inequitable (biased in access) and open to abuse and corruption (McCoy, 2003a).

ADMINISTRATION AND DELIVERY OF CARE

Once patients are selected, further ethical issues such as *what standard of care is applicable* arise at the level of administration of treatment. For example: What minimum infrastructure is required to implement treatment plans and how does this infrastructure affect the quality of care provided to patients? What should the standard of care be for the administration of treatment in poor countries? Should there be uniform standards of treatment globally? Can the "Partners-in-Health" Haiti model (Partners in Health, 2004), which is often cited as the gold standard in the provision of ARV treatment in resource-constrained settings, be successfully replicated in similarly situated developing countries? As stated earlier, one of the major obstacles faced by resource-constrained countries is the poor state of their health and delivery systems. If these systems do not operate efficiently and effectively, the proper delivery and administration of drugs will be difficult or impossible. Problems with these systems arise from a lack of resources, including the inability to procure and sustain affordable drug supplies, the inability to manage complicated laboratory monitoring, a lack of trained personnel, inadequate community education strategies to encourage compliance, corruption at various levels, and the absence of sufficient political will in some countries. The tuberculosis example from Zimbabwe provides a practical and parallel illustration of this problem.

Tuberculosis drugs in Africa cost less than $10 dollars per course, for which the treatment duration is six months. In the 1990s, the Zimbabwean government initiated a national tuberculosis program to treat 50,000 tuberculosis patients annually. Unfortunately, this program has been fraught with problems such as a weak political commitment to tuberculosis control, funding gaps, low access to treatment due to poor infrastructure in new settlements, and limited involvement of communities in tuberculosis control. Consequently, the program has not been able to meet its target goals and Zimbabwean health officials are struggling to meet organizational requirements needed to continue administering the program. A conservative estimate of the number of people in need of antiretroviral therapy in Zimbabwe is 250,000 (Zimbabwe has about 1.5 million HIV infected people). The challenges that the government is encountering as it tries to implement the tuberculosis program will be greatly amplified in ARV scale-up programs unless the underlying infrastructural and political issues are adequately addressed (WHO, 2004).

Tanzania also provides a vivid example of the importance of infrastructure, in this case health care personnel, in the scale-up process. There are fewer than 100 physician specialists in the public sector in Tanzania, serving a population of approximately 32 million. Regional and district hospi-

tals have few or no physicians and are mostly staffed by clinical officers
with only the most basic medical training. It is estimated that if physicians
are required to prescribe ARV therapy, 400 more physicians would be
needed immediately in the country (Marlink, 2003). This presents a difficult challenge for Tanzania, which may have to find other creative ways
(such as recruiting and training traditional healers) to fill the health care
personnel gap. This limited human resources pool poses further ethical
challenges. If all or the majority of doctors and/or health care workers are
recruited to work in ARV scale-up programs, what does that mean for the
entire health care system? Will other critical health care programs be de-
prived of the necessary personnel? Relatedly, if scale-up program responsibilities fall mainly on nongovernmental organizations (NGOs), they will
have to recruit health officers in the country and there is a great danger that
there will be a "brain drain" from public programs to the better-paying
private NGO sector. Safeguards have to be put in place to prevent such
losses to public programs.

In summary therefore, the cost and logistical requirements for delivering, administering, monitoring, and evaluating treatment programs constitute a major obstacle to the implementation of ARV therapy in resource
constrained settings. Because we are dealing with an emergency, there is a
great temptation to expedite the dispensing of drugs to those in need and in
so doing, bypass certain recommended processes. While the desire to expedite treatment is good, it creates an ethical imperative to explore, anticipate, and make concrete provisions for any negative consequences that may
arise due to these expedited actions. In the face of real threats of drug
resistance, this issue is not merely academic. A careful balance has to be
drawn between the ethical imperative to treat the sick immediately and the
need to ensure that the expedited emergency treatment strategies employed
will not fail dramatically for lack of sufficient infrastructure to the detri-
ment of the affected population.

THE NEED FOR OPERATIONAL RESEARCH

Operational research refers to the application of advanced analytical
techniques to help make better decisions and to solve problems. In the
context of ARV programs, it would include the carrying out of observational studies, outcome studies, and cost-effectiveness studies (Quinn,
2004). As mentioned earlier, many scale-up programs are being conducted
in environments where there more questions than answers. For example,
what are the best ARV regimens in a given setting? How can barriers to
adherence be assessed? Who derives the most benefit from ARVs (taking in
to account behavioral factors, stage of disease, and laboratory parameters)
(Quinn, 2004)? How does HIV interact with other endemic diseases and

what is the effect on the patient's response to treatment? How effective is the program in prolonging survival and ensuring quality of care? How can the frequency and predictors of ARV resistance be properly and easily detected (Quinn, 2004)? What are the side effect profiles of ARVs in different populations (Quinn, 2004)? Conducting operations research can therefore help in defining the optimal parameters of care in a variety of ways.

Because there are long- and short-term uncertainties in ARV scale-up programs, there is an ethical obligation on the part of treatment teams to set up the necessary structures to learn from such programs, with a view to improving them. Operations research is thus a critical element to the iterative process of improving quality of care. In addition, monitoring and evaluation measures should not simply focus on process measure, but also the quality measures (personal communication, P. Kelley, Director, Board on Global Health, Institute of Medicine, February 2004). In order to do this, donors and countries have to invest in the creation of information systems to gather, analyze, and manage the relevant data. Because of the sensitivity of the information being gathered including patient records, privacy safeguards will have to be built into the systems.

Without a systematic approach to *learning by doing*, there is a great danger that programs may end up not only wasting limited life-saving resources, but also perpetuating potentially harmful health care practices— an ethically unacceptable state of affairs.

FAIRNESS ACROSS DISEASE GROUPS AND PRIORITY SETTING

Consider this hypothetical case: In a rural family in Kenya, the father, a farmworker, has been diagnosed as HIV-positive and because Kenya is one of the recipients of donor finances to fund treatment for HIV/AIDS, and because the father fits within the eligibility criteria, he is put on a free treatment regimen complete with monitoring and support from the community clinic. The mother suddenly falls ill with malaria, is bedridden, and cannot work. The father's wages are not enough to provide school fees and other necessities for the children. The father, at a complete loss for what to do, decides to sell his HIV treatment in the black market (the drugs will benefit an HIV patient who did not fit into the scale-up program treatment entry criteria). The money he receives from the sale is enough to buy malaria treatment for his wife and to pay for some of his children's needs. In this scenario, what are the health priorities of the family? At a broader level, what priority should the provision of ARV therapy have in relation to the many other competing interests that fall outside of the health care sector in developing countries? (Houston, 2002)

Although HIV/AIDS is an epidemic of unprecedented proportion, people in developing countries suffer from a wide range of devastating ailments, such as malaria and tuberculosis, for which there are not enough resources to provide treatment. Problems also exist at the basic public health level due to a lack of immunization programs and inadequate access to proper nutrition, clean drinking water, and sanitation (Benatar, 2002). In the recent past, more than 14 million people have been at risk of starvation in Zimbabwe, Zambia, Lesotho, Swaziland, Malawi, and Mozambique in southern Africa alone (McCoy, 2003b). Resources in those countries are urgently required for education, nutrition, roads, strengthening local agricultural systems, as well as for industrial and technological developments to compete in the global market (McCoy, 2003b). The above hypothetical case does not suggest that donors should stop funding AIDS programs; rather, donors need to explore how their programs can have synergy with other programs addressing other health and welfare needs and, more broadly, how funding for HIV/AIDS can improve health care infrastructure and development in the long-term. Approaches to expand access to ARV treatment should simultaneously strengthen health systems, interact with treatment, prevention, and health care services, and reach vulnerable groups (McCoy and Loewenson, 2004).

SUSTAINABILITY OF TREATMENT PROGRAMS

The current initiatives to provide funding for treatment are laudable: nevertheless, there needs to be a frank discussion about the sustainability of donor-funded treatment programs. How should poor countries deal with the political question of dependency on rich countries for life-sustaining treatment for their citizens? Is this a sustainable relationship in both political and ethical terms? The sustainability issue is not limited to donor-funded programs, but also to national government-funded initiatives that rely to a large extent on the political will of the day. For example, in February 2004, AIDS activists in Nigeria reported that a government plan to provide cheap AIDS drugs had failed, threatening the lives of people with HIV who had started taking the drugs two years ago. Launched in 2002, the Nigerian scheme was riddled with logistical, financial, and corruption problems that led to treatment centers handing out expired drugs or turning patients away (Associated Press, 2004).

Finally, at the institutional level, technical assistance should be offered to help health and humanitarian organizations and governments that are traditionally designed to deal with health problems on shoestring budgets, to cope with the influx of huge amounts of donor money that could very well transform the nature of their operations.

SOME RECOMMENDATIONS

Ethical problems will be encountered at every turn of the scale-up process. Furthermore, ethical decision making in many countries will be constrained by the prevailing political climate. It bears emphasizing that the manner in which these ethical problems are framed, debated, and decided upon will have serious consequences for the health of people. As the scale-up process unfolds, new ethical issues will emerge requiring guidance based on sound ethical principles. I, however, believe that while deliberation on ethical issues is extremely important, it need not and should not stop or slow down the provision of ARV therapy in resource constrained countries until some ideal or final ethical consensus is reached. Whereas there may be no clearly right or ideal solutions, there can be solutions that are clearly wrong. In that spirit, I believe that ethical decisions should be made in real time and should be further refined by a process of ongoing deliberation that is informed by, and informs, ongoing ARV treatment efforts.

On the question of allocation of treatment, I think it is necessary for donors and international aid agencies involved in providing resources for ARV scale up *to engage* with recipient countries to establish a minimum entry criterion grounded in internationally recognized human rights. I believe that such a criterion is important to create a level of *horizontal equity*, that is, people who are similarly situated should receive similar treatment, and to prevent blatant discrimination against certain classes of persons. This common criterion would also provide some guidance for decision making at the national/local level. It would include broad rights-based elements such as the right not to discriminate on defined grounds like gender, sexual orientation, religion, and ethnic background. Countries would thus ideally be bound by these agreed sets of norms but would still have enough leeway to make ethically defensible decisions on who should get treatment within the set framework, with the full understanding that tragic trade-offs will be made and that decisions arrived at by the countries and communities will vary.

At the national or local level, I think that recipient countries have an ethical imperative to create impartial decision-making bodies to carefully deliberate (in an open and transparent manner) the ethical problems arising in scale-up processes, provide reasoned guidance, and make context specific decisions about how treatment should be distributed and administered (Daniels, 1985). I acknowledge that this is a potentially difficult proposition because such a body would have to have sufficient political leverage to get its decisions enforced, and at the same time be independent enough to take actions that may contradict government policy. I realize that even with all the best decision-making process in place, there will inevitably be problems surrounding representation on such bodies, legitimacy, corruption and sustainability of such processes—however, I believe that if created, such bodies would offer a decent start to solving some of these ethical dilemmas, and they would be able to refine their deliberative processes as ARV scale-up progresses.

Finally, as stated above, the provision of treatment should not be delayed in the name of perfecting the decision-making process or in the name of finding the best ethical theories to support pragmatic decisions. Even if a decision makes moral sense, it may be difficult or impossible to implement it on the ground. I strongly believe that making concrete attempts to anticipate and address ethical problems will make for more effective and equitable programs, as will a commitment to reconsidering and refining these ethical hurdles as the programs progress. However, while ethical principles and ethical deliberation are most important, they should not used as an excuse to delay or prevent the implementation of lifesaving treatment—saving any life is better than saving none.

REFERENCES

Associated Press. 2004. *Lives at Risk as HIV Drug Runs Out.* [Online]. Available: http://www.guardian.co.uk/aids/story/0,7369,1140403,00.html [accessed September 2, 2004].

Attawell K, Mundy J. 2003. *WHO, UK Department for International Development. Provision of Antiretroviral Therapy in Resource-Limited Settings: A Review of the Literature up to August 2003.* [Online]. Available: http://www.who.int/3by5/publications/documents/en/ARTpaper_DFID_WHO.pdf [accessed September 2, 2004].

Benatar S. 2002. The HIV/AIDS pandemic: A sign of instability in a complex global system. *Journal of Medicine and Philosophy* 27(2):163–177.

Calabresi G, Bobbit P. 1978. *Tragic Choices.* New York: W.W. Norton.

Daniels N. 1985. *Just Health Care.* Cambridge, England: Cambridge University Press.

DELIVER. 2002. *The Importance of Logistics in HIV/AIDS Programs, No Product? No Program!* [Online]. Available: http://www.deliver.jsi.com/pdf/factsheets/LogHIV.pdf [accessed September 2, 2004].

Houston S. 2002. Justice and HIV care in Africa: Antiretrovirals in perspective. *Journal of the International Association of Physicians in AIDS Care* 1(2):46–50.

Marlink R. 2003. *The Promise the Fear: Tanzania.* Paper presented at the Harvard School of Public Health Symposium. [Online]. Available: http://www.hsph.harvard.edu/hai/conferences_events/Recurrent/harvard_symposium/hp2_pres_pdfs/marlink.pdf [accessed September 2, 2004].

McCoy D. 2003a. *HIV Care and Treatment in Southern Africa: Addressing Equity.* Harare: Equinet and Oxfam GB. (Equinet Discussion Paper Number 10).

McCoy D. 2003b. *Health Sector Responses to HIV/AIDS and Treatment Access in Southern Africa: Addressing Equity. Health Systems Trust.* (Equinet Discussion Paper Number 10).

McCoy D, Loewenson R. 2004. Access to antiretroviral treatment in Africa: New resources and sustainable health systems are needed. *British Medical Journal* 328(7434):241–242.

Mill JS. 1863. *Utilitarianism.* London: Parker, Sun and Bourn.

Nozick R. 1974. *Anarchy, State and Utopia.* New York: Basic Books.

Partners in Health. 2004. *Learn from Haiti.* [Online]. Available: http://www.pih.org/inthenews/011206nytimes_op-ed/index.html [accessed February 12, 2004].

Quinn TC. 2004. *Specific Questions for Operations Research in the Scale-up of ARV Treatment Programs in Low-Resource Settings.* Paper presented at an Institute of Medicine Workshop on Antiretroviral Drug Use in Resource-Constrained Settings. [Online]. Available: http://www.iom.edu/file.asp?id=18458 [accessed February 28, 2004].

Rawls J. 1971. *A Theory of Justice.* Cambridge, MA: Harvard University Press.

Ssemakula KJ. 2001. Cheaper drugs for HIV/AIDS in Africa: What happens next? Suggested strategies for distributing HIV drugs. *Medlinks.* [Online]. Available: http://medilinkz.org/Features/Articles/CheaperHIVDrugs2P2.htm [accessed September 2, 2004].

UNAIDS (Joint United Nations Programme on HIV/AIDS). 2003. [Online]. Available: http://www.unaids.org/fact_sheets/files/Caribbean_Eng.htm (accessed December 3, 2003).

Veatch R. 1986. *The Foundations of Justice: Why the Retarded and the Rest of Us Have Claims to Equality.* New York: Oxford University Press.

WHO (World Health Organization). 2003a. *Global AIDS Epidemic Shows No Sign of Abating.* [Online]. Available: http://www.who.int/mediacentre/releases/2003/prunaids/en/print.html [accessed December 3, 2003].

WHO. 2003b. *Treating 3 Million by 2005. Making it Happen: The WHO Strategy.* Geneva: WHO/UNAIDS.

WHO. 2004. *Country Profile: Zimbabwe.* [Online]. Available: http://www.who.int/tb/publications/global_report/2004/en/Zimbabwe.pdf [accessed September 2, 2004].

WHO/UNAIDS (World Health Organization and Joint United Nations Programme on HIV/AIDS). 2000. *Key Elements in HIV/AIDS Care and Support.* Draft Working Document. Geneva: WHO/UNAIDS.

WHO/UNAIDS. 2003. *Commitment to Action for Expanded Access to HIV/AIDS Treatment.* [Online]. Available: http://www.who.int/entity/hiv/pub/prev_care/en [accessed August 24, 2004].

Wood E, Braitstein P, Montaner JS, Schechter MT, Tyndall MW, O'Shaughnessy MV, Hogg RS. 2000. Extent to which low-level use of antiretroviral treatment could curb the AIDS epidemic in sub-Saharan Africa. *Lancet* 355(9221):2095–2100.

Appendix
E

Human Resource Requirements for Scaling-up Antiretroviral Therapy in Low-Resource Countries[1]

INTRODUCTION

As drug costs have fallen sharply in recent years and donor funding has risen, ambitious programs are now underway to make the widespread availability of antiretroviral (ARV) treatment for AIDS patients a reality. Through these efforts, the immense benefits of antiretroviral therapy (ART) for individuals and societies alike are becoming within reach. But as the financial barriers to scaling up are relaxed, greater attention is being focused on other potential obstacles to ART expansion.

Against this background, the implications of human resource shortages for the President's Emergency Plan for AIDS Relief (PEPFAR) and other global AIDS initiatives are now receiving increased attention. ART is a new and complicated intervention that is being expanded in settings where there may be only one doctor for every 10 or 20,000 people. It also requires other personnel—nurses, laboratory technicians, pharmacists, and counselors—as well as a capacity to provide supporting services such as voluntary counseling and testing (VCT) and the treatment of opportunistic infections (OIs). Difficulties in developing and retaining a sufficient number of skilled health workers is by no means a new problem, but the sheer scale of the HIV/AIDS epidemic, and its impact on human resources through an array of both supply and demand-side factors, has made the problem much worse.

---

[1]Commissioned paper, by Owen Smith, Abt Associates, Inc.

Furthermore, while HIV/AIDS is a devastating epidemic, it is not the only source of morbidity and mortality faced by the PEPFAR countries. Drawing personnel into ARV provision will mean that fewer workers are available to address other priority health problems. In short, it is possible that in many settings the human resource constraint will be a greater obstacle to program expansion than the financial constraint.

The purpose of this chapter is to provide illustrative estimates of the human resource requirements for achieving the PEPFAR goal of treating 2 million patients with ARVs.[2] There is a rapidly growing literature on the impact of HIV/AIDS on human resources for health, touching on both the complex nature of the problem as well as possible solutions (Aitken and Kemp, 2003; USAID, 2003). The objective here is more narrowly defined: to make a first step toward quantifying the human resource needs for PEPFAR. This exercise can help answer questions such as: How do needs compare with existing capacity? Which countries face the greatest challenge? Which categories of health personnel are in shortest supply? The analysis will also help point the way to potential solutions, although these are not discussed in detail. These issues are most appropriately addressed at the country level, where better data are available and policies can be tailored to local circumstances. The broad approach and illustrative estimates presented here will ideally serve as a starting point for more detailed country-specific work.

In the discussion that follows, the term "human resource requirements" refers to the number of people required to deliver ART-related health services. Making sure that they have the appropriate training to do so is another key aspect of the human capacity development issue that is not addressed here. More broadly still, there is a whole range of critical institutional components to a well functioning health care system—including governance structures, financing arrangements, logistics and information systems, and other issues—that are beyond the scope of this study. The difficulties that many public health systems have experienced in addressing less expensive and less labor-intensive health problems than ART should serve as a reminder that no amount of resources per se, whether financial or human, can guarantee program success in the all-too-frequent absence of these broader "architectural" health system inputs.

---

[2]Human resource needs for other ART initiatives, such as the Global Fund to Fight AIDS, Tuberculosis and Malaria, would be additional to those presented here. Nor does this paper constitute a comprehensive estimate of all PEPFAR human resource needs: VCT and OI services are included, but the treatment of sexually transmitted infections, prevention of mother-to-child transmission, and other services are not.

> **BOX E-1**
>
> Human   =   Number of patients × Annual per-patient time
> resource   requirements for service delivery
> requirement   ———————————————————————————————————————
>   Provider time available to spend with patients each year

The paper is organized as follows. First, the paper outlines the estimation approach and discusses methodological issues related to coverage targets for VCT and OI treatment. Second, it presents the results with respect to two major scenarios, discusses Zambia as a specific country example, and also addresses issues of sustainability. Finally, the paper offers concluding remarks and proposed next steps.

APPROACH

Estimation Approach

The basic calculation undertaken in this paper is to estimate human resource requirements by multiplying the number of patients receiving care by the per-patient time requirements for service delivery, and then dividing by the amount of time that each health worker can spend seeing patients in a year. This is shown in Box E-1. The provision of VCT and OI treatment is also included in the calculations. The result is then compared to the current stock of health workers available in each country.[3] This subsection provides a short discussion of each of the inputs to this equation.

The key variable underlying the number of health personnel required to achieve the PEPFAR treatment goal will be how long different categories of workers spend with each ARV patient to deliver services. In broad terms, the identification of time requirements must balance the limited available

---

[3]The allocation of the 2 million patient target across the 14 countries has not yet been identified under PEPFAR. (Note also that at the time of writing, a 15th PEPFAR country had yet to be identified). It will be assumed here that each country will contribute to the overall target using the number of HIV-infected adults as the weight (data were drawn from Appendix E of the PEPFAR strategy paper [2004]). For example, a country accounting for 10 percent of all HIV infections in the 14 countries would have a target to treat 200,000 of the 2 million patient total. Of course it is unlikely to be this simple in practice, and indeed the issue of human resource constraints is arguably a reason unto itself for expanding services more rapidly in some countries than in others.

stock of health workers (for HIV/AIDS and other health services) with the importance of delivering quality care. There is no "ideal" model of care, but rather a wide range of service delivery options, both with regard to who delivers care (doctors, nurses, community lay workers, etc.) and for how long (per contact as well as the frequency of visits). Existing pilot programs may offer some guidance, but these models of care may not be appropriate for expansion to a national scale. This paper draws on some existing work on time requirements as well as the author's own discussions with providers. Due to the range of options available, two alternative scenarios will be explored. These will be presented in detail in the results section.

The second input is the number of hours per year that health personnel have available to treat patients. To estimate this parameter, the contractual level of effort must be modified to take into consideration holidays, vacation, sick leave, and training activities (all of which will cause absences from the workplace), as well as waiting time, administrative duties, cleaning and maintenance tasks, and other activities that curtail time available to spend with patients even while at work. Especially in high-prevalence countries there is a link between time availability and the epidemic itself, since many health care workers may miss time because they are HIV-positive themselves, because they are the caregiver for someone else who is HIV-positive, or because they are attending the funerals of those who have died from the disease (Aitken and Kemp, 2003).

For all these reasons, the amount of time available to spend with patients may be substantially lower than nominal hours worked. For example, Aitken and Kemp (2003) cite a study that found that laboratory technicians in Malawi work on average about 24 hours per week instead of the expected 44 hours. Kurowski and colleagues (2003) found that in Tanzania less than 40 percent of health worker time was actually spent with patients. Current productivity levels can likely be improved upon through a range of policy interventions (e.g., better remuneration or other measures to improve health worker motivation), and ARV expansion itself implies more patients to treat and therefore possibly less time between patients for providers. However, it should also be recognized that heavy workloads could increase the rate of workforce attrition.

In this paper it will be assumed that all categories of health workers spend 1000 hours per year with patients. This could reflect, for example, an average of about 4 days at work each week (with an average of 1 day per week attributed to holiday, vacation, sick leave, training, etc.) and 5 hours per day spent providing care to patients (with the remaining hours performing other tasks or waiting). Either a greater or smaller number of hours per year could also be justified.

The final major data input used in the analysis, to which the estimation of human resource requirements will be compared, is the current stock of health workers. Up-to-date, internationally comparable data on human capacity for health is virtually nonexistent. The analysis here draws from the World Health Organization's WHOSIS database (WHO, 2004), which relies on country sources. The database states that "estimates of health personnel are extremely difficult to obtain, and those listed here are all that we have available." The data on doctors and nurses may or may not adequately reflect emigration, or the possibility that some qualified personnel hold management or research positions that curtail their time for practice. The extent to which private providers are reflected in the data is also not clear.[4] Finally, information on laboratory technicians is not available.

Even at the national level, accurate data are often very difficult to find. Aitken and Kemp (2003) identified eight different sources of data (mostly government documents) on human resources for health in Malawi, none of which could be fully reconciled with the others. To make matters more difficult, for the purposes of this analysis, the weak information on current stocks of health personnel must also be projected forward to 2008 when PEPFAR goals are to be achieved. The detailed work in Tanzania by Kurowski et al. (2003) predicted some increase in the numbers of doctors and nurses by 2015. However, the reality that in many countries the size of the health workforce has declined in recent years should temper expectations of any sharp increases (Liese et al., 2003). In this paper it is conservatively assumed that there will be no change through 2008 from current data on the number of health workers available.[5]

Supporting Services: VCT and OI Treatment

The expansion of ART requires a capacity to provide supporting services as well, and these will require human resources of their own. The estimates presented in this paper include human resources for VCT and OI treatment. However, unlike for ARV provision, there are no explicit targets for program coverage of these services. This subsection therefore briefly discusses some related methodological issues.

The key entry point to the provision of antiretroviral treatment is VCT services to determine an individual's HIV status. To put the required number of people on ART, a much greater number of people must be tested, since many will turn out to be HIV-negative, while others will be HIV-

---

[4]The database manager believes that the private sector is included for some countries but not for others (personal communication). Whether and how private providers can be engaged in ARV provision will be an important programmatic issue.

[5]PEPFAR proposes to encourage the repatriation of health personnel who have emigrated as well as the importation of foreign health workers, but for the present purpose of estimating the current gap, this potential solution will not be considered in the calculations.

positive but not yet clinically eligible for treatment. Thus, ambitious targets for ARV provision automatically imply ambitious targets for VCT as well, with important implications for human resource needs. VCT also offers important benefits as a prevention tool, and so human resource requirements for VCT should be seen as contributing to the achievement of PEPFAR's prevention goal of averting 7 million new infections as well.

What level of VCT service provision should human resource estimates be based upon? Exactly how many VCT contacts will be required to initiate 2 million people on treatment is very uncertain. People are more likely to seek testing if they have reason to believe that they may have been exposed to the virus, or because they are already developing symptoms. Among those who are tested, therefore, the proportion of individuals who are HIV-positive, and within that group the proportion that is clinically eligible for ART, will be higher than the corresponding population-wide rates. It will be assumed here that the diagnosis rate is two to three times higher than the prevalence rate (depending on the country), and that one-third of those diagnosed as HIV-positive are clinically eligible for treatment.[6] The result is that over 25 million people would need to be tested across the 14 countries to initiate 2 million people on treatment.[7] Human resource requirements for this level of coverage will contribute to both treatment and prevention efforts.

PEPFAR also aims to treat people with opportunistic infections. Since ART provision should reduce a patient's susceptibility to OIs, on the surface it may seem that as ARV programs expand there will be a significant human resource "savings" with respect to OI care. However, for several reasons this may not occur. First, the absolute number of illness episodes per person may not decline because patients will live much longer and ARVs may merely delay the onset of OIs, rather than eliminate them altogether. Second, as the PEPFAR plan recognizes (Office of the United States Global AIDS Coordinator, 2004:36), the goal of expanding the entire continuum of care for HIV/AIDS patients may increase access to health services among certain population groups not previously presenting for the treatment of OIs. Finally, it is important to note that PEPFAR's treatment goal of initiating 2 million people on ARVs by 2008 represents perhaps 20 percent of those who over the next 5 years will be reaching the stage of disease at which they become susceptible to OIs. The need for treatment

---

[6]Anecdotal evidence from VCT clinics in Uganda and Zambia suggested diagnosis rates that were twice the national HIV prevalence rate, although this could vary widely depending on a number of factors. The proportion of HIV-positive individuals who are clinically eligible is usually 10 to 20 percent.

[7]Whether this many people will actually seek testing is a very important issue but is not considered here.

among the other 80 percent will remain unchanged. In sum, overall demand for OI car—and the resulting need for human resources—is unlikely to decline substantially during the course of PEPFAR.

What level of OI service provision should human resource estimates be based upon? PEPFAR has no explicit coverage target for OIs. The plan aims to provide care to 10 million people, but this includes care of orphans and vulnerable children, symptom management, and end-of-life care, in addition to the treatment of OIs. For the present analysis it will be assumed that OI treatment is provided to everyone receiving ARVs (who are much less susceptible to infection than those not receiving ART), as well as to 20 percent of those who are not. This translates into the treatment of OIs for about 3.5 million non-ARV patients over five years, accounting for about one-third of the broader care goal. Four of the most common OIs will be considered: tuberculosis, pneumonia, oral candidiasis, and cryptococcal meningitis (Kombe and Smith, 2004).

RESULTS

This section presents estimates of the number of personnel required in five different service provider categories—doctors, nurses, laboratory technicians, VCT counselors, and community workers—for delivering ARVs to 2 million people by 2008, including supporting VCT and OI services. Other crucial human resource inputs—such as pharmacists, program managers, and logistical workers—are not included. Two scenarios are discussed: the first does not include community workers, while the second adds this cadre and assigns to them certain tasks normally performed by skilled professionals. The case of Zambia is also analyzed to provide a country-specific illustration of key issues. The topic of sustainability is discussed in the final subsection.

Scenario 1: No Community Workers

The assumptions for average per-patient time requirements by personnel category (expressed in annual terms for ARVs and per-episode terms for other services) are shown in Table E-1. Each individual patient in reality will require a different amount of time with health workers depending on a variety of factors. Time requirements for ARV delivery, for example, will be higher for patients who are being initiated on treatment, or for those who are suffering from complications.[8] Models of care may also vary

---

[8]The extent to which second-line treatment regimens are needed will have important implications for human resource requirements—but this is an important unknown for large-scale programs in low-resource countries.

TABLE E-1 Per-Patient Time Requirements in Minutes, Scenario 1

	Doctor	Nurse	Lab Technician	VCT Counselor	Community Worker
VCT, HIV neg (per service)	0	15	0	30	0
VCT, HIV pos (per service)	0	30	0	45	0
ARVs (per year)	90	90	90	0	0
Tuberculosis (per episode)	45	30	60	0	0
Oral candidiasis (per episode)	15	0	0	0	0
Pneumonia (per episode)	15	0	20	0	0
Meningitis (per episode)	30	0	40	0	0

depending on the physical setting (hospital, health center, at home, etc.) in which the service is delivered. But overall human resource requirements will ultimately depend on averages such as those shown in the table.

These estimates are based generally on reserach by Huddart and colleagues (2004), outcomes from a WHO/UNAIDS consensus meeting held in November 2003 (WHO/UNAIDS, 2004),[9] and the author's discussions with providers in Uganda and Zambia. As noted earlier, there is no "ideal" model. A wide range of service delivery options is available and existing models of care may be unrealistic for scaling up to a national level. Note that VCT services are assumed to be performed by a nurse and a VCT counselor but not by a lab technician; in some cases only one person may do everything.[10] For ARV delivery, lab technician time will depend on the number and type of tests to be performed, the technology applied, and even the model of equipment being used. Thus a very wide range is possible; here we will assume that 90 minutes of lab technician time is required per patient per year.

Table E-2 shows the total human resource requirements for this sce-

---

[9]WHO/UNAIDS International Consensus Meeting on Interim Recommendations for Technical and Operational Procedures for Emergency Scaling Up ARV Treatment in Resource-Limited Settings, November 18-21, 2003, Lusaka, Zambia.

[10]A diminished role for lab technicians in VCT delivery should be expected as programs expand, in view of the extreme shortages of this cadre of workers, the increased use of rapid tests, and the plan to offer the service in more nonhospital settings.

TABLE E-2 Total Human Resource Requirements in FTEs, Scenario 1

	Doctors	Nurses	Lab Technicians	VCT Counselors	Community Workers
Botswana	61	71	62	25	0
Cote d'Ivoire	141	198	144	128	0
Ethiopia	400	629	411	512	0
Guyana	4	9	4	10	0
Haiti	50	81	52	68	0
Kenya	483	660	497	416	0
Mozambique	215	301	221	205	0
Namibia	40	52	41	26	0
Nigeria	650	1092	665	944	0
Rwanda	88	127	90	86	0
South Africa	966	1246	990	663	0
Tanzania	263	398	269	293	0
Uganda	101	184	103	173	0
Zambia	206	261	211	133	0

nario, measured as full-time equivalents (FTEs). Note that because per-patient time requirements for ARV delivery were the same for doctors, nurses, and lab technicians at 90 minutes each per year, the overall requirements for these three cadres are similar as well (differences are due to OI treatment). But since all countries have far more nurses than doctors, and often more doctors than lab technicians, the relative burden falls more heavily on doctors and lab technicians. ARV provision is a relatively complicated intervention, and an important implication is that it places a greater burden on more specialized workers. Table E-2 helps to identify where the shortages are likely to be most severe and also points to the potential solution of delegating as much responsibility to nurses and community workers as possible (as will be seen in Scenario 2).

How do the requirements in Table E-2 compare with existing capacity? The fraction of each country's existing doctor workforce required to reach PEPFAR coverage goals under Scenario 1 is shown in Figure E-1. For all countries, approximately 80 percent of the doctor requirements are for ARVs, with the remainder for OI treatment. It is difficult to identify a constraint precisely, since dedicating 100 percent of a country's doctor workforce to HIV/AIDS is obviously not realistic. For four countries (and nearly a fifth), the requirement exceeds 20 percent.

What about the other health worker categories? The burden on the nursing sector is likely to be less serious than in the case of doctors, rarely exceeding 5 percent of existing capacity. However, it is likely to be *more* serious for laboratory technicians. International data for lab technicians are scarce, but the illustrative case of Zambia (which faces a severe challenge) is

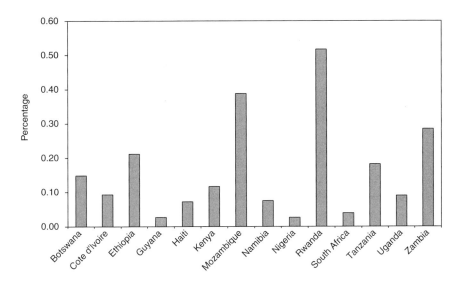

FIGURE E-1 Fraction of existing doctor workforce required under Scenario 1.

discussed below. Finally, there are similarly no international data on existing numbers of VCT counselors. This is the cadre of health workers that could probably be trained most quickly among the four categories, but they may also be subject to the highest burnout rate.

Requirements for all staff categories should be placed in a broader context. As noted earlier, HIV/AIDS is not the only health crisis facing the 14 PEPFAR countries. Devoting personnel to HIV/AIDS will mean fewer are available to contribute, for example, to the reduction in malaria incidence and child and maternal mortality rates as targeted by the Millennium Development Goals (MDGs). Taking a broader view of health sector human resource requirements, Kurowski and colleagues (2003) found that projected human resource availability in Tanzania was "grossly insufficient" for reaching the requirements necessary to scale up priority interventions (including ART) as recommended by the Commission on Macroeconomics and Health (CMI I).

Scenario 2: Adding Community Workers

In recognition of the obstacle to scaling-up posed by inadequate human resources, the PEPFAR plan proposes that alternative service delivery models could ease the burden by shifting certain duties to community workers. The onerous requirements of Scenario 1 discussed above help support the rationale for this devolution of responsibilities.

Table E-3 shows the per-patient time requirements of an alternative service delivery model that makes use of community workers. It is assumed that lab technician responsibilities for ART monitoring and OI diagnosis cannot be reassigned to any other health worker category. The only way to reduce requirements for this job category—where the shortages may be most severe—is to reduce the number of tests.

The resulting human resource requirements are shown in Table E-4. Doctor requirements are reduced by roughly 50 percent compared to Scenario 1. Nurse requirements decline by a narrower margin, since the "savings" generated by allocating some of their responsibilities to community workers are partially offset because they simultaneously adopt part of the doctor's role. Note that in all countries the number of lab technicians required is now higher than the doctor requirement, although many health systems are endowed with more of the latter than the former.

How do these compare to current availability? Figure E-2 shows doctor requirements as a share of existing capacity. For all countries, about 75 percent of the requirements are for ARV provision, while the rest is for OI treatment. Except for Mozambique and Rwanda, all countries are now below the 20 percent threshold. But the requirements in many cases are still substantial. As before, there are no international data on lab technicians and VCT counselors to which comparisons can be made.

As a final comment on Scenario 2, the issue of quality of care should also be considered. Delegating certain responsibilities from skilled health professionals to trained community workers, and scaling back the laboratory monitoring protocol, does introduce a risk that the quality of care will

TABLE E-3 Per-Patient Time Requirements in Minutes, Scenario 2

	Doctor	Nurse	Lab Technician	VCT Counselor	Community Worker
VCT, HIV neg (per service)	0	15	0	15	15
VCT, HIV pos (per service)	0	30	0	30	15
ARVs (per year)	45	60	60	0	75
Tuberculosis (per episode)	30	15	60	0	30
Oral candidiasis (per episode)	15	0	0	0	0
Pneumonia (per episode)	15	0	20	0	0
Meningitis (per episode)	15	15	40	0	0

TABLE E-4 Total Human Resource Requirements in FTEs, Scenario 2

	Doctors	Nurses	Lab Technicians	VCT Counselors	Community Workers
Botswana	33	52	45	16	55
Cote d'Ivoire	77	156	105	72	162
Ethiopia	221	511	304	279	531
Guyana	2	7	3	5	8
Haiti	28	66	38	37	68
Kenya	267	516	367	235	541
Mozambique	120	238	165	114	249
Namibia	22	39	30	15	41
Nigeria	354	895	485	510	926
Rwanda	48	100	66	48	104
South Africa	529	956	726	387	1003
Tanzania	143	318	196	162	331
Uganda	55	153	75	92	158
Zambia	113	200	155	79	210

suffer. ART offers enormous benefits to AIDS patients, but it is not without risks, especially with regard to the development of drug resistance.

The Case of Zambia

The case of Zambia provides one illustration of the potential human resource challenges that lie ahead. The estimates presented earlier assume that Zambia treats about 110,000 individuals with ARVs by 2008 under PEPFAR, based on its share of HIV-infected persons in the 14 countries. But there is a total of about 850,000 HIV-positive Zambians, about half of whom may be eligible for treatment within the next 5 years (and almost all within the next 10 years). Even at this relatively low level of coverage (roughly 25 percent by 2008), however, the human resource requirements will impose a large burden.

The requirement of 206 doctors by 2008, as indicated in Table E-2, represents close to one-third of the existing doctor workforce in the country. The implications of meeting this requirement for the delivery of other priority health services would be substantial. At the same time, however, the requirement of 261 nurses represents only 2 percent of the existing workforce in that category. This serves to highlight the logic underlying proposals to reassign as much of the doctor's role to nurses as possible.

Perhaps the most forbidding constraint, however, is with respect to lab personnel: the need for 211 technicians in Scenario 1 represents about 65 percent of Zambia's 325 public sector lab technicians and technologists (Huddart et al., 2004). The Scenario 2 requirement for lab personnel repre-

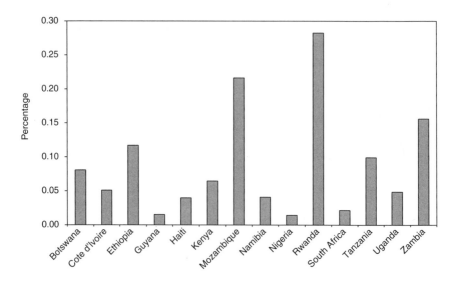

FIGURE E-2 Fraction of existing doctor workforce required under Scenario 2.

sents nearly 50 percent of current capacity. As noted earlier, this job is difficult to reassign to other categories of health personnel or to community workers, and thus the only way to reduce requirements is to reduce the number of tests performed.

A recent study (Huddart et al., 2004) of the HIV/AIDS workforce in Zambia identified two other challenges that may be common elsewhere as PEPFAR activities are scaled up. First, it found that the average loss rate of HIV/AIDS service delivery staff was 30 percent annually. High rates of workforce attrition will make program expansion even more challenging. Second, standards of service delivery in existing programs were found to be low, suggesting that quality of care considerations will become increasingly important as population coverage expands.

Sustainability

As Aitken and Kemp (2003) note, "the impact of HIV/AIDS is devastating and will continue for decades—[and] the response must be on a similar scale and timeframe." As we look further into the future, there will be a greater probability that more health workers can be trained, new interventions and technologies can be developed, or other steps can be taken to ease the human resource constraint.

But the issue of sustainability will remain relevant. PEPFAR aims to treat 2 million patients with ARVs in a group of countries in which about

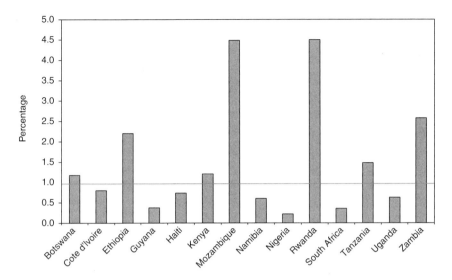

FIGURE E-3 Fraction of existing doctor workforce required for full coverage in 10 years.

20 million HIV-positive individuals currently live. There are millions of people who are seropositive today who still won't be clinically eligible for treatment by 2008, and ultimately they, too, will require human resources for ARV delivery. Also, there are other global initiatives to expand ARV provision, such as the WHO's 3 × 5 initiative and the Global Fund to Fight AIDS, Tuberculosis, and Malaria. These are placing similar demands on human capacity in the health sector but were not included in the estimates presented earlier.

Since virtually all of the 20 million HIV-positive individuals in the 14 countries will become clinically eligible for treatment within the next 10 years, it may be asked hypothetically what the human resource requirements would be if every one of them were actually to receive ARVs at that time.[11] The resulting doctor requirements, assuming the same model of care as in Scenario 1 above, are shown in Figure E-3. In half of the countries, the requirements exceed the entire existing workforce. Even levels above 50 percent, surpassed by four others, are probably not realistic given other health demands. The number of new human resources that would be available 10 years from now is uncertain, but as noted earlier, many countries have suffered recent declines, and so a sharp increase is unlikely.

---

[11]We will disregard the likelihood that some may die in the interim despite receiving treatment.

A more modest pace of expansion would be to duplicate the goals of PEPFAR during the subsequent 5-year period from 2009 to 2013. The human resource needs would be approximately twice the Scenario 1 and 2 results presented earlier. The number of doctors available by then would also need to double just to keep the ratios in Figures E-1 and E-2 constant. Again, this is unlikely. In sum, the human resource challenge applies not only to treating 2 million patients by 2008, but also to initiating treatment for those who will become clinically eligible beyond that year.

CONCLUSION AND NEXT STEPS

The results of the previous section provide an indication of the human resource needs for PEPFAR and how they differ across countries and across different categories of health workers. These are illustrative estimates. Of necessity they are based on general assumptions about what models of care may ultimately be implemented on the ground, and how the overall target of treating 2 million patients will be achieved across countries. Also, the requirements are compared to imperfect data on existing human resource capacity.

However some key findings do emerge. First, the human resource requirements of PEPFAR are substantial. Even providing 90 minutes of doctor time per year to each of the 2 million ARV patients would require about 20 percent or more of the existing doctor workforce in 5 of the 14 PEPFAR countries. Second, the severity of the human resource constraint varies widely among the 14 countries. It is clear that some countries will be much better positioned to rapidly scale up services than others, and indeed this could inform how the overall target of 2 million patients is achieved. Third, the human resource requirements are much more onerous for doctors and lab technicians than they are for nurses and counselors, and models of care need to be designed accordingly.

The results also highlight some important thematic issues. First, the scale of the problem is such that human resource requirements for HIV/AIDS should not be viewed in isolation from other health sector human resource needs.[12] More health personnel for ARVs will mean less for other priority services. Second, while the delegation of responsibilities to community lay workers is a sensible approach to the human resource constraint, these models should also be scrutinized from a quality of care perspective. Quantifying human resource needs—for example, by identifying the aver-

---

[12]More broadly still, human resource requirements for HIV/AIDS cannot be seen in isolation from other (nonhealth related) development needs in low-resource countries.

age number of minutes that an ARV patient spends each year with a doctor —can help inform these discussions. Third, there are millions of people currently infected with HIV who will still not be clinically eligible for ART in 2008, and so issues of sustainability beyond that year should not be ignored.

Ultimately, however, the results presented here should serve as a starting point for detailed country-level work. It is there that the best data and understanding of local circumstances lie. The exercise of quantifying human resource needs by national stakeholders can provide important information before a program expands.[13]

Most important, it can help to inform policy measures that aim to address the human resource constraint. Potential solutions have been discussed in detail elsewhere.[14] They may be pursued on multiple levels simultaneously: within the HIV/AIDS sector, within the health system more broadly, at the national level, or internationally. No single solution will offer a magic bullet to the human resource challenge; countries will need to adopt multipronged strategies to fit local circumstances. But taken together they can help contribute to a more successful program expansion.

REFERENCES

Aitken JM, Kemp J. 2003. *HIV/AIDS, Equity and Health Sector Personnel in Southern Africa*. Equinet Discussion Paper Number 12. [Online]. Available: http://www.equinetafrica.org/Resources/downloads/discussionpaper12.pdf [accessed August 24, 2004].

Huddart J, Lyons JV, Furth R. 2004. *The Zambia HIV/AIDS Workforce Study: Preparing for Scale-up*. [Online]. Available: http://www.qaproject.org/pubs/PDFs/ORMZambia Workforce1.pdf [accessed September 7, 2004].

Kombe G, Smith O. 2004. *The Costs of HIV/AIDS Services within the Basic Health Care Package in Zambia*. Unpublished.

Kurowski C, Wyss K, Abdulla S, Yemadji N, Mills A. 2003. *Human Resource for Health: Requirements and Availability in the Context of Scaling Up Priority Interventions in Low Income Countries: Case Studies from Tanzania and Chad*. London: Health Policy Unit, London School of Hygiene and Tropical Medicine.

---

[13]Country-level work can also better focus on the important issue of geography, which has not been addressed here. There is a strong urban bias to health sector human resource availability in low-resource countries, and this will make program expansion in rural areas even more challenging.

[14]See, for example, Aitken and Kemp (2003), USAID (2003), and Picazo (2003). The PEPFAR plan itself also discusses possible approaches to addressing human resource shortages. See Office of the United States Global AIDS Coordinator (2004).

Liese B, Blanchet N, Dussault G. 2003. *The Human Resource Crisis in Health Services in Sub-Saharan Africa.* [Online]. Available: http://econ.worldbank.org/files/30373_29_ Bernhard_Liese_The_Human_Resource_Crisis_in_Health_Ser.pdf [accessed September 7, 2004].

Office of the United States Global AIDS Coordinator. 2004. *The President's Emergency Plan for AIDS Relief.* [Online]. Available: http://www.state.gov/documents/organization/ 29831.pdf [accessed September 7, 2004].

PEPFAR strategy paper (2004), Appendix E.

Picazo O. 2003. *Deployment and Retention of Health Workers in Africa: A Note on Some Practices and Issues.* Mimeo.

USAID (U.S. Agency for International Development). 2003. *The Health Sector Human Resource Crisis in Africa: An Issues Paper.* [Online]. Available: http://www.dec.org/pdf_ docs/PNACS527.pdf [accessed August 24, 2004].

WHO (World Health Organization). 1998. WHO Estimates of Health Personnel. [Online]. Available: http://www3.who.int/whosis/health_personnel/health_personnel.cfm?path= whosis,topics,health_personnel&language=english [accessed September 7, 2004].

WHO. 2004. WHO Statistical Information System. [Online]. Available: http://www3.who.int/ whosis [accessed September 2, 2004].

WHO/UNAIDS (World Health Organization and Joint United Nations Programme on HIV/ AIDS). 2004. *Report on the Methods Used to Estimate Costs of Reaching the WHO Target of 3 by 5.* [Online]. Available: http://www.who.int/3by5/en/Progressreport.pdf [accessed October 21, 2004].

Appendix
F

Glossary and Acronyms

3TC: Also known as lamivudine. An antiretroviral drug in the class of nucleoside reverse transcriptase inhibitors (NRTIs). Used to treat HIV/AIDS.

Acquired Immunodeficiency Syndrome (AIDS): The most severe manifestation of infection with the human immunodeficiency virus (HIV). The Centers for Disease Control and Prevention (CDC) lists numerous opportunistic infections and cancers that, in the presence of HIV infection, constitute an AIDS diagnosis. In 1993, CDC expanded the criteria for an AIDS diagnosis in adults and adolescents to include CD4+ T-cell count at or below 200 cells per microliter in the presence of HIV infection. In persons (age 5 and older) with normally functioning immune systems, CD4+ T-cell counts usually range from 500 to 1,500 cells per microliter. Persons living with AIDS often have infections of the lungs, brain, eyes, and other organs, and frequently suffer debilitating weight loss, diarrhea, and a type of cancer called Kaposi's sarcoma.

Antenatal: Occurring before birth.

Antifungal: A substance that kills or inhibits the growth of a fungus.

Antimalarial: An antimicrobial drug used to prevent or treat malaria, an infectious disease caused by the genus *Plasmodium*. Malaria is transmitted by mosquito bites. See Malaria.

Antimicrobial: A drug for killing microorganisms or suppressing their multiplication or growth. For the purposes of this report, antimicrobials include antibiotics and antivirals.

Antiretroviral Drugs: Substances used to kill or inhibit the multiplication of retroviruses such as HIV. There are four classes of antiretroviral drugs for the treatment of HIV/AIDS.

Asymptomatic: Having no symptoms.

AZT: Also known as lamivudine. Also known as ZDV. An antiretroviral drug in the class of nucleoside reverse transcriptase inhibitors (NRTIs). Used to treat HIV/AIDS.

CD4 (T4) or CD4+ Cells: 1. A type of T cell involved in protecting against viral, fungal, and protozoal infections. These cells normally orchestrate the immune response, signaling other cells in the immune system to perform their special functions. Also known as T helper cells. 2. HIV's preferred targets are cells that have a docking molecule called "cluster designation 4" (CD4) on their surfaces. Cells with this molecule are known as CD4-positive (or CD4+) cells. Destruction of CD4+ lymphocytes is the major cause of the immunodeficiency observed in AIDS, and decreasing CD4+ lymphocyte levels appear to be the best indicator for developing opportunistic infections. Although CD4 counts fall, the total T cell level remains fairly constant through the course of HIV disease, due to a concomitant increase in the CD8+ cells. The ratio of CD4+ to CD8+ cells is therefore an important measure of disease progression. See CD8 (T8) Cells; Immunodeficiency.

CD8: A glycoprotein found especially on the surface of killer T cells that usually function to facilitate recognition by killer T cell receptors of antigens complexed with molecules of a class that are found on the surface of most nucleated cells and are the product of genes of the major histocompability complex.

Cocci: A spherical bacterium.

Cotrimoxazole: An antimicrobial drug. A bactericidal combination of trimethoprim and sulfamethoxazole that is used to prevent and treat infections in patients with HIV/AIDS.

Cytomegalovirus: A herpes virus that is a common cause of opportunistic diseases in persons with AIDS and other persons with immune suppression. Most adults in the United States have been infected by CMV; however the virus does not cause disease in healthy people. Because the virus remains in the body for life, it can cause disease if the immune system becomes severely damaged or suppressed by drugs. While CMV can infect most organs of the body, persons with AIDS are most susceptible to CMV retinitis (disease of the eye) and colitis (disease of the colon).

D4T: Also known as stavudine. An antiretroviral drug in the class of nucleoside reverse transcriptase inhibitors (NRTIs). Used to treat HIV/AIDS.

Dapsone: An antimicrobial drug. Used to prevent *Pneumocystis carinii* pneumonia in patients intolerant to use of sulfa-containing drugs. Also used to treat leprosy, an infectious disease caused by *Mycobacterium leprae*.

Dual Therapy: The use of two drugs to treat a disease such as HIV/AIDS.

Efavirenz: An antiretroviral drug in the class of nonnucleoside reverse transcriptase inhibitors (NNRTIs). Used to treat HIV/AIDS.

Epidemic: A disease that spreads rapidly through a demographic segment of the human population, such as everyone in a given geographic area; a military base, or similar population unit; or everyone of a certain age or sex, such as the children or women of a region. Epidemic diseases can be spread from person to person or from a contaminated source such as food or water.

Epidemiology: The branch of medical science that deals with the study of incidence and distribution and control of a disease in a population.

Genotype: The internally coded, inheritable information carried by all living organisms. This stored information is used as a blueprint or set of instructions for building and maintaining a living creature. These instructions are found within almost all cells (the internal part), they are written in a coded language (the genetic code); they are copied at the time of cell division or reproduction and are passed from one generation to the next (inheritable). These instructions are intimately involved with all aspects of the life of a cell or an organism. They control everything from the formation of protein macromolecules, to the regulation of metabolism and synthesis.

Gross Domestic Product: A measure of the output produced by factors of production located in the domestic country regardless of who owns these factors.

Hemopoietic: The formation of blood or of blood cells in the living body.

Hepatic: Pertaining to the liver.

Hepatoxicity: Toxic to the liver.

High-Income Country: A country having an annual gross national product (GNP) per capita equivalent to \$9,361 or greater in 1998. Most high-income countries have an industrial economy. There are currently about 29 high-income countries in the world with populations of one million people or more. Their combined population is about 0.9 billion, less than one-sixth of the world's population. In 2003, the cutoff for high-income countries was adjusted to \$9,206 or more.

Highly Active Antiretroviral Therapy (HAART):   The name given to treatment regimens recommended by leading HIV experts to aggressively suppress viral replication and progress of HIV disease. The usual HAART regimen combines three or more different drugs, such as two nucleoside reverse transcriptase inhibitors (NRTIs) and a protease inhibitor (PI), two NRTIs and a non-nucleoside reverse transcriptase inhibitor (NNRTI), or other combinations. These treatment regimens have been shown to reduce the amount of virus so that it becomes undetectable in a patient's blood.

Human Leukocyte Antigens: Marker molecules on cell surfaces that identify cells as "self" and prevent the immune system from attacking them.

Immune Reconstitution: Immune reconstitution is the regeneration of memory and naïve T cells in response to antiretroviral therapy.

Immunodeficiency: Inability to produce normal antibodies or immunologocially sensitized T cells especially in response to specific antigens.

Immunology: A science that deals with the immune system and the cell-mediated and humoral aspects of immunity and immune responses.

In vivo: In the living body of a plant or animal.

Intrapartum: Time during labor and delivery.

Intrauterine: Inside the uterus.

Isoniazid: An antimicrobial drug. Used to prevent or treat tuberculosis infections.

Kaletra: Trade name of an antiretroviral drug in the class of protease inhibitors (PIs). It is a combination of two PI: lopinavir and ritonavir. Used to treat HIV/AIDS.

Lamivudine: Also known as 3TC. An antiretroviral drug in the class of nucleoside reverse transcriptase inhibitors (NRTIs). Used to treat HIV/AIDS.

Lipodystrophy: A disturbance in the way the body produces, uses, and distributes fat. Lipodystrophy is also referred to as buffalo hump, protease paunch, or Crixivan potbelly. In HIV disease, lipodystrophy has come to refer to a group of symptoms that seem to be related to the use of protease inhibitor (PI) and nucleoside reverse transcriptase inhibitor (NRTI) drugs. Also called lipodystrophy syndrome, pseudo-Cushing's syndrome.

Lopinavir: An antiretroviral drug in the class of protease inhibitors (PIs). Used to treat HIV/AIDS.

Low-income country: A country having an annual gross national product (GNP) per capita equivalent to $760 or less in 1998. The standard of living is lower in these countries; there are few goods and services; and many people cannot meet their basic needs. In 2003, the cutoff for low-income countries was adjusted to $745 or less. At that time, there were about 61 low-income countries with a combined population of about 2.5 billion people.

Malaria: An acute or chronic infectious disease caused by parasites of the genus *Plasmodium*. There are four *Plasmodium* species that infect humans. *Plasmodium* infect the red blood cells. The usual cause of malaria is by infection following the bite of a mosquito. Malaria is characterized by periodic attacks of chills and fever that coincide with mass destruction of blood cells and the release of toxic substances by the *Plasmodium* parasite at the end of each reproductive cycle.

Middle-income country: A country having an annual gross national product (GNP) per capita equivalent to more than $760 but less than $9,360 in 1998. The standard of living is higher than in low-income countries, and people have access to more goods and services, but many people still cannot meet their basic needs. In 2003, the cutoff for middle-income countries was adjusted to more than $745, but less than $9,206. At that time, there were about 65 middle-income countries with populations of one million or more. Their combined population was approximately 2.7 billion.

Monotherapy: The use of a single drug to treat a disease such as HIV/ AIDS.

Morbidity: The condition of being diseased or sick; also the incidence of disease or rate of sickness.

Mortality: The number of deaths in a given time or place; also the proportion of deaths to population.

Neuropathy: The name given to a group of disorders involving nerves. Symptoms range from a tingling sensation or numbness in the toes and fingers to paralysis. It is estimated that 35 percent of persons with HIV disease have some form of neuropathy. There are multiple causes of neuropathy, including drug side effects.

Nevirapine: Also known as NVP. An antiretroviral drug in the class of nonnucleoside reverse transcriptase inhibitors (NNRTIs). Used to treat HIV/ AIDS.

Nonnucleoside Reverse Transcriptase Inhibitors (NNRTI):   A class of antiretroviral drugs used to treat HIV/AIDS. A group of structurally diverse compounds that bind to the catalytic site of HIV-1's reverse transcriptase enzyme. Unlike the nucleoside reverse transcriptase inhibitors (NRTIs), the NNRTIs have no activity against HIV-2. As noncompetitive inhibitors of reverse transcriptase, their antiviral activity is additive or synergistic with most other antiretroviral agents.

Nucleoside Analog: An artificial copy of a nucleoside. When incorporated into the DNA or RNA of a virus during viral replication, the nucleoside analog acts to prevent production of new virus. Nucleoside analogs may take the place of natural nucleosides, blocking the completion of a viral DNA chain during infection of a new cell by HIV. The HIV enzyme reverse transcriptase is more likely to incorporate the nucleoside analogs into the DNA it is constructing than is the DNA polymerase normally used for DNA creation in cell nuclei.

Nucleoside Reverse Transcriptase Inhibitors (NRTI):   A class of antiretroviral drugs used to treat HIV/AIDS. A nucleoside analog antiretroviral drug whose chemical structure constitutes a modified version of a natural nucleoside. These compounds suppress replication of retroviruses by interfering with the reverse transcriptase enzyme. The nucleoside analogs cause premature termination of the proviral (viral precursor) DNA chain. All NRTIs require phosphorylation in the host's cells prior to their incorporation into the viral DNA.

Pandemic: A disease prevalent throughout an entire country, continent, or the whole world.

Pediatric AIDS Clinical Trial Group (PACTG): This is the U.S.-based scientific organization that evaluates treatments for HIV-infected children and adolescents and develops new approaches for the interruption of mother-to-infant transmission.

Perinatal: Events that occur at or around the time of birth.

Peripartum: Occurring in or being the period preceding or following birth.

Pharmacokinetics: The processes of absorption, distribution, metabolism, and excretion of a drug or vaccine.

Phenotype: The outward, physical manifestation of the organism. These are the physical parts, the sum of the atoms, molecules, macromolecules, cells, structures, metabolism, energy utilization, tissues, organs, reflexes and behaviors; anything that is part of the observable structure, function or behavior of a living organism.

Plasma viremia: Having virus in the bloodstream.

Pneumocystis: A genus of microorganisms of that are usually considered protozoans or sometimes fungi. One species is *Pneumocystis carinii*. This species can cause pneumonia in immunocompromised individuals.

Prophylaxis: Treatment to prevent the onset of a particular disease (primary prophylaxis), or the recurrence of symptoms in an existing infection that has been brought under control (secondary prophylaxis, maintenance therapy).

Protease inhibitors (PIs): A class of antiretroviral drugs used to treat HIV/AIDS. These drugs act by inhibiting the virus' protease enzyme, thereby preventing viral replication. Specifically, these drugs block the protease enzyme from breaking apart long strands of viral proteins to make the smaller, active HIV proteins that comprise the virion. If the larger HIV proteins are not broken apart, they cannot assemble themselves into new functional HIV particles.

Renal: Pertaining to the kidneys.

Rifampicin: An antimicrobial drug. It is used for the treatment of tuberculosis.

Ritonavir: An antiretroviral drug in the class of protease inhibitors (PI). Used to treat HIV/AIDS. Usually used in combination with another protease inhibitor, lopinavir, to "boost" the effect of lopinavir.

Seroprevalence: As related to HIV infection, the proportion of persons who have evidence of HIV infection in their blood at any given time.

Symptomatic: Having symptoms of a disease.

Teratogenicity: The ability to cause birth defects. Teratogenicity is a potential side effect of some drugs, such as efavirenz, a drug to treat HIV/AIDS.

Toxoplasma: A genus containing the parasite *Toxoplasma gondii.*

Tuberculosis (TB):   A bacterial infection caused by *Mycobacterium tuberculosis.* TB bacteria are spread by airborne droplets expelled from the lungs when a person with active TB coughs, sneezes, or speaks. Exposure to these droplets can lead to infection in the air sacs of the lungs. The immune defenses of healthy people usually prevent TB infection from spreading beyond a very small area of the lungs. If the body's immune system is impaired because of HIV infection, aging, malnutrition, or other factors, the TB bacteria may begin to spread more widely in the lungs or to other tissues. TB is seen with increasing frequency among HIV-infected persons. Most cases of TB occur in the lungs (pulmonary TB). The disease may also occur in the larynx, lymph nodes, brain, kidneys, or bones (extrapulmonary TB). Extrapulmonary TB infections are more common among persons living with HIV.

Undetectable Virus: The threshold at which measurements of plasma HIV RNA levels (viral load) are not detectable depends on the assay used. Common thresholds are <400 copies/ml or <50 copies/ml.

Valganciclovir: An antimicrobial drug used to treat viruses. This drug can be used to treat cytomegalovirus infections that people with HIV/AIDS may develop. It does not cure these infections.

Varicella: Also known as chickenpox. Varicella is caused by the varicella zoster virus, a type of herpes virus. It is an acute contagious infectious disease—especially of children. The infection spreads from person to person by direct contact or through the air from an infected person's coughing or sneezing. The disease is marked by a low-grade fever and a blister-like rash on the body. The rash causes itching. A person with chickenpox is contagious 1-2 days before the rash appears and until all blisters have formed scabs.

Viral Fitness: As HIV obtains certain genetic mutations, its ability to replicate can be diminished compared to that of wild-type strain.

Virologic Failure: Based on U.S. Department of Health and Human Services guidelines, this is defined as detectable HIV virus in the blood after 24 weeks from initiating therapy or changing therapy. HIV RNA level greater 500 copies/ml at 12 to 16 weeks is a good predictor of failure.

Virology: The study of viruses and viral disease.

Zidovudine: Also known as AZT or ZDV. An antiretroviral drug in the class of nucleoside reverse transcriptase inhibitors. It was the first drug approved in the U.S. for treatment of HIV/AIDS. It was approved in 1987.

Appendix
G

Committee and Staff Biographies

James W. Curran, MD, MPH (*Cochair*), an internationally recognized authority on AIDS prevention, was named Dean of the Rollins School of Public Health effective November 1, 1995. Dr. Curran served as the Assistant Surgeon General in the U.S. Public Health Service and Director of the Division of HIV/AIDS Prevention at the U.S. Centers for Disease Control and Prevention (CDC) at the time of his appointment as Dean. He came to the CDC in 1971 after graduating from the University of Michigan Medical School. Dr. Curran directed the CDC Task Force that conducted the initial investigations of AIDS and held various AIDS leadership positions at CDC until joining Emory University. He received his Master of Public Health degree from Harvard University School of Public Health, where he was a resident in general preventive medicine and a fellow at the Harvard Center for Community Health and Medical Care. In 1993, Dr. Curran was elected to the Institute of Medicine (IOM) of the National Academy of Science, one of the numerous awards he has received in medicine and public health. He serves as Chair of the IOM Board on Health Promotion and Disease Prevention, in addition to serving as cochair of the IOM Committee on Antiretroviral Drug Use in Resource-Constrained Settings. Dr. Curran was recently selected as the 2003 winner of the John Snow Award from the Epidemiology Section of the American Public Health Association. He is the author of more than 250 scientific publications. He also serves on numerous boards and committees in research and education including chair-elect of the Associations of Schools of Public Health (ASPH). Dr. Curran's expertise in HIV/AIDS directly strengthens HIV-related projects. In addition, he currently serves as the director and principal investigator for Emory's Center for AIDS Research (CFAR).

Haile Tesfaye Debas, MD (*Cochair*), is Executive Director of UCSF Global Health Sciences and Chancellor- and Dean-emeritus at the University of California, San Francisco. He is a member of the Institute of Medicine and currently serves on Committee for Science, Engineering, and Public Policy of the National Academy of Sciences. He currently serves on the UN Commission for HIV/AIDS and Governance in Africa. He served with distinction as Chair of the UCSF Department of Surgery before he was appointed Dean of the Medical School in 1993. Under his decade of leadership, the School of Medicine saw unprecedented growth in its academic programs with the creation of several multidisciplinary centers and institutes and the implementation of a new curriculum for medical education that has been nationally recognized for its innovations. He is internationally recognized for his scientific contributions in gastrointestinal physiology and numerous other contributions to medicine. Dr. Debas was born in Eritrea and received his MD degree from McGill University Faculty of Medicine in Montreal, Canada.

Solomon Benatar, MB, ChB, FFA, FRCP, FACP (Hon), served as Head of the Department of Internal Medicine at the University of Cape Town and Chief Physician at Groote Schuur Hospital from 1980 to 1999. During the past decade, Dr. Benatar has led the University of Cape Town's Centre for Bioethics, as its founding director. His academic interests have ranged from respiratory medicine, academic freedom, medical ethics, and the humanities in medicine, to human rights, health care systems, health economics and global health—on which topics he has published over 250 journal articles and book chapters. During the 1994 to 1995 academic year he was a Fellow in the program in Ethics and the Professions at Harvard University and Visiting Professor at Harvard Medical School. He has been an invited teacher at many medical schools world-wide. He is an elected Foreign Member of the IOM (1989), and of the American Academy of Arts and Sciences (1994). He is a corresponding member of the U.S. National Academy of Sciences' Committee on Human Rights and has been a consultant to the World Health Organization, UNAIDS, Médecins sans Frontières and the HIV Prevention Trials Network. Since 1999 he has been Visiting Professor in Medicine and Public Health Sciences at the University of Toronto. He is the Program Director of a Fogarty International Center funded capacity building program in International Research Ethics in Southern Africa (2003–2006), Chairman of the South African Interim National Health Research Ethics Committee, and immediate past president of the International Association of Bioethics.

Sally Blower, PhD, is Professor of Biomathematics at the David Geffen School of Medicine at UCLA. Previously she has held faculty positions at the University of California, San Francisco, and at the University of California at Berkeley (School of Public Health). She is a mathematical and evolutionary biologist whose research focuses on developing mathematical models of infectious diseases. She received her undergraduate degree from the University of Edinburgh, and her PhD from Stanford University in 1987. The primary focus of her research is to use models as health policy tools. She uses mathematical models: (1) to design epidemic control strategies, (2) to understand and to predict the emergence of antibiotic and antiviral drug resistance, and (3) to develop vaccination strategies. The overall objective of her research is to develop the study of infectious diseases into a predictive science. She has published over 80 research articles mainly focused on HIV, tuberculosis, and genital herpes. She was the first to publish mathematical models for predicting the potential epidemic-level impact of HIV vaccines, the impact of drug-resistant tuberculosis, and the expected impact of drug-resistant HIV in both developing and developed countries. She introduced uncertainty analysis to the field of infectious disease modeling. These innovative methodologies have transformed infectious disease modeling from description to prediction. She has served as a consultant to the CDC, WHO, RAND, EPA, Burroughs Wellcome, GlaxoSmithKline, Aventis Pasteur, the Frankel Group, and the Global HIV Prevention Group.

J. Brooks Jackson, MD, MBA, is Professor and Chairman of Pathology at the Johns Hopkins Medical Institutions. Dr. Jackson is Director of the clinical HIV Laboratory at Johns Hopkins Hospital and has been involved in numerous clinical HIV therapeutic and prevention trials in the United States, Uganda, and China. He is a funded investigator in the NIAID-sponsored adult and pediatric AIDS Clinical Trials Groups and the HIVNET and HIV Prevention Trials Network. Dr. Jackson is the Protocol Chair of several adult and perinatal HIV prevention trials in the United States and Uganda including the HIVNET 012 perinatal nevirapine trial.

Gilbert Kombe, MBBS, MPH, serves as HIV/AIDS senior technical advisor at Partnership for Health Reformplus Project at Abt Associates Inc. In this capacity, he directs technical assistance and provides leadership to regional and country teams in determining achievable and sustainable strategies to strengthen health systems' capacity to provide effective HIV/AIDS prevention, treatment and care interventions. For many years, Dr. Kombe worked on a number of HIV/AIDS issues including costing and financing of ARVs, designing of service delivery models, and developing national antiretroviral policies in low-resource settings. Recently, he has worked on ARV costing and policy issues in Zambia, Nigeria, and Uganda. Dr. Kombe has worked with numerous donor-funded projects and has been routinely recruited as a consultant to many international organizations including the United Nations Economic Commission on Africa, WHO, The World Bank, and other institutions.

Peter Mugyenyi, MB, ChB, FRCPI, ScD (Hon), is the Executive Director of the Joint Clinical Research Centre (JCRC), a center of excellence that has provided leadership in AIDS care, treatment, research, and prevention in Uganda. The JCRC is a pioneer of antiretroviral therapy (ART) in Africa and currently treats one of the largest numbers of AIDS patients with higly active antiretroviral therapy (HAART) on the continent. He is also the Chair of Africa Dialogue on AIDS (ADAC), and AIDS Care Research in Africa (ACRiA), which are African led initiatives to coordinate HIV/AIDS activities and define best practices for prevention, care, treatment, and research. Dr. Mugyenyi holds other important responsibilities in academic institutions, and national and international organizations involved in planning, review and execution of policies and projects on AIDS treatment and research, HIV vaccines trials, access to drugs, poverty alleviation, and policy formulation and communication. He has provided technical and management expertise to a number of developing countries including his own Uganda Ministry of Health where he is the AIDS Task Force Chairman, responsible for planning and execution of the for national scaling up of ART program.

Nicky Padayachee, MD, has served as the Dean of the Faculty of Health Sciences of the University of Cape Town since January 1999. He previously held the position of Chief Executive Officer of the Greater Johannesburg Metropolitan Council. He is a registered Specialist in Community Health. He obtained his medical degree at the University of Cape Town, and his specialist degree in community health at the University of the Witwatersrand. Dr. Padayachee is the past President of the International Council for Local Environment Initiatives (ICLEI), past President of the Epidemiological Society of South Africa. He is the current Chairperson of the Medical Schemes Council of South Africa, a member of the Medicines Control Council of South Africa (MCC); the National Health Laboratory Services of South Africa (NHLS); the Health Professions Council of South African (HPCSA), and Chair of the Committee of Medical Deans of South Africa.

Nancy Padian, PhD, is a nationally and internationally recognized leader in the epidemiology and prevention of sexually transmitted diseases including HIV. Her work bridges the gap between traditional infectious disease epidemiology and the broader context of women's reproductive health. Dr.

Padian served as a principal investigator on numerous federally and privately funded research projects in high-risk populations. Her domestic research currently addresses adolescent reproductive health among teens in immigrant and minority communities. The major objective of her international research program is to reduce the risk of HIV among young women primarily through use of female-controlled methods of prevention such as microbicides or barrier contraceptives, and through development of programs that foster economic independence and thus reduce reliance on male sexual partners. Nine years ago, in collaboration with colleagues at the University of Zimbabwe, she founded the UZ-UCSF Collaborative Research Program in Women's Health, located in Zimbabwe where she currently has several research projects. She is developing similar programs in India and in Mexico. Dr. Padian is a Professor in the Departments of Obstetrics, Gynecology and Reproductive Sciences, and in Epidemiology and Biostatistics at UCSF. She is also an adjunct Professor in the Epidemiology Program at the School of Public Health at the University of California at Berkeley. Dr. Padian served as vicechair of the University of California task force on AIDS and currently directs international research for the UCSF AIDS Research Institute and is codirector of the UCSF Center for Reproductive Health Research and Policy. Dr. Padian is a frequent participant in annual NIH Office of AIDS Research planning workshops and chaired the committee on international priorities for the last two years. She serves on the NIH AIDS epidemiology study section and is an elected member to the American Epidemiology Society.

Priscilla Reddy, PhD, MPH, is Director of the Health Promotion Research and Development Group at the Medical Research Council of South Africa. She is one of the leading experts in South Africa on behavioral science of HIV, AIDS, and STD. She has been principal investigator on several NIH RO1 grants. She is also Visiting Associate Professor in the Department of Behavioral Science and Health Promotion at the Rollins School of Public Health at Emory University and has been nominated for a full professorship at the University of Cape Town.

Douglas Richman, MD, is staff physician at the VA San Diego Healthcare System and is Professor of Pathology and Medicine at the University of California San Diego. He is Director of the Center for AIDS Research and holds the Florence Seeley Riford Chair in AIDS Research. He trained in infectious diseases and medical virology with research on influenza virus, herpes viruses, and hemorrhagic fever viruses before focusing on HIV in the 1980s. HIV drug resistance was originally recognized in his laboratory in 1988. In addition to his continuing interest in HIV treatment and drug resistance, his research interests have focused on HIV pathogenesis including the issues of viral latency and evolution. Dr. Richman is a Fellow of the American Association for the Advancement of Science, the American Association of Physicians, and the Infectious Disease Society of America. He is a member of the National Institutes of Health AIDS Vaccine Research Working Group.

Bruce D. Walker, MD, is Professor of Medicine and Director of the Division of AIDS at Harvard Medical School, Director of the Partners AIDS Research Center at Massachusetts General Hospital, and a Howard Hughes Medical Institute Investigator. Dr. Walker is a clinician with a specialty in infectious diseases, focusing on the treatment of persons with HIV/AIDS. His basic science research focuses on cellular immune responses to chronic viral infections, particularly HIV and hepatitis C virus. His laboratory has been instrumental in defining the evolution of immune responses in the critical early stages of infection and has shown that immediate treatment of acute HIV infection with potent combination antiviral therapy can enhance functional immune responses to the virus and allow for transient immune control of HIV. He is also involved in vaccine preparedness work through a number of grants and contracts from the NIH. He has also been involved in collaborative research in Africa for over 10 years, and with the University of Natal in Durban, South Africa, for the last 4 years, where he is has been engaged in a collaborative project resulting in the completion of an AIDS Research Center that serves sub-Saharan Africa. He is an Adjunct Professor at the Nelson Mandela School of Medicine at the University of Natal.

IOM Staff

Patrick W. Kelley, MD, DrPH, joined the Institute of Medicine in July 2003 as the Director of the Board on Global Health. Previously he served in the U.S. Army for more than 23 years as a physician, residency director, epidemiologist, and program manager. In his last DoD position, Dr. Kelley founded and directed the presidentially mandated DoD Global Emerging Infections Surveillance and Response System (DoD-GEIS). This responsibility entailed managing approximately $42 million dollars of emerging infections surveillance, response, training, and capacity-building activities undertaken in partnership with numerous elements of the federal government and with health ministries in over 45 developing countries. He also designed and established the DoD Accessions Medical Standards Analysis and Research Activity, the first systematic DoD effort to apply epidemiology to the evidence-based development and evaluation of physical and psychological accession standards. Dr. Kelley is an experienced communicator having lectured in over 20 countries and authored of over 50 scholarly papers and book chapters. He also designed and served as the specialty editor for the two volume textbook entitled: *Military Preventive Medicine: Mobilization and Deployment*. Dr. Kelley obtained his MD from the University of Virginia and his DrPH from the Johns Hopkins School of Hygiene and Public Health.

Stacey Knobler, MPA, is a senior program officer at the Institute of Medicine (IOM) of the National Academies Board on Global Health (BGH). She is currently the Director of the *Forum on Microbial Threats* and a senior program officer for committee activities that include *Scaling Up Treatment for the Global AIDS Pandemic: Challenges and Opportunities in Resource-Constrained Settings* and *Advances in Technology and the Prevention of their Application to Next Generation Bioterrorism and Biological Warfare Threats*. Ms. Knobler previously directed the Board on Global Health's study of *Neurological, Psychiatric, and Developmental Disabilities in Developing Countries* and *The Assessment of Future Scientific Needs for Live Variola (Smallpox)*. She is actively involved in program research and development for the BGH. Previously, she has held positions as a Research Associate at the Brookings Institution, Foreign Policy Studies Program and as a Development and Democratization Consultant for the Organization for Security and Cooperation in Europe at sites in Vienna and Bosnia-Herzegovina. Ms. Knobler has also worked as a researcher and negotiations analyst in Israel and Palestine. She received her baccalaureate, summa cum laude, in political science and molecular genetics from the University of Rochester and her MPA from Harvard University. Ms. Knobler has conducted research and published articles and edited volumes on biological and nuclear weapons control, foreign aid, health policy in developing countries, poverty and public assistance, human rights, and the Arab-Israeli peace process. She is the recipient of the 1999 IOM Einstein Award, the 2001 and 2003 Distinguished Service Award from the National Academies, and the Department of the Army Certificate of Service and Appreciation, 2001, 2002.

Monisha Arya, MD, MPH, is a Christine Mirzyan Science and Technology Policy Intern at the National Academies. She has played a leading role in the research and development for the Institute of Medicine's Board on Global Health report, *Scaling Up Treatment for the Global AIDS Pandemic: Challenges and Opportunities in Resource-Constrained Settings*. Dr. Arya was awarded her MD and Masters in Public Health with a health policy concentration at the George Washington University in Washington, DC in May 2000. During medical school, she was a Health Policy Fellow with the American Medical Student Association and had the opportunity to work in the U.S. Congress and meet with physicians serving as health policy advisors to U.S. Senators. Dr. Arya recently completed her residency training in internal medicine at Georgetown University Medical Center. She earned her BS in psychology from the University of Maryland, College Park. Following the National Academies internship, she will begin a 3-year infectious diseases fellowship program at the Beth Israel Deaconess Medical Center in Boston, Massachusetts.

Marjan Najafi, MPH, is a research associate for the Forum on Emerging Infections in the Board on Global Health. She has also worked with the IOM committee that produced *Veterans and Agent Orange: Update 2000.* She received her undergraduate degrees in chemical engineering and applied mathematics from the University of Rhode Island. Ms. Najafi served as a public health engineer with the Maryland Department of Environment and, later, the Research Triangle Institute. After obtaining a master's degree in public health from the Bloomberg School of Public Health at Johns Hopkins University, she managed a lead poisoning prevention program in Micronesia with a grant from the U.S. Department of Health and Human Services. Prior to joining IOM, she worked on a study researching the effects of cellular phone radiation on human health.

Allison L. Berger is a Program Assistant for the Board on Global Health. She previously served as a Program Assistant for the IOM Board on Neuroscience and Behavioral Health where she worked on two other IOM studies: *Health Literacy* and *Introducing Behavioral and Social Science into Medical School Curricula.* Before joining the IOM staff, she enjoyed a 5-year tenure as an Administrative Assistant for the American Psychological Association, where she assisted the APA Committee on Psychological Test and Assessment, Committee on Scientific Awards, and the Committee on Animal Research and Ethics. She also worked on several funding and grant programs sponsored by the APA Science Directorate.

Leslie A. Pray, PhD, is a science writer and independent consultant for the Institute of Medicine (IOM). She has written extensively on a wide range of genetic, evolutionary biology, emerging infectious disease, public health policy, and graduate education issues for the IOM, the American Association for the Advancement of Science, the American Chemical Society, and elsewhere. Dr. Pray was coeditor on *Biological Threats and Terrorism: Assessing the Science and Response Capabilities* and *Considerations for Viral Disease Eradication: Lessons Learned and Future Strategies.* She received her PhD from the University of Vermont in 1997 and was awarded a National Science Foundation Postdoctoral Fellowship in Biosciences Related to the Environment and an American Society of Naturalists Young Investigator Award for her research in population genetics.